LISA S. LOGAN

D0205765

SANDRITTER'S
COLOR ATLAS AND TEXTBOOK
OF HISTOPATHOLOGY

Seventh English Edition

Sandritter's
Color Atlas and Textbook of
HISTOPATHOLOGY

Seventh English Edition

Carlos Thomas, Dr. med.
Professor of Pathology and Director of
the Center for Pathology, University Marburg

With the assistance of
C. P. Adler, N. Bohm, N. Freudenberg, M. Hagedorn,
Ch. Mittermayer, U. N. Riede, R. Rohrbach and K. Salfelder

Translated and edited by
GOETZ W. RICHTER, M.D.
Professor of Pathology
University of Rochester

Previous English editions by
William B. Wartman, M.D.
Formerly Professor of Pathology
Northwestern University and
University of Virginia

YEAR BOOK MEDICAL PUBLISHERS, INC.
CHICAGO

English-language text copyright © 1984 by Year Book Medical Publishers, Inc. No part of this publication may be reproduced, stored in a retrieval system, or transmitted, in any form or by any means—electronic, mechanical, photocopying, recording, or otherwise—without prior written permission from the publisher except in cases described below. Printed in the United States of America.

This book is an authorized translation from the German edition published and copyrighted 1965, 1967, 1968, 1971, 1975, 1977, and 1983 by F. K. Schattauer Verlag GmbH, Stuttgart, Germany. Title of the German edition: Histopathologie. Lehrbuch und Atlas fur Studierende und Arzte.

0   9   8   7   6   5   4   3   2   1

Library of Congress Cataloging in Publication Data
Sandritter, W. (Walter)
    Sandritter's color atlas and textbook of histopathology.

    Translation of: Histopathologie.
    Rev. ed. of: Color atlas & textbook of histopathology.
6th English ed. 1979.
    Includes index.
    1. Histology, Pathological.   I. Thomas, C. (Carlos),
1931–   . II. Adler, C. P.   III. Richter, Goetz W.,
1922–   . IV. Sandritter, W. (Walter).   Color atlas &
textbook of histopathology.   V. Title.   [DNLM: 1. Histology.   2. Pathology.   QZ 4 S219h]
RB25.S2513   1984   611'.018   84-7515
ISBN 0-8151-8794-7

Sponsoring editor: Susan M. Harter
Editing supervisor: Frances M. Perveiler
Production project manager: Sharon W. Pepping
Proofroom supervisor: Shirley E. Taylor

To the memory of

WALTER SANDRITTER
1920–1980
Professor and Director of the Institute of
Pathology, University of Freiburg in Breisgau
1967–1980

From the Preface to the Ninth German Edition

THE STUDY OF DISEASE includes general, special, and experimental pathology. A subdivision into histopathology and macropathology is undoubtedly a compromise, justified only because of the existence of courses in general and special pathology that include gross and microscopic pathology. In this sense the organization of the two books, *Histopathology* and *Macropathology,* has proved itself. This preface is to serve for both volumes in order to emphasize that they are complementary and are meant to form a single unit.

Instruction in pathology is central to human medicine. The sense of responsibility toward medical students and young physicians, who are relying on the experience of others, must be appropriate. The rapid increase of knowledge confronting us daily imposes excessive demands, not only on students, but also on their teachers. For this reason we need to bear in mind a proven experience: to transmit that factual knowledge which is likely to be valid 5 years hence. In each new edition the author should see to it that the book does not become too big. This was the goal in revising the various chapters (e.g., those on the heart, lung, liver, and kidney). At the same time, new methods of examination, such as immunohistochemistry, and also the international guidelines for nomenclature, classification, and diagnosis of diseases—especially of tumors—were kept in mind. The macroscopic or microscopic picture should, as far as possible, contain the necessary information and be supplemented by a brief text. But in this respect an atlas has its limits, and neither *Histopathology* nor *Macropathology* can replace conventional textbooks of pathology. It is in those books that the reader must look for references to the relevant literature. In this edition we have omitted references, which in the past were mainly in German. The two atlases are meant not only to prepare students for examinations, but, preferably, to help provide practical training for students and young physicians.

Books like these can originate and prove themselves only through the joint efforts of a sizable group. It is a pleasant duty of the principal author to thank all collaborators, both in his own group and at Schattauer Verlag. I owe special thanks to Prof. Dr. h. c. P. Matis, Mr. H. Schwer, Managing Director, Mr. Bergemann (Druckerei Mayr), and Mr. Haub (Grafische Kunstanstalt Brend'amour). The drawings were made by Mr. Tschorner. Finally, I ask readers to remember the name of Walter Sandritter, who created both *Histopathology* and *Macropathology* (first published, respectively, in 1965 and 1970). My task is to develop his concepts further.

CARLOS THOMAS
MARBURG, GERMANY

Preface to the Seventh English Edition

SHORTLY BEFORE HIS SUDDEN and untimely death in 1980, Professor Walter Sandritter suggested that I take over the job of preparing a new English edition of *Histopathologie* on the retirement of Professor William Wartman, the translator and editor of all previous English editions. With the agreement and at the urging of Year Book Medical Publishers, I accepted this challenge.

The seventh English edition is based on the ninth edition of the German text, prepared under the leadership of Professor Carlos Thomas, Director of the Medical Center for Pathology at the University of Marburg, and published in 1983 by F. K. Schattauer Verlag, Stuttgart. Professor Thomas also was co-author of previous German editions.

Color Atlas and Textbook of Histopathology has, in earlier editions, found favor with medical students and aspiring pathologists throughout the world. It has been translated into Spanish, French, Italian, and Japanese as well as into English. Undoubtedly, its success is in considerable measure due to the excellence and relevance of the illustrations, but the simple, direct manner in which the authors have described and explained histopathologic and cellular alterations associated with diseases is also impressive.

This new English edition reflects many changes in the German text. The chapter on diseases of bones and joints has been entirely rewritten. Illustrations and descriptions of neoplasms have been integrated with both General and Systemic Pathology rather than presented in a separate chapter toward the end of the book, as was done before. Other changes are scattered throughout. Many brief references to macroscopic alterations have been retained. However, in the absence of an updated English version of Sandritter's and Thomas' *Makropathologie,* no further attempts at correlation were made in this English edition.

I have revised and adjusted the nomenclature in keeping with current Anglo-American usage but have not made a fetish of such changes. The authors used mainly World Health Organization nomenclature, and this has been retained where doing so seemed advantageous. Drastic changes, such as adoption of SNOMED, would have disturbed the authors' purposes and reduced the didactic value of the book.

My functions as translator and editor have precluded insertion of original material other than a few clarifying statements or revisions. Wherever possible, I have retained the previous translator's text.

The bibliography was dropped in the latest German edition. Accordingly, I have not attempted to provide what could at best only be a highly eclectic list of articles. It seems to me that students should first consult textbooks in which diseases are described more extensively.

Like its predecessors, this new version of "Sandritter-Thomas" bears the stamp of the late Professor Sandritter's highly practical educational and professional ideas, which have now been carried forward by Professor Thomas. May the book be useful and helpful to its readers!

G. W. RICHTER
ROCHESTER, NEW YORK

Contents

Introduction—General Pathology

A certain amount of practical knowledge and skill, particularly with respect to use of the light microscope, is desirable on the part of the reader if he is to get the most good from reading a textbook of histopathology. Profitable use of the microscope requires knowledge of its construction and of the interrelations of its individual parts. Furthermore, it is only possible to interpret a histologic slide after one is informed as to how the tissue has been prepared for cutting and how it has been stained. A solid foundation in normal histology and general pathology goes without saying, for the principles of general pathology are used constantly in special pathology.

Preliminary Technical Remarks

Use of the Microscope

The light source, the lens system with its diaphragms, and the eye must all be correctly aligned with one another in order to obtain optimal information from a histologic section. Artificial light, which consists predominantly of yellowish red light rays, can be corrected by a blue filter so that it will approximate daylight. Köhler's principle is commonly used to adjust the light source, since by using this principle it is possible to illuminate only the object area that is to be examined and that entirely uniformly. With a microscope with a built-in light source, swing in the front lens of the condenser. Focus the microscope on the specimen and stop down the *field diaphragm*. Rack up the condenser as far as possible and then lower it slowly, thus focusing the field diaphragm within the specimen area.

Center the condenser with the two centering screws if necessary (the condensers of many student microscopes are permanently centered so that this step may be omitted). Open the field diaphragm until its shadow disappears from the field of view. The field diaphragm should always be adjusted so that its image just disappears behind the edge of the eyepiece stop. Adjust image contrast and, if necessary, sharpness—but not image brightness—with the *condenser (aperture) diaphragm* by opening it entirely and then closing it down just far enough to remove glare from the specimen. Unstained objects can be seen best when the condenser diaphragm is closed as far as possible or with a phase contrast microscope. With blurred images, reducing the condenser diaphragm will increase the contrast.

The microscopic image is produced by diffraction of the light by the structures in the histologic preparation in the focal plane at the back of the objective (primary image). The secondary image, which is the one observed in the ocular, arises from magnification of the primary image.

Objective and ocular must be properly matched. In usual histologic practice, an ocular with a $10 \times$ magnification is used with the following objectives, in which the first number gives the magnification and the second the numerical aperture of the objective, which is a measure of its resolving power:

1. *Scanning lens:* objective 2.5/0.08—magnification $25 \times$.
2. *Low magnification:* objective 10/0.25—magnification $100 \times$.
3. *High dry magnification:* objective 40/0.65—magnification $400 \times$.

For still higher magnification, especially for examination of smears of cells (blood, lymph node), oil immersion objectives (100/1.25) are available with a magnification of $1,000 \times$ or $1,250 \times$ (with $12.5 \times$ ocular).

1

When using the microscope, the following suggestions will prove helpful. With a monocular microscope, always keep both eyes open, since the adjustment for distance obtained in this way prevents rapid eye fatigue due to constant accommodation.

The lowest magnification should always be used before going to the other objectives because it is easier to orient the various structures under low magnification.

If the image is blurred, you should think of the possibility of the slide being upside down with the cover-slip resting on the stage of the microscope.

Preparation and Staining of Histologic Sections

Sections are prepared from blocks of tissue measuring about 2×2 cm. The selected tissue is usually hardened and fixed in Formol (ordinary 40% commercial Formalin diluted with water 1:9 so that the resulting solution is about 4%). The *hardening* results from coagulation and denaturation of protein, while the *fixation* arrests autolysis and bacterial decomposition. In order to prepare sections 5–10 μ thick, the tissue must have a consistency suitable for cutting. To obtain this, the tissue may either be frozen (at $-20°$ C) with carbon dioxide snow and cut on the frozen-section microtome (this method is used particularly for demonstrating fat or for rapid diagnosis of biopsy specimens at the time of surgery) or the tissue can be processed through a series of alcohols (from 70% to 100%), methyl-benzoate, and benzol into paraffin with a melting point of 56° C. Liquid paraffin at 60° C penetrates the finest tissue spaces and produces a good cutting consistency. After cutting on a microtome, the sections are mounted on microscopic slides and stained, after first being deparaffinized with xylol.

Note: Frozen sections permit demonstration of neutral fat. In paraffin sections the fat is dissolved by alcohol and the droplets of fat appear as optically empty spaces in the tissue.

The methods used for *histologic staining* have been developed empirically and the physicochemical basis for them is not exactly known except in a few cases. Electrostatic binding, among other factors, plays a principal role. Negatively charged groups, for example, nucleic acids (phosphate groups) or proteins ($-COOH$ groups) or the mucopolysaccharides ($-COOH$, SO_4), bind with the basic dye groups, which behave as cations. Acid dyes (e.g., eosin) with electronegative charges bind predominantly with positively charged protein groups (NH_2 groups). Excess and easily soluble dye in the tissue is removed after staining by differentiation in water, alcohol, or weak acid. Finally, the water is removed with 70% and 96% alcohol, the section immersed in a clearing agent (xylol), mounted in Permount or Canada balsam, and covered with a cover-slip.

Histochemistry deals with specific and sometimes quantitative identification of chemical substances in tissues, such as nucleic acids, certain proteins, carbohydrates, enzymes, etc.

Artifacts in histologic sections are caused chiefly by improper fixation, embedding (cracks or tears), or staining (transparent, unstained flaws, or dark spots).

Table 1 reviews the features of some commonly used stains. *Fluorescence microscopy,* in which tissues are stained with fluorescing dyes and examined under ultraviolet light, allows detection of dyes in low concentrations because the ultraviolet light rays (e.g., 350 nm) liberate secondary rays in the visible range. Some substances show autofluorescence, e.g., lipids, porphyrins, and elastic fibers.

TABLE 1.—STAINING METHODS

METHOD	RESULTS			REMARKS
Hematoxylin-eosin	**Blue** *Hematoxylin* Basophilic cytoplasm, nuclei, bacteria, calcium	**Red** *Eosin* Cytoplasm, connective, and all other tissues		Figs 1–15, 1–16
van Gieson's	**Yellow** *Picric Acid* Cytoplasm, muscle, amyloid, fibrin, fibrinoid	**Red** *Fuchsin* Connective tissue, hyalin	**Black** *Iron Hematoxylin* Nuclei Fig 1–6	
Elastica stain	**Black** *Resorcin-fuchsin* Elastic fibers	**Red** *Nuclear fast red* Nuclei		Fig 2–14
Elastica-van Gieson's	Used in combination			Fig 2–7
Azan	**Red** *Azocarmine* Nuclei, erythrocytes, fibrin, fibrinoid, acidophilic cytoplasm, epithelial hyalin	**Blue** *Aniline blue, Orange G* Collagen fibers, basophilic cytoplasm, mucus		Fig 2–10
Silver stain	**Black** *Ammoniacal AgNO₃* Reticulum fibers, nerve fibers			Collagen fibers brown
Fat stain	**Red** *Sudan III, Scarlet Red* Neutral fat	**Blue** *Hematoxylin* Nuclei, cytoplasm		Fig 2–6
Congo red	**Red** *Congo red* Amyloid	**Blue** *Hematoxylin* Nuclei		Fig 6–7
Weigert's fibrin stain	**Blue** *Lugol's solution, Crystal violet* Fibrin, bacteria	**Red** *Nuclear fast red* Nuclei		Not specific for fibrin Fig 3–29
Prussian blue reaction	**Blue** *Calcium ferrocyanide* Hemosiderin Fe^{III}	**Red** *Nuclear fast red* Nuclei		Fig 3–9
Giemsa (May-Grünwald-Giemsa)	**Blue** *Methyl violet* Nuclei, all basophilic substances	**Red** *Azur-eosin* Eosinophils, cytoplasm and its granules, collagen fibers		Metachromatic: mast cells violet melanin green Fig 16–2
Ladewig	**Blue—gray-blue** *Aniline blue* Parenchyma Mesenchyma	**Orange red** *Acid fuchsin-gold-orange* Muscle Fibrin	**Black** *Iron hematoxylin* Nuclei	
Mason-Goldner	**Orange-red** *Azofuchsin* Parenchyma Fibrin	**Green** *Light green* Mesenchyma	**Black** *Iron hematoxylin* Nuclei Fig 6–9	

TABLE 1.—STAINING METHODS (continued)

METHOD	RESULTS		REMARKS
Spielmeyer's myelin stain	**Blue-black** *Iron-alum* *hematoxylin* Myelin, erythrocytes		Figs 14–14, 14–17
Ziehl-Neelsen	**Red** *Carbofuchsin* Acid-fast rods, Tb bacilli, lepra bacilli	**Blue** *Hemalum* Nuclei	
Periodic acid-Schiff reaction (PAS)	**Red** *Schiff reagent* Adjacent hydroxyl groups and amino- alcohols		Neutral and acid polysaccharides Fig 4–28 Demonstration of fungi, parasites
Levaditi	**Black** *AgNO₃-reduced* *Pyrogallic acid* Spirocheta pallida Listerella monocytogenes		Fig 15–3 Fig 5–16
Thionine, toluidine blue	**Blue** Basophilic cytoplasm	**Blue** Nuclei	Metachromasia (mucins, lipids)
Staining of smears (Papanicolaou)	**Blue-violet** *Hematoxylin* Nuclei, bacteria	**Orange-red** *Orange-G* Cellular glycogen, keratin Blue-green/green/rose *E.A. 36 dye mixture* Cytoplasm of basophilic cells: (blue-green) Cytoplasm of acidophil cells: (rose-colored) Mucus: (green)	

Histologic Interpretation and Diagnosis

A famous physician (Franz Volhard) once said: *"The Gods have put diagnosis before therapy—man must put careful observation and interpretation before diagnosis." Analysis must precede synthesis* as it does in all other branches of knowledge. Analysis begins with the examination of the subject with a clear-cut objective in mind. *Careful observation* of similarities and dissimilarities, the separation of the typical and the atypical, the general from the special, all contribute to the desired knowledge of the subject. The arrangement, color, size, and form of the tissue elements and their relations to one another all help to determine the essential characteristics of the various structures under consideration. As such observations cannot be obtained without adequate preparation, a thorough theoretical grounding and a certain amount of experience become essential.

The beginning student will find it helpful in getting exact histologic details either to make drawings or to set down his observations in abbreviated outline form. The student is thus forced to emphasize the essential features and to deemphasize unessential ones.

After first carefully making the necessary observations, it is then possible to take the second step, that is, to synthesize the observations and make a diagnosis. On the other hand, hasty, careless examination will often lead to an incorrect opinion. In order to arrive at a *diagnosis,* the histologic observations need to be classified in some logical manner, usually one which has been reached through a compromise of experience and hypothesis. But, by its very nature, no diagnosis can be considered final, since it can change with the progress of scientific knowledge. Thus, it is understandable that an exact description retains its validity indefinitely, even when the interpretation and diagnosis of a section have already been revised.

The student will therefore be well advised to put his chief effort into a careful description of a microscopic section. In examinations, this is always graded higher than a diagnosis unsupported by accurate description.

In practice, the first step in examining a histologic preparation is to look at the section with the *unaided eye.* The shape and the various components of the tissue structures— easily recognized by differences in staining—often provide essential topographical information and have an important influence on the next step in the analysis of the section. *An inverted ocular used as a scanning lens* will provide an overall view of the tissue at very low magnification. Ordinary *low-power magnification* can then be used to examine in greater detail the structures already seen with the inverted ocular. In this way, a rough overall picture of the essential elements of the lesion is formed. Further details can also be distinguished with *low magnification,* such as the size and position of the nuclei and the structure of the cytoplasm. This magnification is probably the most useful of all, for at a magnification of about one hundred-fold, all the essential structures are well seen without losing the overall architectural relationships. A drawing at this stage of the examination will fix the typical findings firmly in mind. Practically all histologic preparations can be diagnosed with low magnification. *High magnification* is used only to clarify individual details, such as the shape and division of nuclear chromatin, mitoses, and so forth.

Such a methodical approach is an essential prerequisite for profitable observation and correct diagnosis. In studying histopathologic slides the student acquires the knowledge necessary to separate essential from nonessential observations—knowledge that a physician uses at the bedside.

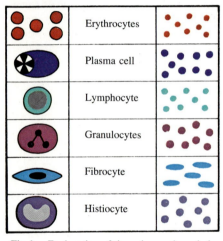

	Inflammation Necrosis		Hyalin
	Exudate Edema		Fibrin, fibrinoid Thrombus
	Pus		Fatty degeneration Fat
	Collagen fibers Scar		Vascularization (granulation tissue)
	Nucleus		Cytoplasm Parenchyma, Muscle

	Erythrocytes		
	Plasma cell		
	Lymphocyte		
	Granulocytes		
	Fibrocyte		
	Histiocyte		

Fig 1.—Explanation of the colors and symbols used to depict lesion components and pathologic processes.

Notes on General Pathology

These brief, almost stenographic, introductory remarks about general pathology are intended only as a means of making it easier to understand the complexities of special pathology. Reference to the appropriate illustrations of the book permits its use as a guide to the principles of general pathology.

In the schematic diagrams and tables the same symbols and colors are used for similar pathologic processes throughout the book (Fig 1). The individual components of a lesion or process are indicated by colors or symbols based, unless otherwise noted, on the gross (e.g., pus—greenish yellow) or microscopic appearance (e.g., collagen fibers—curly lines).

A knowledge of general pathology is an excellent foundation for the study of disease. The knowledge so obtained can be applied in nearly all special situations, since *the host in reacting to the many different pathologic stimuli that may affect it has only a limited number of possible responses available*. These originate essentially from either transient or permanent increase *(anabolism)* or decrease of metabolism *(catabolism)* or from *work failure*. In addition, complex tissue responses occur in *circulatory disturbances*, the various forms of *inflammation*, and in *tumors*.

In theory, pathologic stimuli can reach the cells and tissues in various ways (Fig 2):

(1) *directly* (e.g., trauma, radiant energy); (2) by way of the *bloodstream* or the *lymphatics* with resultant direct cell injury (e.g., toxins, alterations of the vascular contents as in thrombosis); (3) *indirectly*, when the stimulus acts on the *vessel walls*, a secondary circulatory disturbance then causing the cell injury (e.g., nervous derangement of permeability); (4) the pathologic stimulus can come from conduits such as the *alimentary tract*. Finally, primary (e.g., inborn) defects of metabolism may cause secondary cellular reactions.

The following diagram sets out the possible reactions of the organism to pathologic stimuli in simple fashion (Fig 3).

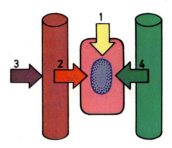

Fig 2.—See text for explanation.

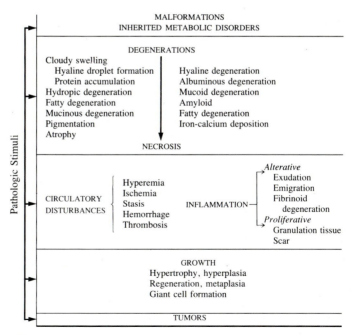

Fig 3.—Schematic survey of possible host reactions to pathologic stimuli.

Malformations: Inherited Metabolic Disorders

Malformations or *metabolic disorders* can develop in the embryonal (up to the third month of pregnancy) and fetal periods (after the third month) either because of hereditary errors in the genetic material or of the action of pathologic stimuli (e.g., teratogens). These manifest themselves, for example, either in *agenesis* (absence of enzymes, e.g., galactosemia; defective organ formation) or *aplasia* or *hypoplasia* (faulty development of existing organs). A great number of different manifestations can be produced in this way.

Degenerations

The different sorts of *degeneration* are morphological manifestations of metabolic disturbances either of cells (left-hand column of Fig 3) or of intercellular substances (right-hand column of Fig 3).

Cloudy swelling and hydropic degeneration (Fig 4) result from disturbance of the metabolic systems that maintain the ionic environment of cells (so-called ion pumps). When these regulatory mechanisms fail, then sodium and water flow into the cells and potassium leaves them. As a result, the mitochondria swell and the cytoplasm appears to be filled with fine "protein granules" *(cloudy swelling)*. The resulting cloudiness is due to increased scattering of light *(Tyndall effect)*. The mitochondria may also be transformed into water-filled vesicles *(hydropic transformation* of mitochondria). The water may accumulate in the cytosol or in the cisternae of the endoplasmic reticulum (hydropic degeneration). Compare Figs 6–1, 6–2 (light photomicrographs); Table 4, Fig 1–22 (electron micrographs).

Nuclei may also show swelling *(degenerative nuclear swelling)*. This must be distinguished, however, from physiologic or *functional nuclear swelling,* which is often accompanied by enlargement of the nucleolus and is a reflection of increased metabolic activity.

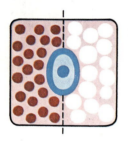

Fig 4.—Cloudy swelling *(left);* hydropic degeneration *(right).*

Hyalin droplet degeneration (protein accumulation) should be distinguished from cloudy swelling (Fig 5). The microscopic appearances of the two conditions can be similar, but in hyalin droplet degeneration active work is performed by the cell (anabolism) with accumulation of protein in cytoplasmic organelles, for example, the reabsorption of protein in the renal tubules. Such reabsorption of material is accomplished by pinocytosis, in which small vesicles are formed by constriction of the cell membrane. Phagocytosis, on the other hand, is the process by which the cytoplasm takes up large, formed materials, such as bacteria (see Figs 10,A and 19 and 20).

See also Figures 6–2 (light photomicrograph) and 6–12 (electron micrographs).

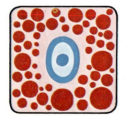

Fig 5.—Hyalin droplet regeneration (protein reabsorption).

The term *fatty degeneration* (perhaps better called fatty change or fatty metamorphosis) describes the appearance of microscopically visible fat, either in the form of fine (Fig 6, right) or large (Fig 6, left) droplets. The size of the droplets depends on the proportion of neutral fat to phospholipid (large droplets contain little phospholipid). Normally, fat is taken up in the form of fatty acids, which is accomplished through pinocytosis. The fatty acids are synthesized to triglycerides, bound to phospholipids and proteins, and delivered to the blood as lipoproteins. Any disproportion between the amounts of triglycerides (e.g., increased alimentary supply) and protein or of phospholipids (e.g., choline deficiency) or failure of energy coupling (oxygen or enzyme deficiencies) leads to accumulation of fat, i.e., to fatty degeneration.

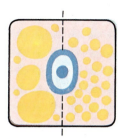

Fig. 6.—Fatty degeneration: *left*, large droplet form; *right*, fine droplet form.

See Figure 1–8 (light photomicrograph) and Figure 5–48 (electron micrographs).

Fat phanerosis may develop in *necrobiosis* (perceptible, slow cell death) in which structurally intact fat tissue is broken down into microscopically visible droplets.

In disordered carbohydrate metabolism, glycogen droplets may appear (e.g., in the kidney in diabetes), or mucinous degeneration may develop (production of mucopolysaccharides but without secretion) as, for example, in mucinous carcinoma (signet ring cells, Fig 7).

See Fig 4–32

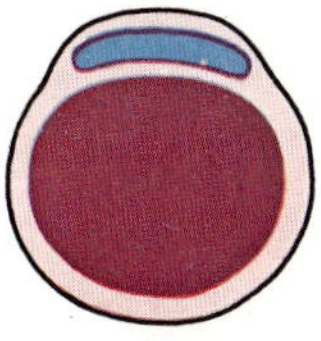

Alteration of the character of mucin secretion may also result in obstruction of excretory ducts (e.g., cystic fibrosis of the pancreas).

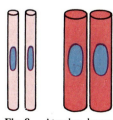

Fig 7.—Signet ring cell.

See Fig 4–51

Glycogen storage disease is caused by an *inborn error* of carbohydrate metabolism.

Pigments are naturally colored materials that are laid down in either diffuse or granular fashion. They usually have as a chief component either *protein* (e.g., melanin), *lipid* (lipopigments, e.g., lipofuscin) or derivatives of *hemoglobin* (hemosiderin or siderin, hematoidin, bile pigment). In addition, a number of *exogenous pigments* may be seen.

See the following:

Lipofuscin Table 2, Fig 1–3   Bile pigment, Fig 5–4
Melanin, Fig 9–24   Malaria pigment, Fig 5–3
Hemosiderin or siderin, Figs 3–9,   Exogenous pigments, Table 2, Fig 11–27
5–36
Hematoidin, Table 2, Fig 11–25

Table 2 lists the most important differential characteristics of various pigments.

Atrophy of cells (Fig 8) results from inactivity or chronic malnutrition, is manifested by reduction in cell size *(simple atrophy),* and eventually results in reduction of cell number *(numerical atrophy).* Hypertrophy connotes enlargement of cells, with increased function.

Degeneration of the connective and supporting tissues affects chiefly the *ground substance.* It may result in unmasking of the fibers, infiltration of fat and mucin, and deposition of foreign substances.

Fig 8.—Atrophy; hypertrophy.

9

TABLE 2.—PIGMENTS

SUBSTANCE	COMPONENTS	LOCATION	IRON REACTION	FAT STAIN	H_2O_2	ACID	BASE	PAS*	Ag NO$_3$†	FLUORESCENCE‡	GMELIN TEST
Lipofuscin (Fig 1–3)	Unsaturated oxidized, fatty acids	Parenchymal cells	–	(+)	(+)	–	–	+	+§	+	–
Ceroid	Unsaturated oxidized, fatty acids	Intracellular (mesenchymal)	–	+	–	–	–	+	±	+	–
Melanin (Pigmented Tumors, chap. 9)	Tyrosine derivatives	Intracellular	–	–	+	–	(+)	–	+‖	–	–
Siderin Hemosiderin (Figs 3–9, 5–36)	Iron glycoprotein	Intracellular	+	–	–	+	–	+	+	–	–
Hematoidin (Fig 11–25)	Bilirubin	Extracellular	–	–	–	+	+	–	–		+
Bile pigment (Fig 5–51)	Bilirubin Biliverdin	Intra- and extracellular	–	–	–	+	+	–			+
Malarial pigment (Fig 5–3)	Hemoglobin derivative	Intracellular	(+)	–	+	+	+				
Formalin pigment (Fig 11–26)	Protoporphyrin	Extracellular	–	–	–	+	+	–	–	–	
Exogenous pigments (Fig 11–27)	e.g., carbon silver, etc.	Intra- and extracellular	–	–	–						–

*Periodic acid-Schiff reaction for demonstration of polysaccharides (α-glycol).
†Reduced silver.
‡Primary fluorescence without staining.
§Brown.
‖Black.

Albuminous or granular protein degeneration and mucoid degeneration of the connective tissues (Fig 9) result from disintegration of the ground substance with precipitation of protein in cartilage or other tissues having a low metabolic rate. Protein complexes appear in the ground substance, or there is an increase in mucopolysaccharides. The collagen fibers are exposed in the process (Felty degeneration of cartilage) and finally destroyed, with the result that cysts are formed (*mucocystic degeneration, e.g., in a meniscus*).

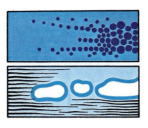

Fig 9.—Albuminous or granular protein degeneration *(top)*; mucocystic degeneration *(bottom)*.

Fig 10.—A, distinguishing characteristics of ''hyaline'' hyalin, fibrinoid, and amyloid (eosinophilic, homogeneous, refractive substances).

KIND	LIGHT MICROSCOPIC STRUCTURE	ELECTRON MICROSCOPIC STRUCTURE	CHARACTERISTICS	OCCURRENCE
Epithelial hyalin			H & E, azan: red; van Gieson's: yellow; protein produced in cells and secreted into extracellular spaces (e.g., gland lumens)	Thyroid colloid; prostatic secretion; parotid mixed tumor
Cellular & hematogenous hyalin			H & E, azan: red; van Gieson's: yellow; protein produced in cells (e.g., plasma cells) intracytoplasmically or after cytolysis of extracellular deposits	Mallory bodies; Russell bodies
			H & E: red; van Gieson's: yellow; heterophagocytosis of protein with intracytoplasmic storage in lysosomes	Hyalin droplets; protein storage in renal tubule cells
			H & E: red; van Gieson's: yellow; necrotic cellular material Hyaline thrombi Blood plasma Fibrin	Councilman bodies; shock lung Kidney; hyaline kidney casts; lung edema; lung hyaline membrane
Connective tissue hyalin			van Gieson's: red; azan: blue; quaternary structure of the collagen maintained; tangled arrangement of fibrils with deposition of acid mucopolysaccharide between them and noncollagenous protein	Pleural hyalin; capsular hyalin of spleen (sugar icing)

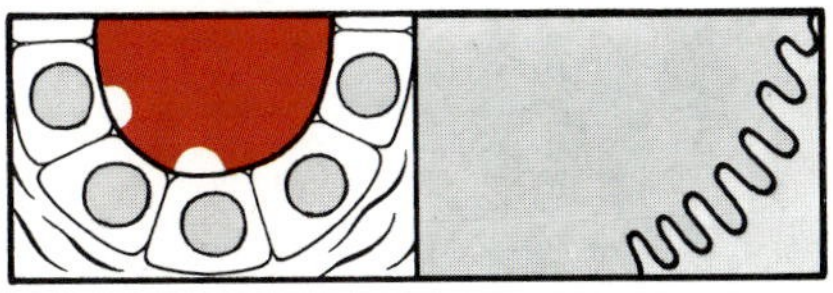

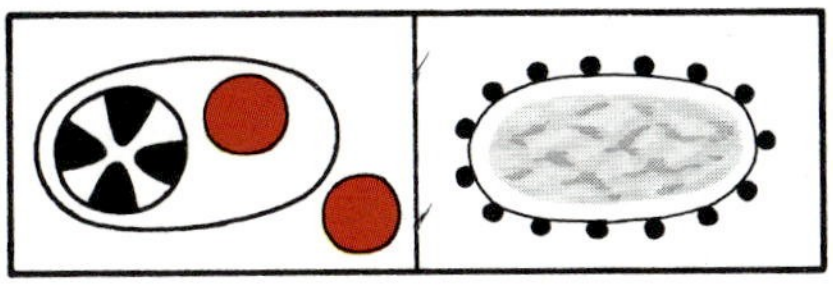

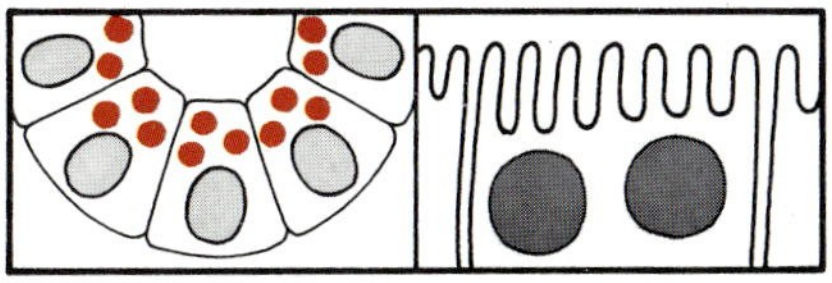

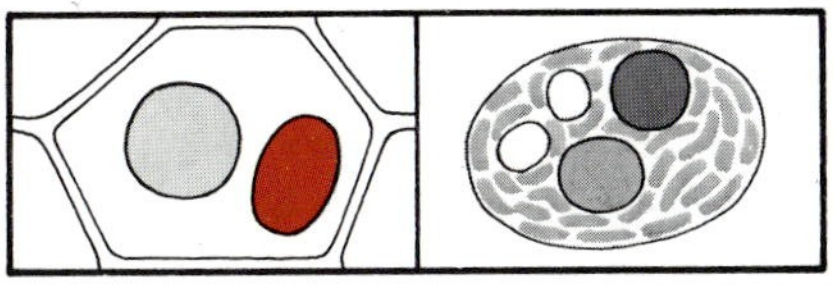

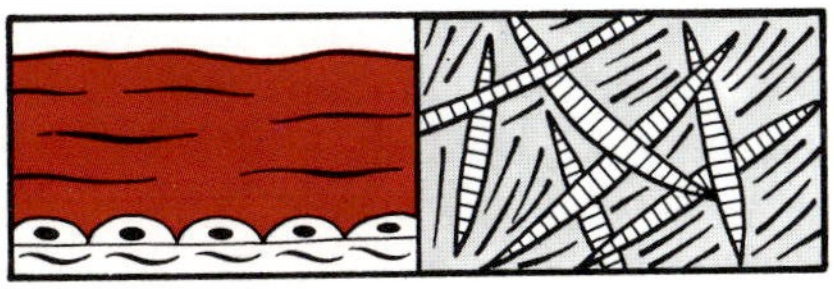

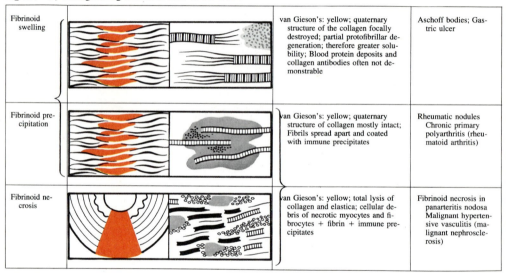

KIND	LIGHT MICROSCOPIC STRUCTURE	ELECTRON MICROSCOPIC STRUCTURE	CHARACTERISTICS	OCCURRENCE
Vascular hyalin			van Gieson's: red/yellow; blood protein; lipoproteins and immune precipitates and cell detritus; on glomerular mesangial matrix and basal membranes	Hyalinization of arterioles; Kimmelstiel-Wilson hyalin in glomeruli
Amyloid			van Gieson's: yellow; Congo red: red; cellular synthesis of glycoproteins and immunoglobulins (light chain); intra- and extracellular aggregates of rod-shaped proteins	Amyloidosis

Fig 10.—**B,** distinguishing characteristics of fibrinoid.

Fibrinoid swelling			van Gieson's: yellow; quaternary structure of the collagen focally destroyed; partial protofibrillar degeneration; therefore greater solubility; Blood protein deposits and collagen antibodies often not demonstrable	Aschoff bodies; Gastric ulcer
Fibrinoid precipitation			van Gieson's: yellow; quaternary structure of collagen mostly intact; Fibrils spread apart and coated with immune precipitates	Rheumatic nodules Chronic primary polyarthritis (rheumatoid arthritis)
Fibrinoid necrosis			van Gieson's: yellow; total lysis of collagen and elastica; cellular debris of necrotic myocytes and fibrocytes + fibrin + immune precipitates	Fibrinoid necrosis in panarteritis nodosa Malignant hypertensive vasculitis (malignant nephrosclerosis)

Hyalin

"Hyalin" is a catch-all word used to describe a variety of lesions of diverse causes and development that have a similar appearance when examined with the light microscope. Hyalin was first observed and described in the mid-19th century when only the light microscope was available for examination of diseased tissues; and since the lesion appeared homogeneous and was light refractive, in this respect resembling the microscopic appearance of hyalin cartilage, it was called "hyalin." It is used to indicate any lesion in either tissues or cells that stains red with eosin, is homogeneous in appearance, and has a high refractive index. Hyalin has various sites of localization, and recent electron microscopic and biochemical studies have shown that the structure and chemical composition of hyalin may be different in different sites and under different conditions. The following sorts of hyalin are recognized: *epithelial hyalin,* produced by epithelial cells, e.g. colloid; *cellular hyalin,* resulting from retention of cellular secretion, e.g., retention of antibodies in plasma cells, the so-called Russell bodies, or the Mallory bodies in liver cells of alcoholics, or the hyalin droplets of reabsorbed protein in renal tubules. In a wider sense, the large homogeneous areas of eosinophilic necrosis found for example in myocardial infarcts or in the isolated necrotic cells sometimes found in liver and known as Councilman bodies, are also described as hyalin. Other examples are hyalin casts formed in proteinurea, hyalin membranes in the lung, and hyalin thrombi in shock, which are sometimes called hematogenous hyalin. *Connective tissue hyalin* has a porcelain white gross appearance, e.g., hyalinization of the pleura or capsule of the spleen. The lesions result from a little understood disturbance of formation and orderly deposition of collagen fibers. In *vascular hyalin* (hyalinization of arterioles—a special form of arteriosclerosis) the hyalin material lies between the intima and atrophic media and consists of blood proteins, lipids, immunoglobulins (IgG, IgM), necrotic medial muscle, and mucopolysaccharides. Glomerular hyalin is produced by the mesangial cells (mesangial matrix).

Amyloid is a hyalin substance that stains specifically with Congo Red dye and when examined with the electron microscope is found to be composed of fibers without definite periodicity. Recent studies show that amyloid is produced by cells of the reticuloendothelial system and is deposited extracellularly. The usual sites of deposition are spleen, liver, kidney, adrenal, and intestines.

The different sorts of fibrinoid cannot be separated histologically since all appear homogeneous and eosinophilic. In contrast to connective tissue hyalin, fibrinoid is invariably accompanied by an inflammatory reaction in the tissues, as for example in Aschoff nodules or the extracardiac nodules of rheumatic fever or panarteritis. In Aschoff nodules the collagen fibrils are split and show loss of cross-striations (fibrinoid swelling). In the extracardiac nodules of rheumatic fever, accumulations of blood protein and fibrin lie between the fibrils (fibrin stains are positive, *fibrin precipitation*). In panarteritis there is necrosis of blood vessel walls or of adjacent tissues with fibrolysis of collagen bundles which are splintered and no longer show cross-striations (*fibrinoid necrosis*).

TABLE 3.—DISTINGUISHING CHARACTERISTICS OF HYALIN,
AMYLOID, FIBRINOID, AND FIBRIN

STAIN	HYALIN	AMYLOID	FIBRINOID	FIBRIN	REMARKS
Hematoxylin-eosin	**Red,** homogeneous	**Red,** homogeneous	**Red,** homogeneous	**Red,** fine fibers or homogeneous	
van Gieson's	**Red***	**Yellow**	**Yellow**	**Yellow**	
Congo red	–	**Red**	–	–	
Methyl violet	–	**Red**	–	–	Metachromatic red
Azan	**Blue†**	**Red**	**Red**	**Red**	
Weigert's fibrin stain	–	–	±	±	Depending on the fixative used and on the age of the fibrin
Digested by trypsin	–	–	+	+	
Pepsin	–	–	–	–	
Tissue reaction	–	Occasional giant cells	Slight acute inflammation, granulation tissue, histiocytes	Granulation tissue	

Note: Hyalin—no tissue reaction. *Fibrinoid*— almost always a tissue reaction: granuloma, e.g., Aschoff nodules (Figs 1–28, 1–29), or granulation tissue (periarteritis Fig 2–9).
*Epithelial hyalin: yellow.
†Epithelial hyalin: red.

Necrosis

Necrosis (focal death of tissue) is recognized morphologically by destruction of cell nuclei (pyknosis = nuclear shrinkage, karyolysis = nuclear dissolution, karyorrhexis = fragmentation of nuclei, Figs 11 and 21), homogenization of the cytoplasm, and distinctly increased eosinophilia (see also Figs 1–13, 1–14, and 1–20).

In the early or acute stages, denaturation of proteins occurs and evokes a leukocytic reaction. Later, the necrotic tissue is resorbed by granulation tissue and finally a scar is formed. There are, however, various other paths that differ from this ordinary sequence of events, as shown in Figure 12. In occasional cases, regeneration occurs with complete restitution of tissue integrity (e.g., liver, especially in young persons).

Electron Microscopy

The advances in the field of electron microscopy have added a new dimension, that of ultrastructure, and it is essential to consider the significance of this fact with respect to general pathology. The advancing edge of this new dimension is closing the large gap between light microscopy and biochemistry. Electron microscopy, and in particular histochemical electron microscopy, is making visible for the first time those cellular structures that are the morphological bases of metabolic processes. This new knowledge has greatly

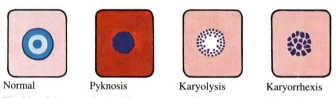

Normal   Pyknosis   Karyolysis   Karyorrhexis

Fig 11.—Diagram of the different manifestations of nuclear destruction.

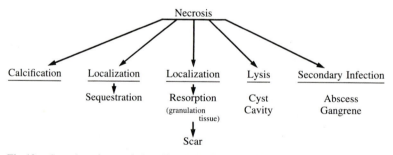

Fig 12.—Sequelae of necrosis (see Figs 1–13 through 1–18).

increased our understanding of disease. Structure and function are no longer to be conceived of as antagonists, but rather as parts of a whole.

The electron micrographs that follow on the next pages have to do with certain problems of general pathology. Those illustrating special pathology are placed under the sections on the respective organs.*

In attempting to present the electron microscopic basis of general pathology in tabular

---

*The rule shown in the electron micrographs is one micron in length unless otherwise indicated.

Ultrastructure of a Normal Liver Cell

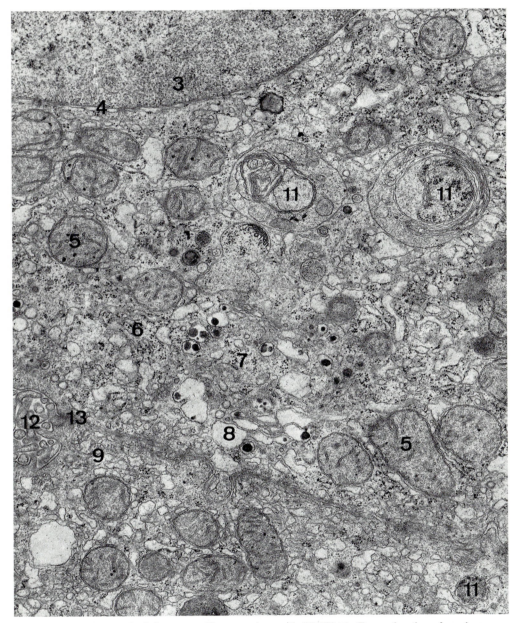

Fig 13.—Normal liver cell of the mouse. Electron micrograph (20,600×). For explanation of numbers, see legend to Figure 14.

form (Table 4), it is realized that the brevity of the tabular form imposes severe restrictions. Only the barest outline of the alterations of cell organelles can be indicated. However, the juxtaposition achieved in the table makes it clear that at the level of ultrastructure, as well as at the level of light microscopy, there are no *specific* cellular lesions and the most widely different injurious agents may call forth quite similar reactions.

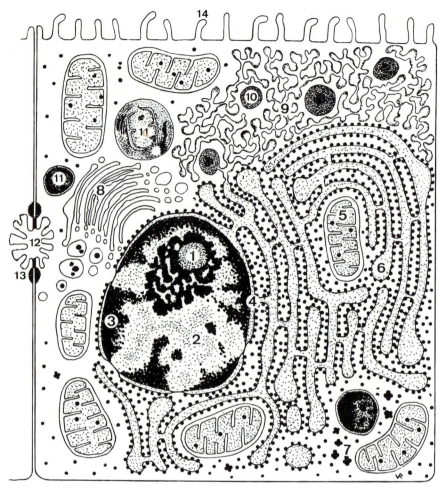

Fig 14.—Diagram of the electron microscopic appearance of a normal bipolar liver cell: 1. *Nucleolus* (synthesis of precursors of ribosomes) with pars amorpha and nucleolonema. 2. *Loose chromatin* (euchromatin: synthesis of messenger and transfer RNA). 3. *Dense chromatin* (heterochromatin: genetically inactive). 4. *Perinuclear, cistern with clear pore,* transition to rough endoplasmic reticulum (RER). 5. *Mitochondria* with cristae (citric acid cycle, respiratory enzymes, part of fatty acid synthesis) and *matrix granules* (lipoprotein with cations, calcium depot). 6. *RER* with outer border of *ribosomes;* transitions of RER into smooth endoplasmic reticulum (SER). 7. Protein is synthesized on the ribosomes *(polysomes)* with the help of messenger RNA. In the cisternae of the RER protein transport occurs. The *Golgi apparatus* (8) serves as a condensation and packaging station. 9. *SER.* Tubular cisternae without ribosomes. The RER and SER together form a membrane system (the *endoplasmic reticulum* is the same as the biochemist's microsome fraction) with organ-specific enzymes. SER contains organ-specific enzymes such as glucose-6-phosphatase (glycogen metabolism) hydroxylase, demethylase, etc. for detoxification. 10. *Peroxisomes.* These contain catalase and counteract internal storage of peroxidase. 11. *Lysosomes* with absorbed organelle constituents. They contain acid hydrolases such as acid phosphatase, β-glucuronidase, cathepsin, collagenase, etc. 12. *Bile capillary* with microvilli. The products of disintegration in lysosomes are excreted here. Situated near the apical or biliary pole of the cell. 13. *Desmosomes.* These bind the liver cells to each other. 14. *Microvilli* on the surface of the liver cell extending into the space of Disse. Basal or vascular pole of the cell.

TABLE 4.—PATHOLOGIC ALTERATIONS OF CELL ORGANELLES

NORMAL	PATHOLOGIC	REMARKS
1	a. Swelling mitochondria Normal (1) Matrix type Crista type (2)	**Swelling:** *Histologically* this is the matrix type of cloudy swelling. The crista type is unremarkable histologically. Swelling may progress to degeneration of cytoplasm. *Causes:* O_2 deficiency. Uncoupling of oxidative phosphorylation. Toxins. Substrate deficiency. *Metabolic effect:* reduced oxidative phosphorylation.
2	b. Structural changes	**Structural changes:** *Histologically*—no equivalent. Giant mitochondria can appear deceptively like Mallory bodies. Structural changes accompanied by hyperplasia of mitochondria cause cytoplasmic oxyphilia (oxyphile cells in hyperthyroidism). *Occurs with:* hypovitaminosis, chronic alcoholism, disturbance of protein synthesis. *Metabolic effect:* disturbance of citric acid cycle and/or oxidative phosphorylation.
3	c. Membrane changes (3)	**Membrane changes:** No *histologic* equivalent. Myelin-like degeneration of external membrane. Proliferation of cristae. *Causes:* Chronic O_2 deficiency. Increased CO_2 or O_2 tension (lung), muscular exercise, tumors, cholestasis.
4	d. Matrix changes (4)	**Matrix changes:** Amorphous thickening of mitochondrial matrix. *Causes:* Malnutrition, hypovitaminosis, methylcholanthrene application, alcoholism. Dense matrix aggregates (with calcium). *Occurs with:* tissue necrosis, nephrocalcinosis. Loss of matrix granules. *Occurs with:* calcium deficiency, ischemia and necrosis. Crystalline inclusions: *Occurs with:* alcoholism, Wilson's disease, polymyositis, lipid nephrosis, cholestasis, dehydration, and hypovolemic shock.

5	**Rough endoplasmic reticulum**
	
	(5) a) → b) a. Vesiculation
	  b. Lysis of ribosomes
	c) → d) c. Vacuolation
	  d. Ballooning
	electron microscope / light microscope / reversible
		Rough endoplasmic reticulum: *Histologically* the first sign is vacuolization and ballooning.
		Occurs with ischemia, toxins and end stages of many different cell injuries.

6	(6)	**"Fingerprint" degeneration:** *Occurs* in chronic intoxication (hydrocarbons), excessive regeneration, carcinogenesis, disturbed protein metabolism. Sometimes manifested *histologically* by basophilic nodules (so-called cytoplasmic "nebenkerne").
	e f	**Collapsed cisternae (e):** manifestation of membrane injury by peroxidation (e.g. CCl_4). Reduced synthetic output (hypothyroidism). **Blocked cisternae (f):** with accumulation of products of synthesis. *Occurs in:* plasma cells as Russell bodies, in cartilage cells in chondrodystrophy.

TABLE 4.—PATHOLOGIC ALTERATIONS OF CELL ORGANELLES *(cont.)*

NORMAL	PATHOLOGIC	REMARKS
7		**Ribosomes** Polysomes (aggregates of 80 S-ribosomes) disappear. 50 S- and 30 S-ribosomes appear. *Histologically:* Swollen, basophilic cytoplasm (RNA). Diffuse basophilia. *Occurs* with: CCL_4 poisoning, antibiotics, nutritional deficiency, carcinogenesis, ischemia. *Metabolic effect:* decreased protein synthesis.
8		**Smooth endoplasmic reticulum** **Hyperplasia and proliferation.** *Histologically:* cells appear milky (milk glass)—hyperplastic cells with hyalinized cytoplasm. *Causes:* barbiturate, antiepileptic, antidepressant drugs. Resorcin. Hydrocarbons. Carcinogens. Alcoholism. Jaundice. Virus hepatitis B. **Vacuolization and ballooning** similar to that in rough endoplasmic reticulum.
9		**Golgi apparatus** a. Hypertrophy due to swelling. *Occurs* in: Oxygen deficiency, Vitamin E deficiency b. Intracisternal accumulation. *Occurs* in various sorts of secretory disturbances.
10		**Peroxysomes:** *Function:* degradation of toxic cell peroxides (catalase). a. Hypoplasia in necrosis, malignant changes in a tumor (hepatoma). b. Hyperplasia due to antihyperlipidemic agents, salicylates, antihistamines.
11		**Lysosomes:** *Autolysosomes:* Absorption and digestion of cellular cytoplasmic constituents (organelles, glycogen etc.) = autophagocytosis. *Occurs* in all cells with a moth-eaten appearance in sublethal cell injury. Hunger, atrophy of inactivity, senile involution of organs. Product of degradation = lipofuscin granules. *Heterolysosomes:* Absorption and digestion of foreign bodies by phagocytosis. Digested materials: fibrin in Schwartzman phenomenon, hemosiderin from hemorrhage, bacteria and viruses in infections, protein or hemoglobin. Nuclear fragments, mononuclear cells in typhus. Cellular fragments in Kupffer cells in hepatitis.
12	a b	**Hyaloplasm** a. *Amyloid* (special stains). b. *Fatty degeneration:* Histologically there are cytoplasmic fat droplets.

Phagocytosis—Pigments

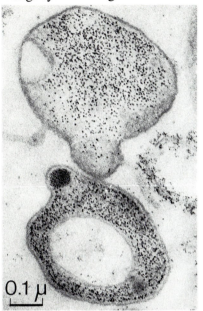

Fig 15.—Macrophage after injection of iron showing siderosomes with both large particles (siderin) and finely granular ones (ferritin, 55 Å) (50,000×). (Jones-Williams)

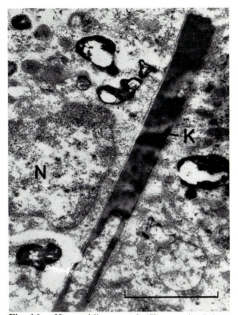

Fig 16.—Hematoidin crystal *(K)* contained in a macrophage and surrounded by invaginated cell membrane (→). *N,* nucleus (25,000×). (Gieseking)

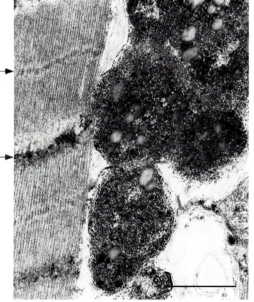

Fig 17.—Lipofuscin in hypertrophied human heart muscle. 1→, Z band; 2→, M band (30,000×).

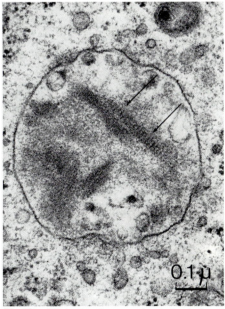

Fig 18.—Fibrin showing cross bands (typical periodicity →) lying in a cytoplasmic vacuole in a Kupffer cell following administration of endotoxin ("fibrin-clearing" mechanism in the Schwartzman phenomenon) (71,000×). (Prose)

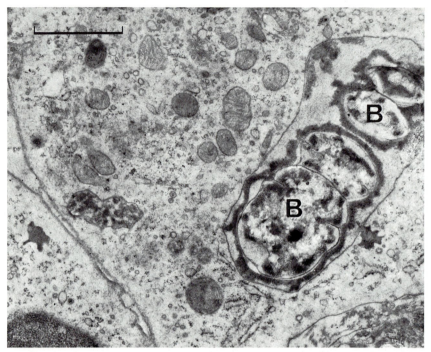

Fig 19.—Phagocytosis of bacteria in the blood by a macrophage (24,000×). (Staubesand)

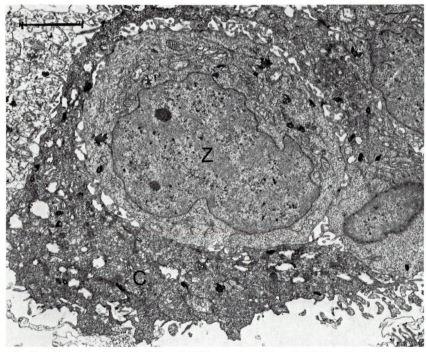

Fig 20.—Phagocytosis of one Hela cell (Z) by another Hela cell. The cytoplasm *(C)* of the phagocytizing cell has completely surrounded the other cell (8,000×). (Staubesand and Wittekind)

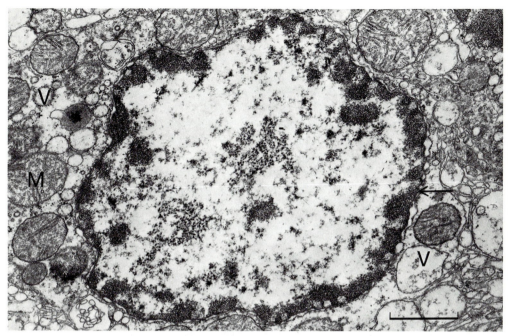

Fig 21.—A, ischemic necrosis of epithelium of a proximal renal tubule with hyperchromatic nuclear wall, i.e., increased margination of chromatin on the nuclear membrane plus pallor of the interior. *V,* vacuole in endoplasmic reticulum (vascuolar degeneration); *M,* swollen mitochondria (17,000×). (Totovic)

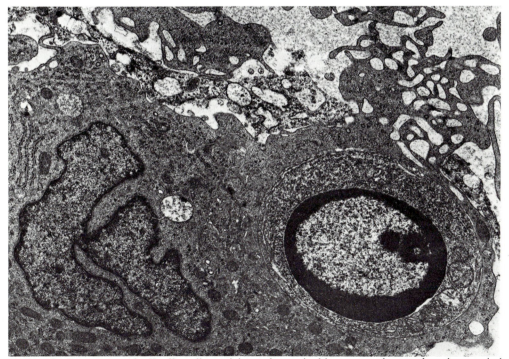

Fig 21.—B, fine structure of a Kupffer cell containing a phagocytized hepatocyte whose nucleus shows typical margination of chromatin (15,000×).

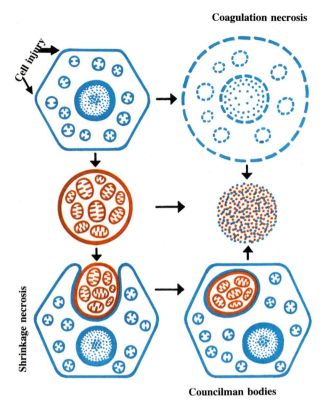

Fig 22.—Pathogenesis of coagulation necrosis and shrinkage necrosis.

Cell Necrosis

Depending on the severity of an injury and the length of time that it acts, different sorts of cellular necrosis are observed (Fig 22). If the injury is short acting (i.e., acute) and lethal, coagulation necrosis occurs. This starts with damage to membranes and leakage of fluid so that the cells become hydropic with marked swelling of mitochondria and leads to total disintegration of the cellular constituents and breakup of the cell (Fig 21,A, B). As a rule, coagulation necrosis involves groups of cells.

If the injury is long acting (i.e., chronic) and sublethal, the affected cells appear much shrunken (shrinkage necrosis). Nuclei and cytoplasm are mostly shriveled and dense. In the initial stages, mitochondria remain intact both morphologically and functionally. This sort of necrosis as a rule involves single cells (e.g., in viral hepatitis). In the liver, such shrunken necrotic cells are frequently phagocytosed by other cells (hepatocytes, Kupffer cells) and on light microscopy are seen as eosinophilic hyaline bodies, the so-called Councilman bodies. After being completely broken down by lysosomes they are eliminated by the cell.

Circulatory Disturbances

The *circulatory disturbances,* like inflammation, involve complex processes in a variety of tissues. These processes take place in the terminal circulatory channels, the arterioles, meta-arterioles, capillaries, and venules. Even under normal conditions, there is a changing interplay of hyperemia (in activity) and anemia (at rest) which, under pathologic conditions, change to *passive* (stasis of blood) or *active hyperemia* or to *ischemia. Stasis* indicates stagnation of the blood current with hemoconcentration. If the stasis persists, necrosis will result. Depending on local factors, there will develop either an *anemic infarct* (coagulation necrosis: in organs supplied with end-arteries, e.g., heart, kidney, spleen, etc.) or a *hemorrhagic infarct* (necrosis and hemorrhage, e.g., in lung, intestine).

Hemorrhage may occur for various reasons (e.g., injury of capillary walls, deficiency of platelets, deficiency of fibrinogen). Derangement of the coagulation mechanism, together with slowing of the blood stream and endothelial injury, results in formation of a thrombus which either breaks off *(embolus),* becomes organized, calcified, or softened interiorly *(putrid softening),* or is dissolved *(fibrinolysis).*

See the following Figures:
Congestion, Figs 3–9, 3–10, 5–11   Hemorrhagic infarct, Fig 3–5
Stasis, Figs 3–11, 3–27   Hemorrhage, Figs 14–5, 14–6
Anemic infarct, Fig 6–21   Thrombosis, Figs 2–20, 2–21, 2–22

Inflammation

Inflammation consists of a series of complex reactions by vascular and connective tissue elements to a tissue injury. In the acute phase, there is *hyperemia, fluid exudation* (if chiefly blood serum, *serous inflammation;* if chiefly fibrinogen, *fibrinous inflammation;* if accompanied by hemorrhage, *hemorrhagic inflammation*) and *emigration* of leukocytes *(purulent inflammation).*

Figure 23 shows the intensity of the response of some tissue reactions in both acute and chronic stages of inflammation.

See the following Figures:
Serous inflammation, Figs 25, 3–25   Hemorrhagic inflammation, Fig 3–33
Fibrinous inflammation, Figs 1–35, 1–36, 3–25,   Purulent inflammation Figs 1–23, 3–19, 3–25,
3–29   4–46, 5–14, 6–38

Intensity

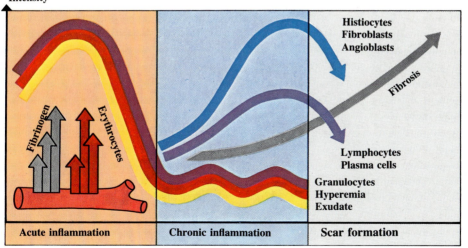

Fibrinogen · Erythrocytes

Histiocytes
Fibroblasts
Angioblasts

Fibrosis

Lymphocytes
Plasma cells

Granulocytes
Hyperemia
Exudate

| Acute inflammation | Chronic inflammation | Scar formation |

Fig 23.—Schematic representation of the tissue reactions to inflammatory stimuli.

In the *chronic stages,* proliferation of connective tissue cells, histiocytes and capillaries predominate *(granulation tissue).* Different morphological appearances and functional disturbances are produced, depending upon the duration of the injury, the amount of denatured protein (necrotic tissue, fibrin) deposited or the presence of foreign bodies in the tissue. Essentially, there is proliferation of *fibroblasts,* young connective tissue (fibrosis → scar), *histiocytes* (phagocytic function) [now thought to come from blood monocytes!] and *new capillaries* (nutritional function). There are also varying numbers of lymphocytes, plasma cells, mast cells and polymorphonuclear leukocytes.

On the basis of the cell type, some authors separate a *cellular form of proliferating granulation tissue,* which is rich in lymphocytes and histiocytes, from *granulation tissue in a narrow sense* (only capillary twigs and fibroblasts), and from an *infiltrating form of granulation tissue* which appears between the local tissue elements and may be transformed into them.

Among the chief functions of granulation tissue the following may be mentioned:

1. *resorption,* e.g., the resorption of necrotic tissue, thrombi or fibrin;

2. *tissue replacement,* e.g., replacement of defects in the skin or mucous membranes (Fig 9–10);

3. *localization,* e.g., walling off of an abscess.

The result is always the formation of a *scar* to replace the defect caused by loss of local parenchymatous tissue.

See Figs 1–19, 1–20, 4–27

Macroscopic: Immature granulation tissue: red. Scar tissue: white, glistening, fibrous and tough.

See Figs 3–39, 3–41, 3–44

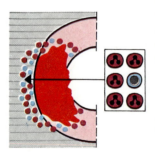

Fig 24.—Fibrinoid necrosis in an artery.

Fibrinoid degeneration or necrosis (Fig 24) develops after severe acute disturbance of vascular permeability with subsequent sudden leakage of blood plasma into the vessel wall and the surrounding connective tissue. Because of this, the vascular tissues are either obscured or destroyed (see Table 3). The blood plasma proteins may combine chemically with collagen or the tissue mucopolysaccharides. Fibrin is often demonstrable with both the light and electron microscopes. A slight, fleeting leukocytic reaction or secondary proliferation of histiocytes (e.g., Aschoff nodules in rheumatic fever) or granulation tissue (e.g., in polyarteritis (panarteritis) nodosa) may follow, with consequent resorption of the fibrinoid.

Circumscribed nodules of granulation tissue are seen in granulomatous inflammation (histiocytic granuloma, e.g., Aschoff nodules; foreign body granuloma; epithelioid granuloma of tuberculosis, etc.).

See Figs 3–39, 3–41, 3–44

By the term "specific inflammation" is meant a tissue reaction distinguished by a characteristic (specific) morphological appearance that suggests the etiologic agent, e.g. tuberculosis, which shows a typical arrangement of cells and tissues (often with necrosis). It should be noted, however, that such lesions are specific only in a limited sense, since epithelioid cell granulomas, for example, may occur in diseases of different causes (tuberculosis, syphilis, brucellosis, histoplasmosis, sarcoid, etc.).

Acute Inflammation

In *serous inflammation,* fluid leaks from the blood vessels. Figure 27 shows what happens. The tight adhesion between the endothelial cells (normally desmosomes) is lost. Through these pores (0.1 to 0.8 μ) blood serum escapes and collects under the basement membrane or the pericytes (Fig 27). *Leukocytes, lymphocytes, monocytes,* and *erythrocytes* also pass through these pores (Figs 25 through 27). Exudation of *fibrinogen* is thought to take place in a similar fashion. Once outside the vessels, it polymerizes to fibrin. Because a thick layer of fibrin may be deposited on and be bound to the collagen fibers, a homogeneous, eosinophilic microscopic appearance results that is referred to as *fibrinoid swelling* or *degeneration.* Lysosomal enzymes and the acid pH of the inflamed area cause the collagen fibers to loosen (tuftlike splintering). In addition, fibrin may be deposited between the protofibrils *(fibrinoid necrosis).* Leukocytic proteolytic enzymes often cause tissue liquefaction (abscess), during which process the collagen fibers disintegrate and probably can form hyalin (Fig 35, *reconstituted hyalin*).

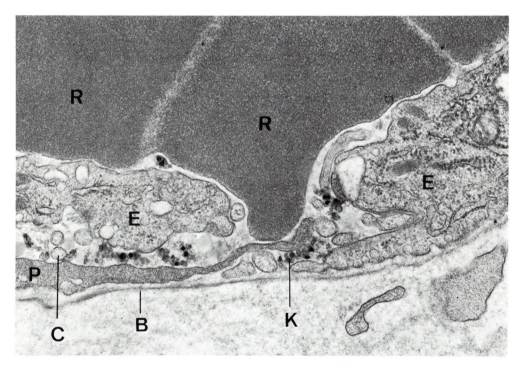

Fig 27.—Serous inflammation: wall of a venule in rat skeletal muscle following local injection of histamine and carbon. A gap has formed between endothelial cells *(E)* through which carbon *(K)* as well as chylomicrons *(C)* from the blood have passed. Part of an erythrocyte *(R)* has also passed through the gap. The erythrocytes are tightly packed—a sign of blood stasis. *P,* cytoplasmic process of a pericyte; *B,* basal lamina (47,500 ×). (I. Joris)

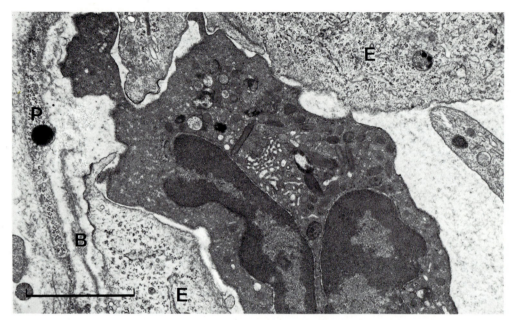

Fig 25.—Early stage of leukocyte emigration from a venule in acute inflammation of rat omentum. A polymorphonuclear leukocyte has pushed between the two endothelial cells *(E)*. *B,* basement membrane; *P,* cytoplasm of a pericyte (27,500×). (I. Joris)

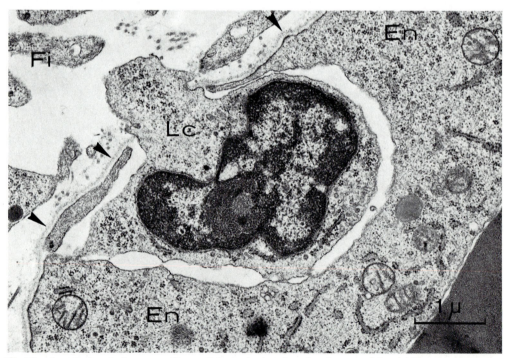

Fig 26.—Lymphodiapedesis, postcapillary venule in the lymph node of a normal fetus 165 mm crown-rump length. *En,* endothelial cell; *Lc,* lymphocyte; *Fi,* process of a fibroblast. Note erythrocyte in the venule lumen. Note also the defect in the basement membrane *(arrows),* which is continuous elsewhere, and the place of egress of the lymphocyte. (Magnification about 19,600×.) (G. Kistler)

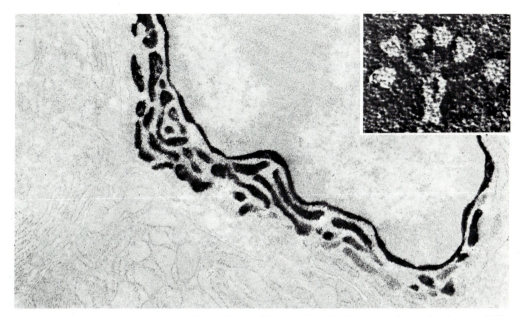

Fig 28.—Site of specific antibody formation (antihorseradish peroxidase) in the ergostoplasm of a plasma cell (6 days after first injection) (24,000×). (Cottier) *Insert:* Human complement factor C1 with six binding sites (1,100,000×). (Villiger)

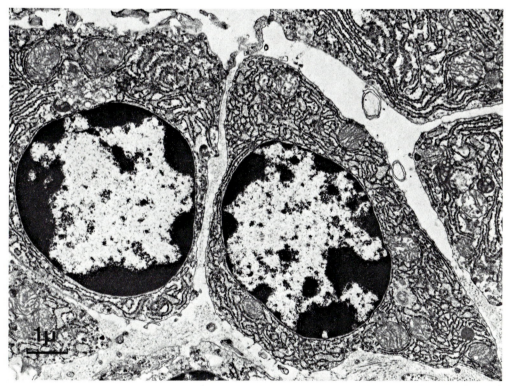

Fig 29.—Plasma cells from a bronchogenic carcinoma. Note structure of the nucleus as well as the distended rough endoplasmic reticulum. (Magnification about 10,500×.) (Kistler)

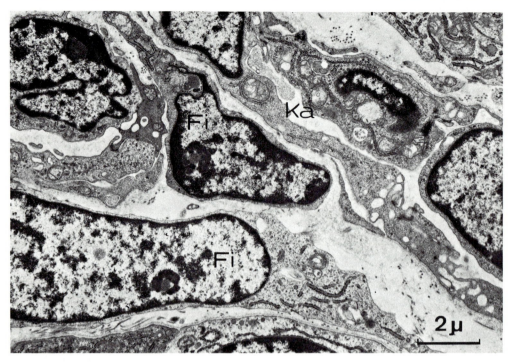

Fig 30.—Fibroblasts *(Fi)* and capillaries *(Ka)* in the interstitial tissue of a fetus 180 mm crown-rump length (about 8,500×). (Kistler)

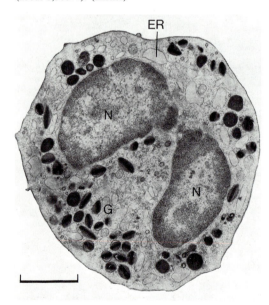

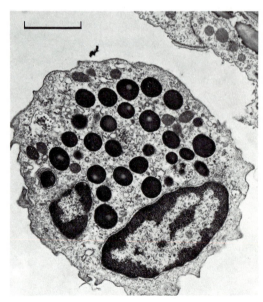

Fig 31.—Eosinophilic granulocyte from rat bone marrow. *G,* eosinophilic granules with crystalline inclusions (lysosomes); *N,* lobulated nucleus; *ER,* endoplasmic reticulum (7,000×). (Staubesand)

Fig 32.—Mast cell (rat) with intracytoplasmic granules containing histamine and serotonin (13,000×). (Staubesand)

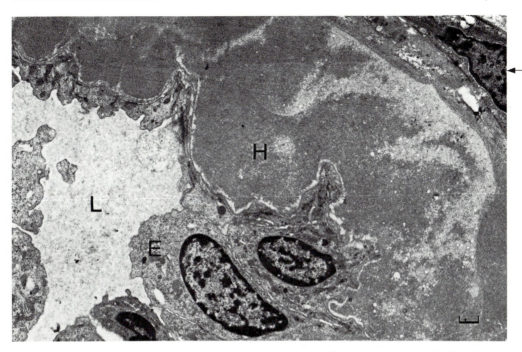

Fig 33.—Hyalinized afferent arteriole of renal glomerulus (human) in hypertension. *L,* lumen of arteriole; *E,* intact endothelium; *H,* amorphous hyaline material; → necrotic muscle of media (8,500 ×).

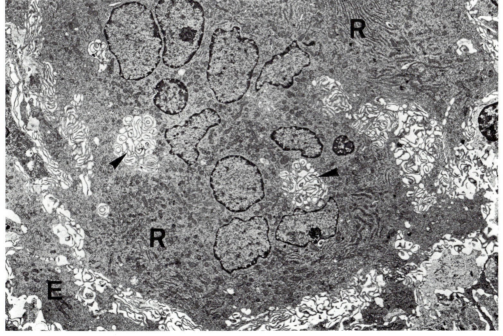

Fig 34.—Langhans' giant cell *(R)* in a lymph node. Note the numerous cell processes with microvilli and the invaginations of membranes *(arrowheads)*. *E,* epitheliod cells (about 1,700 ×). (Kistler)

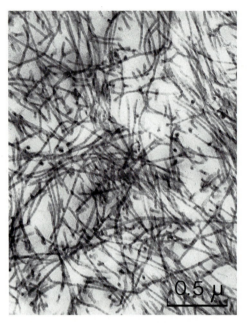

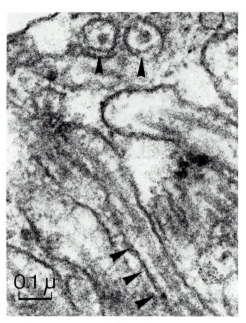

Fig 35.—Hyaline transformation of collagenous fibrous tissue showing cross-striations (reconstituted hyalin) (30,000×). (Gieseking)

Fig 36.—Persistent chronic hepatitis B in a 38-year-old person with a kidney transplant. Note smooth endoplasmic reticulum of a liver cell with hepatitis B surface antigen in longitudinal and cross sections *(arrows)* (about 11,500×). (Kistler)

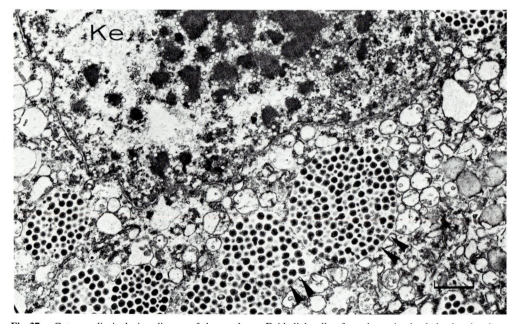

Fig 37.—Cytomegalic inclusion disease of the newborn. Epithelial cells of renal proximal tubule showing immature virus particles in the nucleus *(Ke)* and vacuolar swelling of the endoplasmic reticulum with mature (encapsulated) cytomegalic viruses *(arrowheads)* (about 10,700×). (Kistler)

Growth and Tumors

Increase in metabolic work finds morphological expression in enlargement of cells and nuclei (hypertrophy, Fig 8) or in increased numbers of cells (numerical hypertrophy or hyperplasia) (see Chap. 1, Part II, Introductory Comments). Formation of equivalent specific organs and tissues is called regeneration. In addition, one sort of tissue can be transformed to another sort, e.g., columnar epithelium to squamous epithelium, a process called metaplasia. The basal cells of the epithelial tissue in this example have differentiated to epithelium that is foreign to the site (Fig 7–10).

Giant cells appear under various conditions and in a variety of forms (Fig 39). Frequently, they are the result of the increased work of resorption (e.g., Langhans' giant cells, foreign body giant cells, osteoclasts). They result from fusion of cells or from nuclear division without cytoplasmic division (amitotic division). In many cases, giant cells develop from capillary twigs (e.g., giant cells in an epulis). Touton giant cells are found in chronic resorbing inflammation in fat tissue.

See the following Figures: Figure 9–9, foreign body giant cell; Figure 3–41, Langhans' giant cell; Figure 4–3, giant cells in an epulis or brown tumor; Figures 1–28 and 1–29, giant cells in an Aschoff nodule; Figure 9–8, Touton giant cells; Figures 11–13 and 11–14; Hodgkin and Reed-Sternberg giant cells; Figure 13–25, osteoclasts; Figure 7–23, placental giant cell; Figure 9–36, 13–29, tumor giant cell.

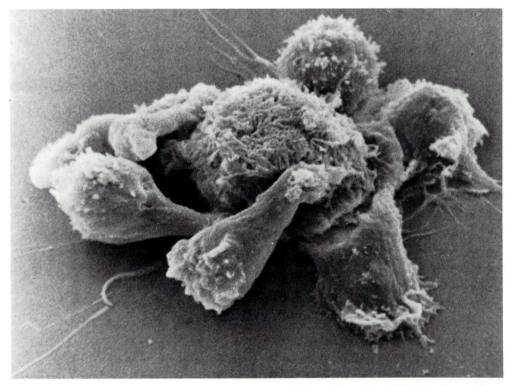

Fig 38.—Cellular aggression against a rounded-off cancer cell (HeLa cell) by cativated killer lymphocytes (scanning electron micrograph; 5,500 ×). (Paweletz, Cancer Center, Heidelberg)

Giant Cells

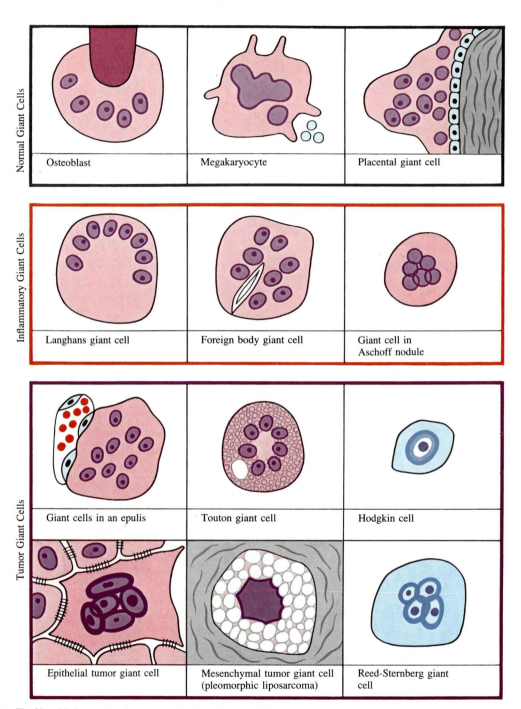

Fig 39.—Various sorts of normal and pathologic giant cells.

Tumors (synonyms: neoplasm, new growth, blastoma) *are abnormal tissue masses, which arise by autonomous, progressive and excessive proliferation of the body's own cells.*

For useful *diagnosis* and *classification* of a tumor it is necessary to consider several individual factors, especially the morphology (microscopic structure) and the histogenesis (recognition of the parent tissue from which the tumor arises). It is desirable not only to make an *accurate diagnosis* of a tumor but also to give an opinion of the *prognosis* and of the *appropriate therapy*. The most important consideration in classifying a tumor, without doubt, is its *biologic behavior*. It should be borne in mind, however, that the terms *benign* and *malignant* are anthropomorphic rather than scientific concepts of tumor. There are tumors that are truly benign (e.g., cutaneous warts) and others that are unquestionably malignant (e.g., malignant melanoma). For *locally malignant tumors* that have a locally destructive growth pattern and recur but do not metastasize the term *semimalignant* is used. Basal cell carcinoma, cylindroma, carcinoid, and salivary gland tumors belong to this group. In the current WHO nomenclature basal cell carcinoma and cylindroma are considered as basal cell carcinoma or as adenoidcystic carcinoma and so are unequivocally counted among malignant tumors. Carcinoids behave differently, depending on their location: carcinoids of the appendix are often benign, carcinoids of the ileum may metastasize to the liver. Today salivary gland tumors are placed with pleomorphic adenomas, since they recur only after incomplete surgical removal.

The diagnostic assessment of a tumor demands the collection and evaluation of numerous individual pieces of clinical and pathologic information. Thus it must be remembered that the final diagnosis of any pathologist is the result of his experience and that he predicts the possible final outcome of the disease from the static appearance of the fixed tissue submitted to him. The most important pieces of information are summarized in Table 5. In practice one is always faced by the question, *is the tumor still benign or already malignant?* We know that a malignant tumor (e.g., a carcinoma) does not arise directly from a normal cell but is rather the end stage of a series of changes that may progress from the normal cell through regenerative changes and benign tumors to malignant tumors. This course is termed *progression*. Thus it is possible that a tissue sample may be of a transitional phase or intermediate stage of a tumor and the question of its behavior cannot be definitely settled. Such cases are called *borderline* tumors.

In recent years it has been observed repeatedly that the *prognosis of a tumor*—measured in terms of 5- or 10-year survival—depends on certain well-established pathologic-anatomical facts which are taken into account either by the **TNM system** or by tumor grading. In the **TNM system** (*T,* tumor; *N,* node; *M,* metastasis) the macroscopic findings, such as tumor size, its localization, spread, involvement of lymph nodes, and the presence of distant hematogenous metastases, are taken into account. At present attempts are being made to provide a code for tumors arising in each organ. In **tumor grading** the prognosis of a tumor is estimated from its histologic structure and degree of differentiation, well-differentiated tumors as a rule having a better prognosis than undifferentiated tumors (see carcinomas of the thyroid).

TABLE 5.—DIFFERENCES OF BEHAVIOR OF BENIGN AND MALIGNANT TUMORS

CHARACTERISTICS	BENIGN TUMORS	MALIGNANT TUMORS
	Clinical Findings	
Sex	Not significant	Not significant
Age	Chiefly in young persons	Chiefly in older persons
Location of tumor	Both benign and malignant tumors occur in all organs: tumor characteristics may be determined by localization: a histologically benign tumor can have a malignant behavior because of its location (e.g., in the brain)	
Clinical symptoms	Rather slight, nonspecific (many exceptions, e.g., endocrine tumors)	Marked, often detected first in advanced stages
Duration of illness	Long (years or decades)	Rather short (months)
Specific cell function	Chiefly normal	Mostly lacking
Growth	Expanding, displacing	Infiltrating, invasive
Metastases	Lacking	Common
Recurrence	Can occur	Common
	Pathologic Findings	
Organ changes	Pressure atrophy	Destruction
Tumor capsule	Present	Lacking
Consistency	Variable	Mostly soft
Cut surface	Uniform	Variegated (red hemorrhages, yellow necrosis)
Tissue type (compared to parent tissue)	Homologous, mature	Heterologous, immature
Cellularity	Often poorly cellular	Richly cellular
Cell size and shape	Regular, isomorphous	Irregular, polymorphous
Cell atypia	Lacking	Common
Mitoses: number and type	Rare, typical	Common, atypical
Chromatin	Regularly distributed	Irregular: partly dense partly vesicular
Chromosomes (DNA content)	Euploid	Chiefly aneuploid with chromosomal aberrations
Nucleolus	Similar to parent cells	Variable size; often prominent
Nucleus/cytoplasm ratio	Normal	Displacement in favor of nucleus
Cytoplasmic staining	Normal	Often increased by increase in RNA; slightly basophilic
Enzyme content of cells	Normal	Often deficient

Tumors—Electron Microscopy

There is no one specific ultramicroscopic feature by which a cancer cell can be invariably recognized. There are, however, certain recognizable morphological changes that differentiate a normal cell from a tumor cell.

In animals, oncologic viruses can be detected in certain tumors, for example, breast carcinoma, leukemia, and other tumors. In man, viruses have been *identified* only in certain papillomas and cutaneous warts. It is true, nonetheless, that similar particles have been *observed* in human leukemia cells and a few other cancer cells.

Electron microscopic evaluation of the **nuclear membrane** is of special importance. Marked infolding of the nuclear membrane is typical of certain tumor cells, e.g., mycosis fungoides cells (Fig 41) or Reed-Sternberg cells in Hodgkin's disease, although the changes usually can only be identified with certainty in semithin sections (thickness less than 1 μ).

The **cytoplasm** also shows ultrastructural alterations. Certain tumors, such as oncocytoma, show pathologic changes of *mitochondrial* DNA. The cells are filled with plump, functionally defective mitochondria (histologically oxyphilic, pale, granular cytoplasm). Tumors of a high grade of malignancy, by comparison, are mostly *poor in mitochondria* or show *dystrophic giant mitochondria*. The *endoplasmic reticulum* is likewise indicative of the degree of differentiation of a tumor. The cells of a benign tumor (adenoma) or of a well-differentiated liver cell carcinoma (Fig 44), for example, possess well-developed capacities for synthesis and secretion of proteins. Consequently these cells contain well-developed endoplasmic reticulum. In a rapidly growing malignant hepatoma, on the other hand, the tumor cells lose their *metabolic capability:* smooth endoplasmic reticulum is absent. In sarcoma cells the content of endoplasmic reticulum diminishes with decreasing cell differentiation.

Study of the ultrastructure of tumors can contribute to *differential diagnosis* and histogenetic classification. *Desmosome-like intercellular bridges* are typical of a squamous cell carcinoma (Fig 46). In other carcinoma cells the *microvillus-like differentiation of the outer cell membrane* indicates derivation from cells that line a lumen, viscus, or a body cavity (glands, respiratory tract, mesothelium). The recognition of *intracytoplasmic granules* with a zigzag internal structure suggests a melanoma. In spindle cell sarcomas an accurate histogenetic classification is often possible only after electron microscopic investigation. The presence of a sarcomere-like *arrangement of myofilaments* suggests a rhabdomyosarcoma (Fig 42); of *heavy bundles of filaments,* a leiomyosarcoma.

Electron microscopy can also give information about the *spread of a tumor,* especially in regard to the *tumor-stroma relationship.* In these cases the ultrastructural findings (e.g., the basement membrane, Fig 47) contribute to better demarcation of invasive from preinvasive stages and of early cancer changes.

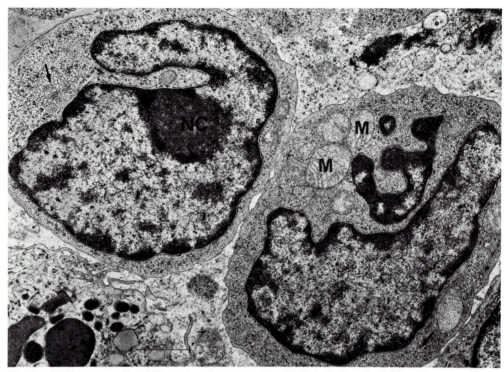

Fig 40.—Burkitt tumor cells. Malignant lymphoma occurring chiefly in the jaws in children. It consists of lymphoblasts with scanty cytoplasmic margins and distinctly polymorphous nuclei, irregular, clumplike divisions of heterochromatin, and large nucleolus *(NC)*. The cytoplasm is rich in free ribosomes and polysomes (→) but poor in mitochrondria *(M)* (10,000×). (Bernhard)

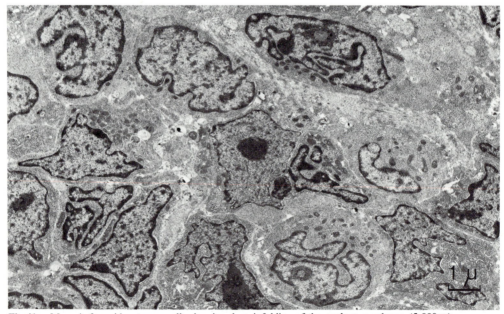

Fig 41.—Mycosis fungoides; tumor cells showing deep infolding of the nuclear membrane (5,000×).

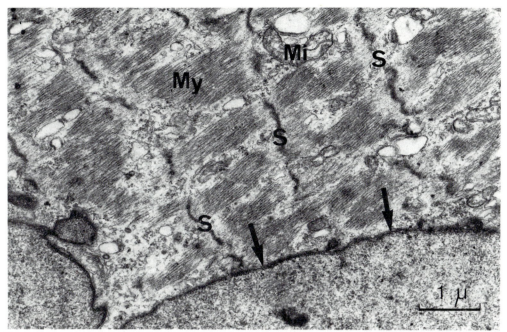

Fig 42.—Section of rhabdomyosarcoma cell. Myofilaments *(M)* are clearly shown and have a sarcomere-like arrangement *(S)*. *Mi*, mitochondria. The *arrows* point to the nuclear membrane (12,000×).

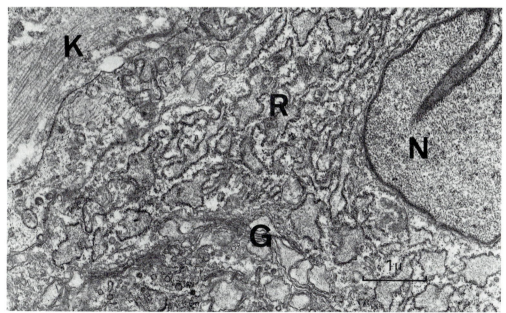

Fig 43.—Section of a fibrosarcoma cell. The cell is surrounded by primitive collagen fibrils *(K)* and has a lobulated nucleus *(N)* and well-developed rough endoplasmic reticulum *(R)* and Golgi apparatus *(G)* (12,000×).

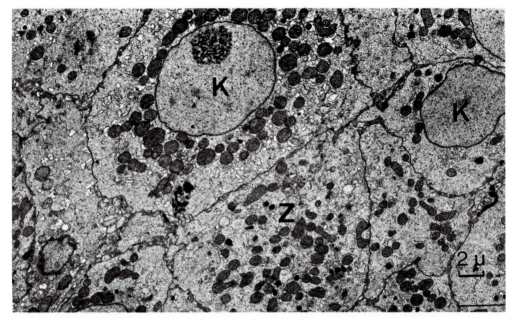

Fig 44.—Section of a moderately fast growing Morris hepatoma. The cytoarchitecture of the tumor cells for the most part resembles that of normal hepatocytes. The orderly lobular pattern is lacking. *Z*, cytoplasm; *K*, nucleus. Note the large nucleolus (7,500×).

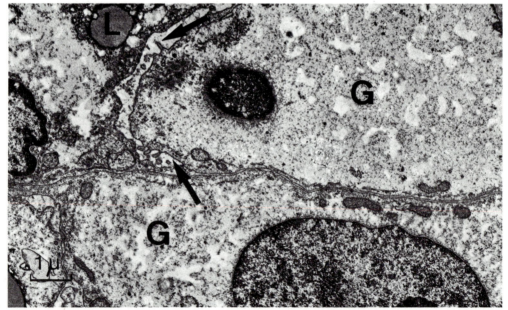

Fig 45.—Section of a clear cell from a hypernephroma (renal clear cell carcinoma). The cytoplasm contains large amounts of glycogen *(G)* and lipid droplets *(L)*. The *arrows* point to villous differentiation of the cell surface (10,500×). (Kistler)

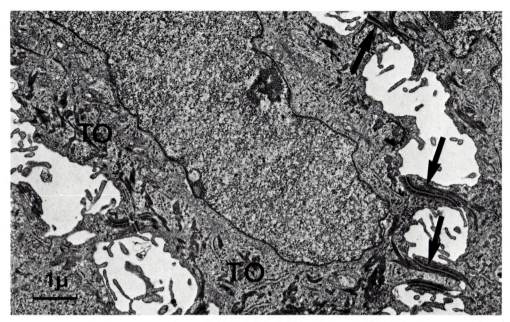

Fig 46.—Section of a tumor cell from a squamous cell carcinoma of the bronchus. The typical intercellular bridges are clearly seen with their desmosome-like structures (→), which are characteristic of squamous epithelium. The cytoplasm is rich in tonofibrils *(TO)* (12,000×). (Kistler)

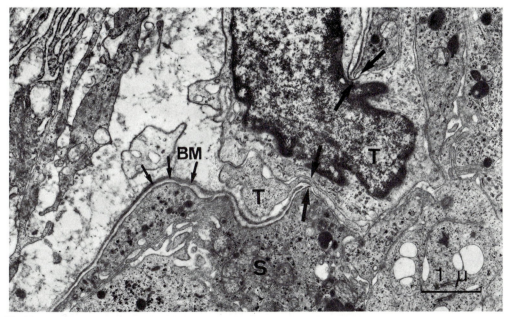

Fig 47.—Epithelial-stromal junction of a mammary duct carcinoma. The intraductal tumor cell is bounded by a basement membrane *(BM)*. Tumor cells *(T)* penetrate the stroma through a break in the basement membrane (→) (15,000×). (Ozello and Sanpitak)

39

Classification of Tumors

1. **Primary tumors**

    1.1 Epithelial Tumors (subdivided by morphological criteria)
    1.1.1 Benign tumors
    Adenoma (polyp): trabecular, follicular, tubular, alveolar, oncocytic, clear cell, acidophile
    Papilloma: squamous epithelial, transitional epithelial
    Cystoma
    1.1.2. Malignant tumors (carcinomas): solid, medullary, scirrhous, glandular (adenocarcinoma), mucinous, trabecular, tubular, follicular, acidophile, oncocytic, clear cell, cribriform, adenoid cystic (cylindroma), signet ring, adenoacanthoma, squamous cell, transitional cell, mucoepidermoid, papillary, intraductal, lobular, etc.

    1.2. Mesenchymal tumors (subdivided by tissue of origin)

    1.2.1. Benign tumors: fibroma, leiomyoma, chondroma, etc.
    1.2.2. Malignant tumors: fibrosarcoma, leiomyosarcoma, chondrosarcoma, etc.

    1.3. Neurogenic tumors (subdivided by tissue of origin): neurinoma, neurofibroma, meningioma, glioma (astrocytoma, oligodendroglioma, glioblastoma multiforme), ependymoma, medulloblastoma, neuroblastoma, pheochromocytoma

    1.4 Mesothelial tumors: benign and malignant mesotheliomas

    1.5 Pigmented tumors: pigmented nevus (nevus cell nevus, blue nevus), malignant melanoma

    1.6 Mixed tumors
    1.6.1 Benign tumors: fibroadenoma, mature teratoma, cystadenofibroma
    1.6.2 Malignant tumors: cystadenosarcoma, immature teratoma, lymphoepithelioma

    1.7 Tumors classified by organ (location): hepatoma, cholangioma, small cell bronchial carcinoma, endometrial carcinoma, Brenner tumor of ovary, granulosa-theca cell tumor, gonadoblastoma, chorionepithelioma, sweat gland tumors, odontomas, Wilms' tumor of kidney, Ewing's sarcoma (bone), carcinoids of intestine, etc.

2. **Secondary tumors** (metastatic)

3. **Malignant systemic diseases**
    3.1 Hemopoietic system: leukemias, plasmacytomas
    3.2 Malignant lymphomas: Hodgkin's disease, non-Hodgkin's lymphomas

Benign Epithelial Tumors

Benign epithelial tumors (Fig 48) can arise from a mucous membrane (*fibroepithelial exophytic growth* = papilloma or polyp) or from a solid, parenchymatous organ (*endophytic growth* = adenoma).

Chronic irritation or inflammation can cause circumscribed thickening of a mucous membrane. In **leukoplakia** (Fig 48,a) there is acanthotic thickening of the epithelium with superficial parakeratotic cornification (cornified lamellae containing nuclei) and an inflammatory infiltrate in the depths of the stroma. Leukoplakias of oral mucous membrane, lip, tongue, larynx, and of the urinary bladder are considered precancerous lesions. In contrast, simple hyperkeratosis *(leukoplakic thickening)* of the esophagus or uterine cervix is harmless.

Pseudopolyps (Fig 48,b) arise by expansion of a submucosal tumor. Example: submucous or subcutaneously situated lipoma.

Papillomas (Fig 48,c) are benign, broad-based, epithelial new growths that develop on squamous or transitional epithelial surfaces. They occur in the urinary bladder, skin, or oral cavity and as villous polyps in the colon, where they are demarcated by the muscularis mucosae (48,e). Invasion is a sign of malignant transformation (Fig 48,f).

Tubular adenomas (adenomatous polyps, Fig 48,d) are benign epithelial new growths with a narrow base and a long stalk. The surface is covered by glandular epithelium. Example: adenomatous polyp of the colon.

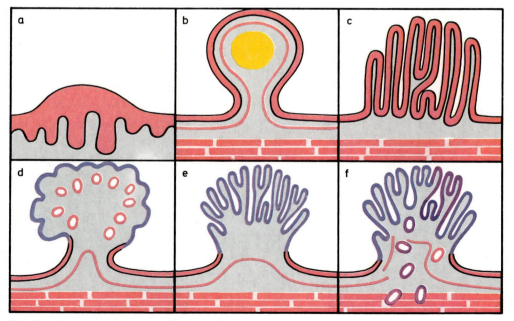

Fig 48.—Schematic depiction of papillomas and polyps.

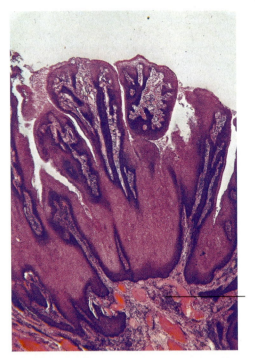

Fig 49.—Condyloma acuminatum (hematoxylin-eosin; 20×).

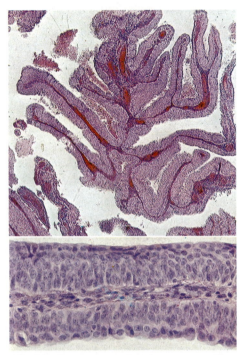

Fig 50.—Low-power and high-power magnification of a papilloma of the urinary bladder (hematoxylin-eosin; 30× and 150×).

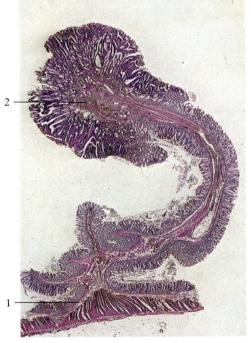

Fig 51.—Tubular adenomatous polyp of the rectum (hematoxylin-eosin; 8×).

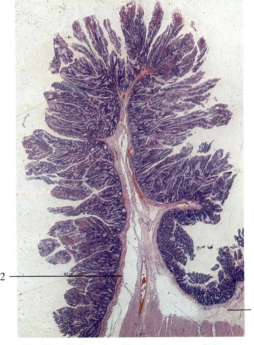

Fig 52.—Villous (papillary) adenoma of the rectum (hematoxylin-eosin; 6×).

Papillomas—Adenomas (polyps)

Condyloma acuminatum (Fig 49). *A benign, broad-based fibroepithelial new growth, chiefly occurring in the perianal and periurethral regions, or on the penis or external female genitalia.* Histologically the lesion consists of a papilloma resting on connective tissue of variable thickness and covered on the surface by a thickened layer of squamous epithelium (stratum spinosum shows many mitoses). The basal stroma is inflamed and vascular.

Condyloma acuminatum is a virus-caused hyperplasia of mucous membrane induced by chronic irritation— occasionally as an accompaniment of some other disease (e.g., gonorrhea). The lesion tends to recur but not to become malignant. It must be differentiated from syphilitic *condyloma latum*.

Urinary tract papilloma (Fig 50) *is a* **histologically** *benign, exophytically growing, fibroepithelial tumor of the upper urinary passages and bladder which, however, frequently recurs and shows malignant transformation. It is therefore* **clinically** *considered at least an obligate precancerous lesion or even a well-differentiated transitional cell carcinoma (grade 1).* Low magnification (Fig 50, top) shows the many-layered transitional epithelium. It is a papilloma with a broad cellular layer (more than 7 cell layers), cell atypia (variable sizes of cells and nuclei), as well as mitoses which are signs of marked proliferation or malignant transformation, although signs of invasive growth in the material examined may be entirely lacking.

Papillomas of the urinary bladder commonly develop in men 60—70 years old. Recurrences occur in about 70% of cases and are seldom as low grade as the primary tumor. In 10% of papillomas evidence of invasive growth is present. Proliferating cells showing all the cytologic criteria of malignancy but with an intact basement membrane are designated *carcinoma in situ* and tend to spread superficially.

Polyps of the Colon (Figs 51, 52)

Polyps of the gastrointestinal tract are benign exophytic new growths occurring chiefly in the colon and infrequently in the gastric mucosa and small intestine. Both clinically and pathologically the following types are recognized: (1) Solitary *retention polyps*. These usually develop in children under 6 years, are localized in the rectum, and are benign. (2) Solitary *adenomatous polyps* (Fig 51) occur in adults and very rarely become malignant. (3) Large (over 3 cm in diameter), solitary, *villous, rectal polyps,* by contrast, more commonly become carcinomas. (4) *Polyposis coli* shows many mucosal polyps that are of adenomatous type histologically but become malignant early (young men under 36 years of age). (5) In *polyposis intestini (Peutz-Jeghers syndrome)* benign polyps with long stalks develop in the gastrointestinal tract accompanied by prominent, flecklike melanin pigmentation of the lips and oral mucous membranes. Polyps also occur in the *Gardner* and *Cronkhite-Canada* syndromes.

Figures 51 and 52 show the prognostically important differences in structure between an adenomatous and a villous polyp of the rectum. An *adenomatous rectal polyp* (Fig 51) has a narrow site of attachment ($\rightarrow$ 1), a long, thin stalk and a thick, knoblike head. The stroma arises from the muscularis mucosae, submucosa, and blood vessels. Near the surface ($\rightarrow$ 2) there are collections of erythrocytes and macrophages containing hemosiderin (sign of bleeding). The superficial layer is made up partly of pale mucus-containing epithelium and partly of dark regenerating and hyperplastic epithelium. A *villous rectal polyp* (Fig 52) on the other hand, has a broad-based papillary structure and the pattern of the superficial epithelium has changed to a hyperplastic adenomatous one. The tumor-free submucosa ($\rightarrow$ 1) and the intact muscularis mucosae exclude malignancy in this case.

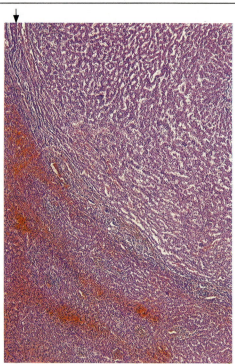

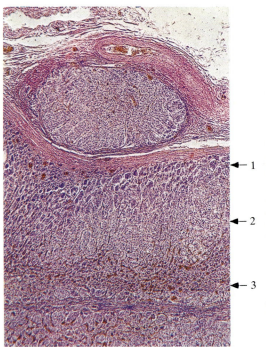

Fig 53.—Adrenal cortical adenoma (near top of picture). Below it, normal adrenal cortex (hematoxylin-eosin; 35×).

Fig 54.—Benign liver cell adenoma (hematoxylin-eosin; 40×).

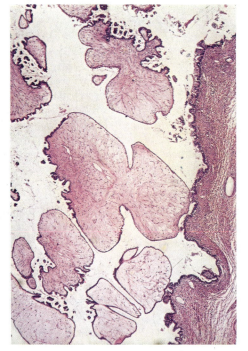

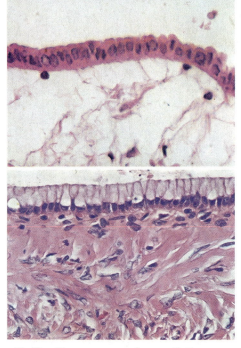

Fig 55.—Papillary serous cystadenoma of ovary (hematoxylin-eosin; 30×).

Fig 56.—Top, serous cystadenoma. Bottom, pseudomucinous cystadenoma of ovary (hematoxylin-eosin; 250×).

Adenoma—Cystoma

An **adenoma of the adrenal cortex** (Fig 53) *is a well-circumscribed, encapsulated, benign neoplasm arising from the adrenal cortex.* Since these and similar tumors in the endocrine organs are an expression of augmented hormonal demand, they are sometimes spoken of as adaptation hyperplasia. This means that—at least at the beginning—both growth and function are under hormonal control. The figure shows an adenoma lying in the capsule of the adrenal and isolated from the underlying adrenal, which shows the normal cortical layers (lower half of figure): *zona glomerulosa* (→1), *zona fasciculata* (→2), and *zona reticularis* (→3).

Adrenal cortical adenomas are frequently multiple in patients with hypertension *(nodular hyperplasia of adrenal cortex)*. They also occur as true autonomous adenomas and can be hormonally silent or active (Conn or Cushing syndromes). These adenomas are especially rich in lipids (yellow cut surface).

Hepatoma (Fig 54) *is a benign new growth arising from proliferating hepatocytes.* Histologically it is a circumscribed but not encapsulated nodule (→) composed of cells having a trabecular arrangement. Under high magnification the tumor is seen not to be bounded by normal liver cells. The adjacent tissue at the periphery shows pressure atrophy and is bloody.

Hepatomas develop with special frequency in cirrhosis of the liver and in the advanced stages of the disease cannot be differentiated from *regenerative nodules*. Isolated hepatomas develop in normal liver but only occasionally and are thought to be tumor-like malformations *(hamartomas)*. Well-circumscribed *benign cholangiomas* are also regarded as hamartomas. They consist of proliferating glanduloalveolar bile duct epithelium supported by fibrous stroma.

Cystadenoma (cystic adenoma, cystoma) (Figs 55, 56). Cystadenomas occur chiefly in the ovary and rarely in other organs (e.g., pancreas). They consist of *single or multilocular cysts* lined by flattened or papillary, simple or pseudomucinous epithelium and contain, respectively, thin, yellow or mucinous fluid. On the basis of these features there are *unilocular or multilocular, simple or papillary, serous or pseudomucinous cystadenomas.* This classification has both prognostic and therapeutic significance. **Serous ovarian cystadenomas** develop in both ovaries in about 50% of cases and tend to have the same percentage of malignant transformation. By contrast, **pseudomucinous cystadenomas** are solitary and only occasionally show malignant change (less than 5% of cases). They may rupture and cause **pseudomyxoma peritonei** (rupture → mucinous and tumor adhesions develop in the peritoneum → implantation metastases → further mucin production and spread of intraperitoneal adhesions, especially of the small intestines).

Serous papillary **cystadenoma of the ovary** (Figs 55, 56, top) consists of a cyst lined with cuboidal epithelium. In the cavity of the cyst there are papillary structures having a loosely arranged fibrous stroma and a superficial layer of epithelium. Higher magnification (Fig 56, top) reveals cuboidal cells with eosinophilic cytoplasm and centrally situated nuclei. Commonly there are small concentrically layered calcium deposits in the stroma (psammoma bodies).

Pseudomucinous cystadenoma of the ovary (Fig 56, bottom) consists of a single layer of cylindrical epithelium with basally placed nuclei and apical cytoplasmic mucous vacuoles. These cells resemble the goblet cells of large bowel mucosa. The cysts contain PAS-positive mucus (*pseudomucin* because it is not precipitated by acetic acid).

Ovarian cysts are derived from germinal ovarian epithelium. Differentiation between benign and malignant cysts is often very difficult. In such *borderline tumors* there is often beginning invasion of stroma by clumps of cells showing glandular differentiation.

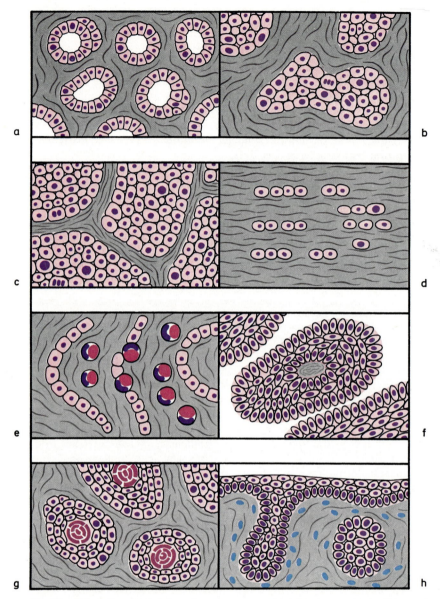

Fig 57.—Schematic representation of carcinomas: *a*, gland-forming carcinoma (adenocarinoma); *b*, solid carcinoma; *c*, medullary carcinoma; *d*, scirrhous carcinoma; *e*, signet ring cell carcinoma; *f*, transitional cell carcinoma; *g*, squamous cell carcinoma; *h*, basal cell carcinoma.

Carcinoma—Malignant Epithelial Tumor

Carcinomas *are epithelial tumors which both clinically and pathologically show signs of malignancy.* They are classified according to the parent tissue from which they come (e.g., hepatocellular carcinoma) or according to their cellular and tissue differentiation (e.g., squamous carcinoma or signet ring cell carcinoma).

Carcinomas which arise from a glandular parenchymatous organ are called **adenocarcinomas.** Such tumors may show advanced **glandular differentiation,** e.g., follicular, alveolar, cystic, or cystic papillary structures (Fig 57,a).

Undifferentiated adenocarcinomas are classified on the basis of the proportion of tumor cells to stroma:

1. In **solid carcinoma simplex** (Fig 57,b) tumor cells and stroma are present in about the same proportion (1:1 ratio). Figure 58 shows small carcinoma deposits comprised of 10—20 tumor cells and surrounding collagenous connective tissue stroma. Mitoses and cellular atypia are common, in contrast to carcinoid.

2. **Medullary carcinoma** (Fig 57,c) typically shows a predominance of the epithelial tumor component and only scanty stroma. Figure 59 is a completely undifferentiated carcinoma traversed only by occasional septa of connective tissue. Near the right margin of the photograph one can see rests of local connective tissue.

3. In **scirrhous carcinoma** (Fig 57,d) the collagenous connective tissue stroma clearly predominates. Enclosed in the stroma are single tumor cells or small strands and clusters of tumor cells *(tumor cells in goose step).* These neoplasms have an especially firm, compact consistency and were formerly called *linitis plastica.*

All three types of tumor are especially common in stomach and breast.

Signet ring cell carcinoma (Fig 57,e) shows a special sort of cell differentiation. The cells are round and the cytoplasm contains a large PAS-positive vacuole of mucin which pushes the nucleus to the periphery of the cell. Signet ring cells are observed in mucinous carcinoma of the breast and in early carcinoma of the stomach.

Among carcinomas of surface epithelium are *transitional cell carcinoma* (Fig 57,f: urinary bladder and passages) and *squamous epithelial carcinoma* (squamous carcinoma, Fig 57,g) which can arise either from normal pavement epithelium or by squamous metaplasia. Malignant epithelial tumors developing from basal cells are called *basal cell carcinoma* (Fig 57,h, see skin tumors).

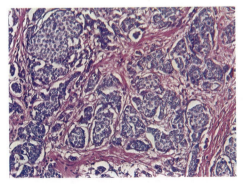

Fig 58.—Solid carcinoma simplex of the breast (hematoxylin-eosin; 80×).

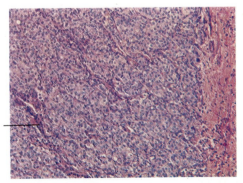

Fig 59.—Medullary carcinoma of the breast (hematoxylin-eosin; 80×).

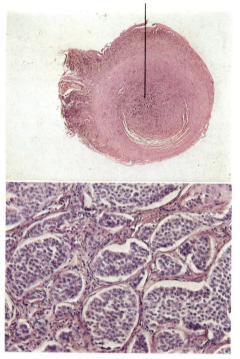

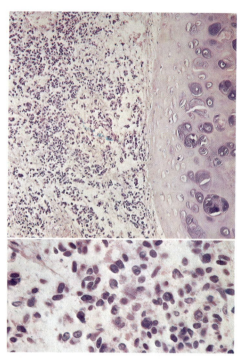

Fig 60.—Carcinoid of the appendix (**top:** scanning lens; 8×; **bottom:** higher magnification, hematoxylin-eosin; 100×).

Fig 61.—Small cell carcinoma of the bronchus (**top:** scanning lens; 80×; **bottom:** higher magnification, hematoxylin-eosin; 320×).

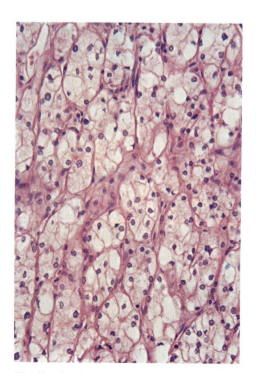

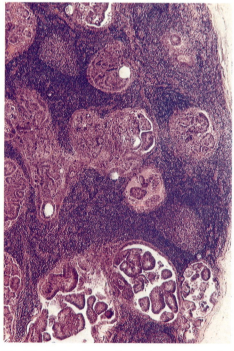

Fig 62.—Renal hypernephroma (clear cell adenocarcinoma) (hematoxylin-eosin; 200×).

Fig 63.—Metastatic carcinoma in a lymph node (hematoxylin-eosin; 50×).

Histology of Special Tumors

Carcinoid of the vermiform appendix (Fig 60). The term "carcinoid" arose because of the similarity of this tumor to a true carcinoma. A **carcinoid** *is a solid, infiltrating tumor that arises from the enterochromaffin system and rarely metastasizes (exception: carcinoid of the ileum).* Figure 60 shows a cross section of an appendix. The lumen is obstructed by a scar and is thickened. With a scanning lens the diffuse infiltration (→) of the organ is easily seen. Higher magnification (Fig 60, bottom) shows the ball-like arrangement of uniform tumor cells. Mitoses are rare.

Carcinoids occur chiefly in the appendix (incidental finding at appendectomy), occasionally in a bronchus or the ileum. They produce serotonin and kallikrein which are decomposed in the liver. When a metastasis develops in the liver these substances are released into the bloodstream and provoke a *carcinoid syndrome.* Carcinoid syndrome may also occur with other tumors, e.g., in bronchial carcinomas.

Small cell carcinoma of the bronchus (Fig 61) *is a malignant epithelial tumor composed of lymphocyte-like cells.* Low magnification—adjacent to a still preserved bronchial cartilage—shows tumor invasion. Higher magnification (Fig 61, bottom) shows a mixture of round (lymphocyte-like) and elongated nuclei (oat cell carcinoma). There is only a sparse stroma.

Bronchial small cell carcinomas are especially malignant tumors which produce distant metastases very early. Since serotonin granules can be demonstrated by electron microscopy in the cytoplasm, it is thought these tumors are malignant variants of carcinoids.

Renal hypernephroma (adenocarcinoma, clear cell carcinoma, Grawitz tumor, Fig 62) *is a malignant kidney tumor comprised of water-clear, plantlike cells with an alveolar or trabecular arrangement, clear, optically empty cytoplasm (glycogen), and round nuclei.* Indications of malignancy in hypernephromas are: size over 3 cm diameter, atypical and polymorphic cells (sarcoma-like growth).

Wilms' tumor (adenomyosarcoma, Fig 64) is a special form of malignant kidney tumor that occurs in young children. Histologically it is a mixed tumor with sarcomatous stroma and pseudotubular (→ 1) as well as pseudoglomerular (→ 2) structures.

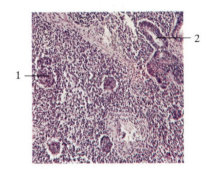

Fig 64.—Wilms' tumor (hematoxylin-eosin; 160×).

Lymph node metastases (Fig 63). *As a rule the discovery of epithelial tissue in a lymph node indicates metastatic carcinoma.* However, benign ectopic epithelial tissue (e.g., of salivary glands, thyroid, or endometrial tissue) does occur occasionally. Figure 63 shows a lymph node invaded by small eosinophilic deposits of metastatic carcinoma.

The appearance of lymph node metastasis can have diagnostic (the first clinical manifestation of an occult carcinoma), prognostic (bad sign), and therapeutic significance.

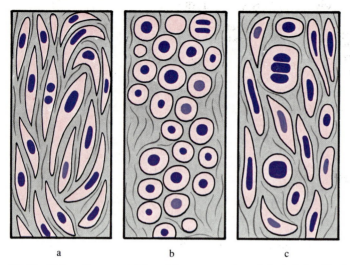

a   b   c

Fig 65.—Schematic representation of the sarcomas (morphological classification): *a,* spindle cell carcinoma (leio-myosarcoma, fibrosarcoma); *b,* round cell sarcoma (lymphosarcoma, immunoblastic sarcoma); *c,* polymorphocellular (pleomorphic) sarcoma (rhabdomyosarcoma, liposarcoma, undifferentiated spindle cell sarcoma).

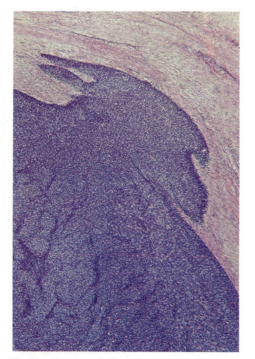

Fig 66.—Invasive spindle cell sarcoma (hematoxylin-eosin; 20×).

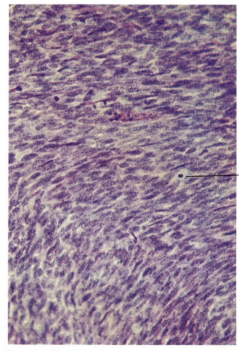

Fig 67.—Undifferentiated spindle cell sarcoma (hematoxylin-eosin; 320×).

Sarcoma—Malignant Mesenchymal Tumor

Sarcomas *are malignant tumors of mesenchymal tissues.* They can be classified either according to morphological or histogenetic criteria. For the pathologist a morphological classification has the advantage of simplicity: it separates **round cell, spindle cell,** and **polymorphous (pleomorphic) sarcomas** (Fig 65).

It is also known that tumors with similar tissue patterns may have very different prognoses. Thus there are spindle cell sarcomas that metastasize early and are particularly malignant. However, other spindle cell sarcomas are locally invasive and recur but produce distant metastases late. A histogenetic classification (according to the parent tissue of derivation) allows separation, for example, of a particularly malignant leiomyosarcoma from a so-called fibrosarcoma.

A histologic classification gives rise to difficulties with respect to undifferentiated tumors. Histologic examination commonly reveals no differences in cell structure or intercellular substances so that it is possible only to make a diagnosis of undifferentiated spindle cell carcinoma (Figs 66, 67). In such cases special studies may be helpful, as for example: electron microscopy, immunohistology, or histochemistry. Electron microscopy frequently allows identification of primitive cellular structures such as myofilaments (leiomyosarcoma) or sarcomeres (rhabdomyosarcoma, Fig 42). Myosin in muscle sarcoma cells can be detected immunohistologically by anti-myosin serum. These methods, however, are expensive and as a rule require unfixed material.

Figures 66 and 67 show scanning lens and high-magnification views of an **undifferentiated spindle cell sarcoma.** The tumor is richly cellular with peg-shaped extensions invading the neighboring eosinophilic connective tissue. The marked basophilia of the tumor is caused by the close proximity of the nuclei. High magnification reveals elongated, parallel lying cells with hyperchromatic nuclei. Mitoses (→) are plentiful (Fig 67). There is no intercellular substance (collagen fibers) between the tumor cells. Poorly differentiated spindle cell sarcomas (few or no collagen fibers between the tumor cells) recur (75%) and metastasize (24%) more frequently than collagen–forming, so-called fibrosarcomas, which have locally invasive growth, recur (40%), but do not metastasize.

Pseudosarcoma. Occasionally there are fast growing new growths that morphologically resemble a sarcoma, but—as their later course shows—have a good prognosis. Histologically they correspond to a fibrosarcoma or lymphosarcoma and are grouped together under the general heading of **pseudosarcoma.**

Pseudosarcomatous nodular fasciitis (Fig 68) *is a benign, rapidly developing disease, probably virus induced, that is characterized by sarcoma-like proliferation of fibroblasts in the deeper layers of the subcutaneous fat tissue.* Histologically there is infiltrative growth of fascial fibroblasts (→ 1) with distinctly pleomorphic nuclei and mitoses. In the periphery of the lesion there is inflamed granulation tissue (→ 2). Metastases do not occur.

Pseudosarcomas with a lymphocyte-like pattern are called **pseudolymphomas.** They have been described for several organs, chiefly in the gastrointestinal tract. Histologically they resemble a lymphoblastic lymphoma. However, their long course over years or decades suggests a benign lesion.

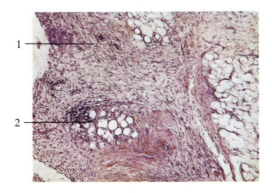

Fig 68.—Pseudosarcomatous fasciitis (hematoxylin-eosin; 32 ×).

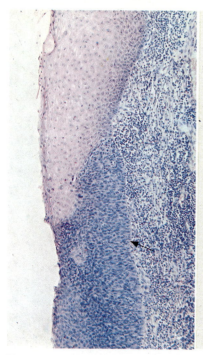

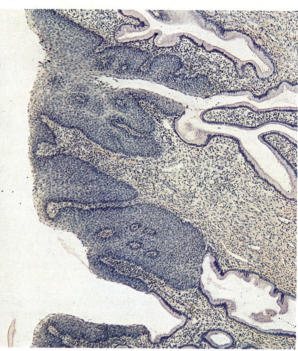

Fig 69.—Carcinoma in situ with simple replacement of surface epithelium (hematoxylin-eosin; 100×).

Fig 70.—Carcinoma in situ with simple replacement of cervical glands (hematoxylin-eosin; 80×).

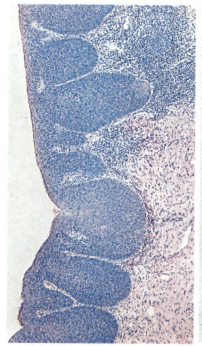

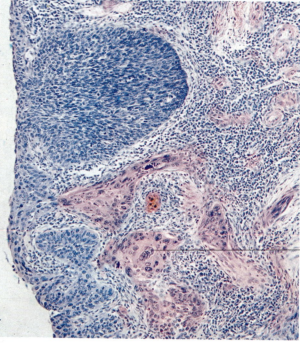

Fig 71.—Carcinoma in situ with bulky growth (hematoxylin-eosin; 80×).

Fig 72.—Carcinoma in situ with early invasion of stroma (hematoxylin-eosin; 120×).

Precancerous Lesions—Carcinoma In Situ

Precancerous lesions *are those tissue lesions or disease entities that during their late stages often become carcinoma.* If the malignant transformation develops in a relatively short time (less than 5 years) and in a specially high percentage of cases (20%–50%), it is called an *obligate precancer. Facultative precancer,* on the other hand, changes to cancer after a longer course and in less than 20% of cases.

The term **carcinoma in situ** was first used for the changes in the mucosa of the uterine cervix (Broders, 1932), in which the cytologic signs of malignancy were present but the basement membrane was still intact. That is, these mucosal alterations that histologically appear to be carcinoma lacked the most important sign of malignancy: invasive growth. At a later date carcinomas in situ were described in other organs. Today we distinguish:

1. **Carcinoma in situ,** which develops in the cervix and is clearly precancerous. If untreated, an invasive carcinoma develops in about 60% of cases.

2. **Carcinoma growing in situ** (superficial carcinoma, mucosal carcinoma) is, in contrast, a carcinoma from the beginning. At first it spreads in the mucosa, later—as a rule—breaks through the basement membrane of the mucosa and so becomes an invasive carcinoma (example: surface carcinoma of the colon).

Early carcinoma of the stomach is a special form of carcinoma in situ (see Fig 4–28, superficial carcinoma, "early cancer"). The tumor cells are located in the mucosal stroma, or even in the submucosa. Even though there is stromal invasion, and thus evidence of invasive carcinoma, it occupies a special position because over 90% of treated patients live more than 5 years.

Additional examples of precancerous tissue changes or diseases: Skin *(Bowen's disease, senile keratosis, lentigo maligna or melanosis circumscripta preblastomatosa of Dubreuilh, intraepidermal epithelioma of Borst-Jadassohn),* vulva *(Bowen's disease, extramammary Paget's disease),* breast *(lobular carcinoma in situ),* uterine cervix *(carcinoma in situ, moderate and marked dysplasia),* endometrium *(adenomatous hyperplasia, carcinoma in situ),* penis *(erythroplasia of Queyrat),* larynx *(proliferative leukoplakia),* colon *(villous polyps, ulcerative colitis),* liver *(cirrhosis),* etc.

Carcinoma in situ (epidermoid carcinoma in situ) of the cervix of the uterus (Figs 69 through 72). *This is a precancerous lesion of the squamous epithelium of the cervix in which the cytological signs of malignancy are present but the basement membrane has not been breeched.* In simple replacement of surface epithelium (Fig 69) there is in addition to the normally layered acidophilic squamous epithelium (upper part of figure) atypical, markedly basophilic epithelium. The normal layering of cells is broken up. The cells have nuclei of variable size and scanty cytoplasm. Mitoses are common. An intact basement membrane (→) separates the carcinoma in situ from the inflamed stroma. Figure 70 shows **simple replacement of a cervical gland by carcinoma in situ.** To the right in the figure there are still intact glands with lumens lined by cylindrical epithelium. To the left is the carcinoma in situ which has already filled the necks of the glands and looks as if it had invaded the stroma, but here also the basement membrane of the surface epithelium as well as of the cervical glands is intact. **Bulky growth** may be a further manifestation of carcinoma in situ (Fig 71). The lesion arches itself against the underlying stroma without infiltrating it. Figure 72 shows transition to an **invasive stage** where besides the bulky growth (left side of figure) there are small, markedly acidophilic epithelial pegs showing distinct nuclear pleomorphism (→). Such cases are spoken of as **early infiltration** or **invasion. Net-like infiltration** (interlacing carcinomatous strands in the stroma) is spoken of as microinvasive carcinoma when it is not over 5 mm in depth. The *progression to carcinoma,* from normal cell to clinically manifest, invasive squamous cell carcinoma, extends from moderate to marked dysplasia* to carcinoma in situ, to early infiltration and microinvasive carcinoma.

---

*Dysplasia: cells showing dyskeratosis and disturbed cellular polarity.

Appendix

The student and young physician can easily forget that the pathologist has an important function to play in the preservation and care of the state of health. In practice, this function is often manifestly concerned with the examination of *biopsy material,* since frequently the decision between life and death for the patient depends on the pathologists diagnosis. The clinical examiner can contribute to an unobjectionable histologic diagnosis by observing a few simple but essential technical rules. The interpretation of histologic appearance is, in many cases, significantly dependent on clinical findings, the site of biopsy, and the age and sex of the patient. This information is often essential for pathologic diagnosis. For this reason, it is important that the form accompanying the request for examination of an important biopsy specimen be completely filled out by the person submitting it. Likewise, the fixation of the biopsy specimen must be just right (aqueous 40% Formalin diluted 1:9, the ratio of specimen to volume of fixative at least 1:20, thickness of tissue block not more than 1 cm). As to the biopsy itself, it is essential that *both normal and diseased tissue be removed,* so that the two can be compared in the histologic preparation. In the case of polyps and papillomas, the tissue in the deepest part of the lesion should be included in the specimen and most carefully examined in order to discover possible invasion.

The use of frozen sections, which can be cut on the cryostat and stained in a few minutes, enables the pathologist to make a quick diagnosis during a surgical operation. This allows the surgeon to plan his operation, for example, in a case of suspected carcinoma of the breast—to decide the necessity of removing the axillary lymph nodes. The accuracy of a diagnosis made from a frozen section by a competent pathologist is almost as good as that made from a paraffin section. But there are limitations to the use of rapid frozen sections for diagnosis and certain questions cannot be answered. The method is only rarely helpful in diagnosing nonmetastatic diseases of lymph nodes.

Every piece of tissue removed from a patient should be examined histologically—a requirement that the physician in his own best interests should never neglect, even when the macroscopic appearances seem ever so plain.

If a physician takes to heart these simple rules, he cannot fail to help his patients.

Unfortunately, physicians are prone to overestimate the reliability of their diagnoses. It is a fact that only 40% of clinical diagnoses in fatal diseases are entirely correct. Another 40% are almost correct, i.e., one of the listed diagnoses is proved to be correct (for example, myocardial infarct, pulmonary embolism, cerebral infarct); 20% of diagnoses are insufficient or wrong. The accuracy of clinical diagnoses is quite significantly improved when an excision biopsy specimen or fine-needle biopsy specimen is examined histologically.

Histologic examination of tissue and the autopsy are essential to quality assurance in medicine. This principle applies as much to treatment of tonsils, gallbladders, and appendices as it does to treatment of grossly cancerous tissue. The rise in the number of malpractice suits should also be borne in mind in this relation.

Systemic Pathology

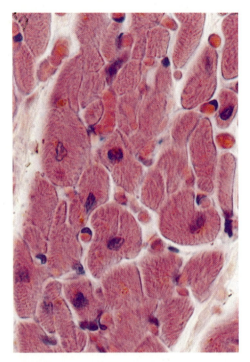

Fig 1–1.—Normal heart muscle cells (hematoxylin-eosin).

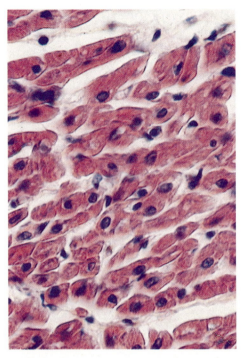

Fig 1–2.—Growing heart muscle cells in a child (hematoxylin-eosin).

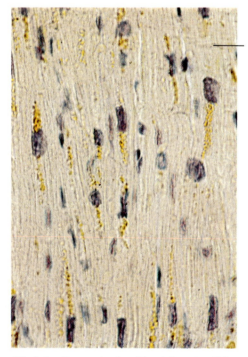

Fig 1–3.—Brown atrophy of heart (hematoxylin).

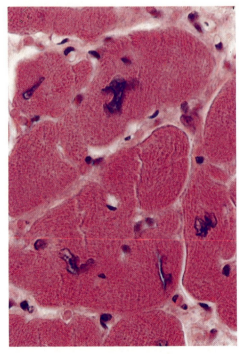

Fig 1–4.—Myocardial hypertrophy (hematoxylin-eosin).

1. Heart

Cardiac Hypertrophy—Cardiac Atrophy—Polyploidy

Photomicrographs 1–1 through 1–4 have been taken at the same magnification in order to permit comparison of diseased heart muscle with the normal. The changes can be appreciated by comparing the width of muscle fibers, the size and shape of their nuclei, and the number of nuclei per unit area. Compared to normal myocardium (Fig 1–1: normal adult heart weighing 300 gm), growing heart muscle has thin muscle fibers with small, round nuclei that have condensed chromatin (Fig 1–2: heart from 6-year-old child). In cardiac atrophy (Fig 1–3: weight of heart 200 gm) there is a relative increase in the number of nuclei per unit area that is a consequence of the smaller size of the muscle fibers (numerical atrophy). One also finds an increase in cytoplasmic content of finely granular, yellow-brown lipofuscin pigment (brown atrophy), which occurs mainly near cell nuclei. In cardiac hypertrophy (Fig 1–4: weight of heart > 600 gm), muscle fibers are thickened twofold to threefold over normal; the number of nuclei per unit area is decreased and the nuclei are enlarged and misshapen, with an increase in chromatin (increase in DNA content). In cross-sectioned sarcoplasm one can see thickened myofilaments that are increased in number.

Polyploidy (Fig 1–5): The DNA content of heart muscle cells depends on the age of the person and on cardiac function. Up to the 12th year diploid nuclei predominate (2c: lower right of the diagram); in adults, tetraploid nuclei predominate (4c: right center). With increasing cardiac load, in connection with myocardial hypertrophy, polyploidy increases (DNA content 8c to 32c: upper right in Fig 1–5). This is morphologically manifested by enlarged, hyperchromatic nuclei.

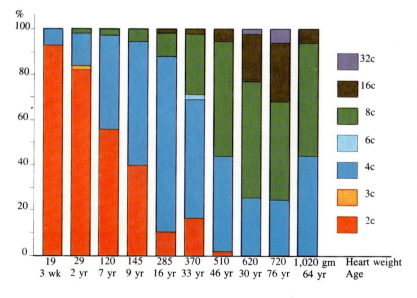

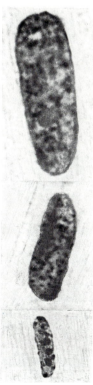

Fig 1–5.—Pattern of development of polyploidy in human heart muscle. **Right:** heart muscle nuclei (Feulgen reaction to show DNA): *bottom,* a diploid nucleus (2c); *middle,* a tetraploid (4c); *top,* an octoploid nucleus (8c).

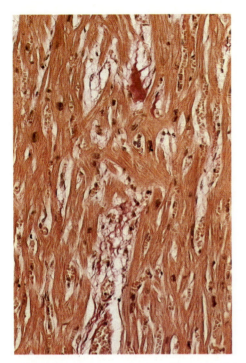

Fig 1–6.—Cardiomyopathy (van Gieson's stain). (Prof. Knierem)

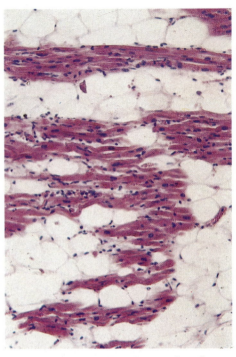

Fig 1–7.—Fatty infiltration of myocardium (hematoxylin-eosin).

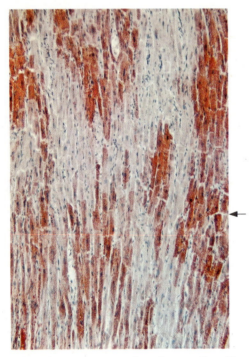

Fig 1–8.—Fatty degeneration of myocardium (tigering) (Sudan-hematoxylin).

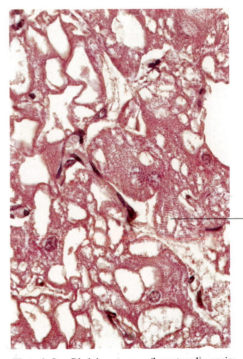

Fig 1–9.—Rhabdomyoma (hematoxylin-eosin; 250×).

Cardiomyopathy—Fatty Infiltration—Fatty Degeneration—Rhabdomyoma

Cardiomyopathy is a collective term encompassing different diseases that are characterized by functional disturbance and enlargement of the heart and that are not due to hypertension, sclerosis of coronary arteries, or valve defects. If a cause can be demonstrated, the cardiomyopathy is of secondary type (inflammatory, toxic, nutritional, metabolic, neuropathic, or myopathic, or due to tumors). The pathogenesis of primary, idiopathic cardiomyopathy is unknown. Four sorts can be distinguished: hypertrophic with or without obstruction; congestive, with dilated ventricles; obliterative, as in endomyocardial fibroses; and a restrictive form (myocardial deposits in metabolic disturbances, for example in amyloidosis).

In **hypertrophic cardiomyopathy** (Fig 1–6) the histologic pattern is distinctly abnormal. The muscle fibers are hypertrophied and do not run parallel to each other: they form a network.

In **fatty infiltration** or fatty heart (Fig 1–7) there is an increase in fat cells in the myocardium, such as is normally present to a small degree in the anterior portion of the right ventricle and occurs markedly in generalized obesity. At first there is an increase in subepicardial adipose tissue; later typical fat cells (round cells with clear cytoplasm and peripheral nuclei) are also situated between myocardial fibers that may be somewhat atrophic.

Fatty degeneration of the heart muscle (tigering) (Fig 1–8). Chronic oxygen deficiency leads to fatty degeneration of the myocardium. Low-power magnification shows tiny, Sudan-positive, orange-red fat droplets in the cytoplasm of altered muscle fibers. Typically, these fibers run parallel to and between unaltered fibers. The arrow in the picture indicates postmortem fragmentation of heart muscle fibers.

Rhabdomyoma of myocardium (Fig 1–9). This is a rare tumor of the heart that occurs mainly in small children and is thought to be a hamartoma, i.e., an abnormal mass of tissue of a kind that is normally present. Histologically there are irregular muscle cells of variable size, containing glycogen and possessing cross-striations in the cytoplasm (→).

Primary tumors of the heart are very rare (0.01% of necropsies). Benign tumors predominate. These include intracavitary myxomas (mainly in adults) that are true neoplasms, as well as rhabdomyomas, which occur almost exclusively before age 16. Other primary tumors of the heart are fibroma, lipoma, hemangioma, mesothelioma, and papillary fibroelastomas.

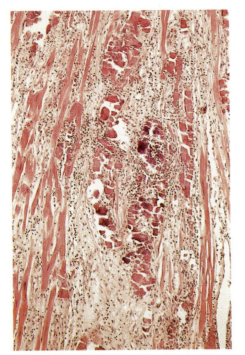

Fig 1–10.—Metastatic calcification of myocardium (hematoxylin-eosin; 100×).

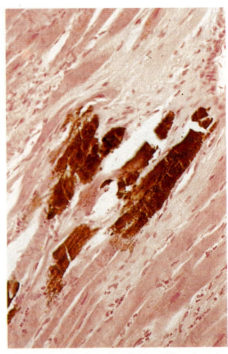

Fig 1–11.—Calcium deposits (von Kossa's stain; 100×).

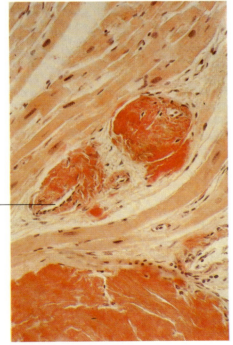

Fig 1–12.—Amyloidosis of myocardium (Congo red stain; 100×).

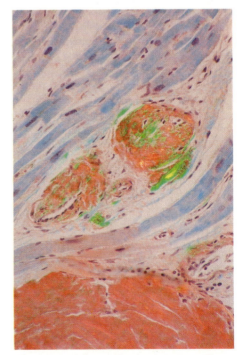

Fig 1–13.—Amyloidosis of myocardium (Congo red stain; green birefringence in polarizing light; 100×).

Calcification, Amyloidosis, and Siderosis of Myocardium

Calcification of myocardium (Figs 1–10, 1–11). Extensive calcification of the myocardium occurs in hypercalcemias together with necrosis, for example in hyperparathyroidism. In sections stained with hematoxylin-eosin there are fragmented muscle fibers with blue-stained calcium deposits. Eventually such muscle fibers disintegrate. There is interstitial inflammation and fibrosis. Von Kossa's stain for calcium reveals brown masses (Fig 1–11). Similar changes may be found in the lungs and in the gastric mucosa.

Amyloidosis of heart (Figs 1–12, 1–13). All forms of systemic amyloidosis can lead to deposits of amyloid in the heart. However, isolated cardiac amyloidosis is most frequent and occurs mainly in patients over age 70 (senile amyloidosis). It is associated with diffuse enlargement of the heart (secondary cardiomyopathy). At first there are only focal, subendocardial deposits of amyloid. Later the walls of coronary arteries are also involved. Microscopy reveals homogeneous Congo red–positive, metachromatic deposits of amyloid (Fig 1–12). In polarizing light the Congo red–positive material shows green birefringence (Fig 1–13). In Fig 1–12 one can see two blood vessels with deposits of amyloid: the arrow indicates a slitlike lumen that is lined by endothelial cells.

Siderosis of heart muscle (Fig 1–14). Deposits of iron-containing pigment inside of myocardial fibers occur in hemachromatosis and severe hemosiderosis. Sections stained with hematoxylin-eosin (Fig 1–14, top) reveal finely granular, brown cytoplasmic pigment that stains blue with the Prussian blue reaction (Berlin blue reaction) (Fig 1–14, bottom) and can therefore be identified as hemosiderin.

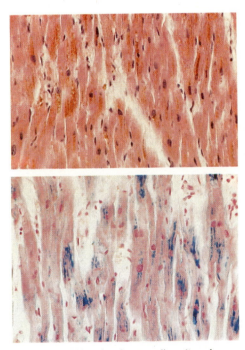

Fig 1–14.—Siderosis of myocardium (**top,** hematoxylin-eosin; **bottom,** Prussian blue; 100×).

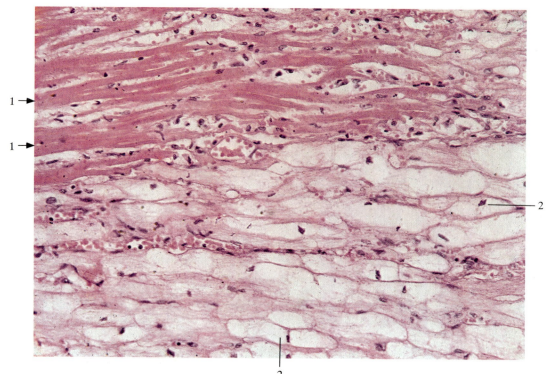

Fig 1–15.—Fresh necrosis of heart muscle showing sarcolysis (hematoxylin-eosin; 225×).

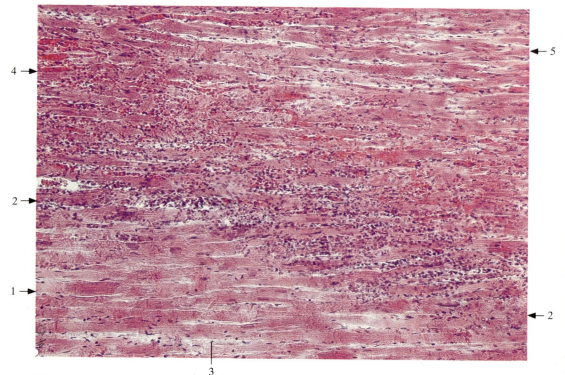

Fig 1–16.—Fresh necrosis of heart muscle surrounded by leukocytes (hematoxylin-eosin; 70×).

Infarct of the Heart

Infarcts of the heart show ischemic coagulation necrosis resulting from lack of oxygen due to obstruction of the coronary arteries (arteriosclerosis, thrombosis, which are common, or embolism, or narrowing of the orifices of the coronary arteries by syphilis).

Table 1–1 shows the *time sequences* of the macroscopic and microscopic changes and of some of the clinical events.

TABLE 1–1. TIME SEQUENCE OF EVENTS IN HEART INFARCTS*

TIME	MACROSCOPIC	MICROSCOPIC	OTHER CHANGES
15 sec	. . .	. . .	ECG changes (experimental)
30–60 min	. . .	Edema of fibers	Electron microscopic changes; H_2O uptake
2 hr	. . .	Hyalinization of fibers (homogeneous, eosinophilic)	Calcium loss up to 24 hr
3 hr	. . .	Clumping of sarcoplasm Fatty degeneration	Increased sodium content Decreased enzymes of the citric acid cycle in infarct
4 hr	TTC reaction negative	Necrosis	Infarct enlarging and elevated serum CPK
6 hr	Slight pallor	Leukocytic reaction	
9 hr	Yellow, dry, firm	Fully developed necrosis	
18–24 hr	Yellow, dry, firm	Fully developed necrosis	Increased enzymes in serum
2–3 wk	Red granulation tissue	Granulation tissue	
5 wk	Scar	Scar tissue	
2 mo	White, firm, fibrous		

*TTC reaction: triphenyltetrazolium chloride reaction (for detection of succinic dehydrogenase). CPK, creatine phosphokinase.

Figure 1–16 shows a **new infarct** with fresh muscle necrosis that is about 8 hours old (→ 1) and bordered by a broad zone of leukocytic infiltration (→ 2). At the edge of the infarct, in adjacent myocardium, there is a zone of recent hemorrhage (→ 4), beyond which the myocardium is normal (→ 5). Muscle fibers in the necrotic area lack nuclei and have homogeneous cytoplasm. Notice that the nuclei of the interstitial connective tissue are preserved (→ 3).

Fresh Myocardial Necrosis Showing Sarcolysis. Microscopic examination of the necrotic myocardium with high magnification shows very clearly the homogenization of the sarcoplasm (Fig 1–15; see also Fine Structure of the Myocardium, later this chapter) and the absence of cross-striations (→ 1). The depth of staining with eosin is also noteworthy. Myocardial nuclei have disappeared, although nuclei of the interstitial connective tissue cells are still present. The illustration also shows advanced sarcolysis, or dissolution of necrotic sarcoplasm, leaving only the empty shells of the sarcolemma (→ 2) (myocarditis in diphtheria). Essentially the same process, but with clumping of the sarcoplasm, is seen in Figure 1–24. Capillaries, some collapsed and others dilated, can be recognized in the interstitial tissue. Remnants of the sarcolemma may persist in the scar of an infarct for long periods.

Macroscopic appearance: A circumscribed, lemon yellow, dry, firm area.

Complications of myocardial infarcts: Rupture of the ventricle with pericardial tamponade, rupture of a papillary muscle (mitral insufficiency may develop), mural thrombosis with arterial embolism, fibrinous pericarditis, acute or chronic ventricular aneurysms, cardiac shock.

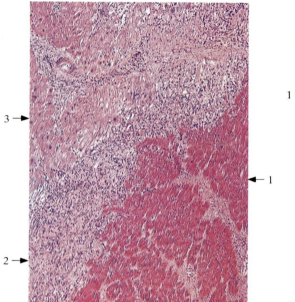

Fig 1–17.—Organization taking place in a some-what older myocardial infarct (hematoxylin-eosin; 41×).

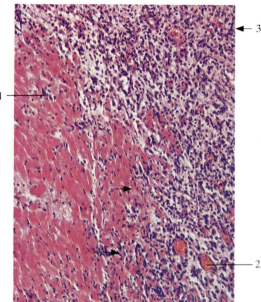

Fig 1–18.—Organization taking place in a some-what older myocardial infarct (detail) (hematoxy-lin-eosin; 120×).

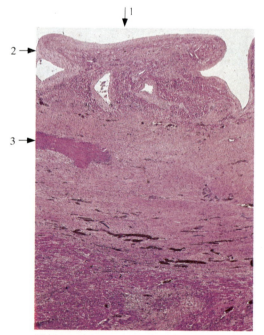

Fig 1–19.—Subendocardial myocardial scar (he-matoxylin-eosin; 15×).

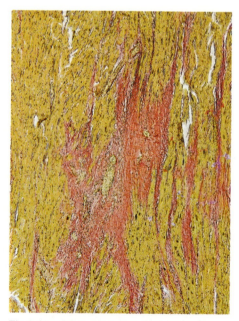

Fig 1–20.—Myocardial scars due to coronary ar-tery insufficiency (van Gieson's stain; 39×).

Necrotic heart muscle will largely be reabsorbed by granulation tissue during the course of 2–3 weeks, depending on the size of the infarct. In such an **organizing infarct** (Fig 1–17), examination of a microscopic section with the unaided eye or at low magnification shows an irregularly shaped, intensely red area which is the *necrotic zone* (→ 1), a richly cellular layer (blue appearing) bordering the necrotic zone (*granulation tissue* → 2), bordered in turn by the less deeply eosin-stained *normal heart muscle* (→ 3). Medium magnification reveals the essential alteration, namely, necrotic muscle fibers that have lost their nuclei. Higher magnification shows the loss of cross-striations. The cytoplasm of the myocardial fibers is homogeneous and eosinophilic. In addition, the nuclei of the interstitial tissue have nearly completely disappeared. In adjacent granulation tissue, capillaries can be seen with medium magnification as small, empty, round or ovoid spaces between which there are round cells (lymphocytes, histiocytes), fibroblasts, and connective tissue fibers having a distinctive smooth, straight shape. The cellular infiltration seen in the granulation tissue extends only slightly into the uninjured myocardium, in which well-preserved nuclei can be clearly seen.

Macroscopic: Red granulation tissue intermixed with remnants of yellow necrotic tissue.

Figure 1–18 is a detail under higher magnification of another somewhat *older infarct in the process of organization* showing the line of division between necrosis and granulation tissue. In the necrotic zone on the left-hand side of the picture are seen once again anuclear muscle fibers with homogeneous, intensely red eosinophilic sarcoplasm. The nuclei of the interstitial connective tissue are partially preserved, and in some places wandering histiocytes can already be seen (→ 1). The granulation tissue is richly cellular and contains dilated capillaries (→ 2). The earliest wandering cells to infiltrate the granulation tissue (→ in picture) are histiocytes with large round to oval nuclei and basophilic cytoplasm. In the upper right-hand part of the figure (→ 3) the granulation tissue is less cellular. A delicate background of fine collagen fibers has appeared between the small rod-shaped nuclei of the fibroblasts.

The final outcome of a myocardial infarct is a **scar of the heart muscle.** Figure 1–19 is from a section of myocardium taken perpendicular to the endocardium, so that the trabeculae (→ 1) of the inner ventricular surface can be seen. The endocardium is thickened by connective tissue (→ 2) and beneath it the muscle fibers are for the most part preserved, since they are nourished from inside the heart chambers. Next to the myocardium there is a broad layer of practically acellular collagenous tissue: the scar. At the lower margin of the picture, normal myocardium can be seen interspersed with small islands of scar tissue. Within the large scarred area there is a red area (→ 3): fresh necrosis of a surviving remnant of myocardium (recurrent infarct).

Macroscopic: White scar tissue, sometimes intermixed with yellow areas of necrosis.

Myocardial Scars in Coronary Insufficiency (Fig 1–20). *Coronary insufficiency develops because of a disproportion between the amount of oxygen needed by the myocardium and the amount of oxygen available to it* (for example, in cardiac hypertrophy with mild coronary arteriosclerosis or diminished oxygen tension in the absence of coronary arteriosclerosis). The essential difference from a myocardial infarct can be seen on naked-eye examination. Instead of a large necrotic area or a large scar in the heart muscle, there are small disseminated, flecklike scars which in sections stained by van Gieson's method are colored bright red. Heart muscle stains yellow.

Macroscopic: Firm, fibrous, glistening, white scar tissue.

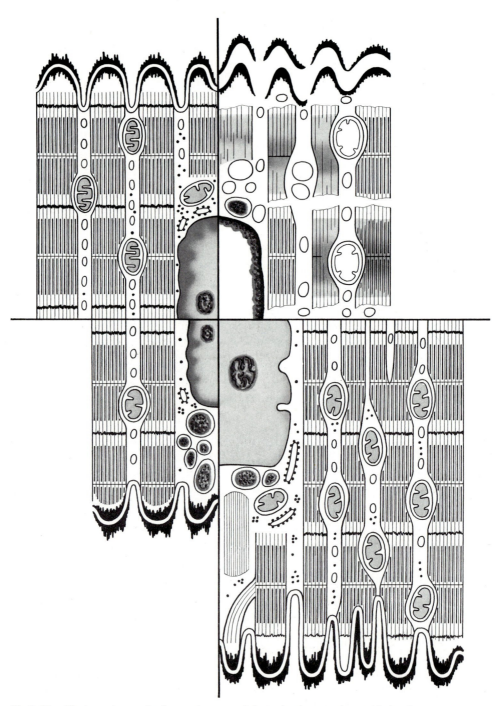

Fig 1–21.—Electron microscopic changes in myocardial atrophy, hypertrophy, and ischemia.

Fine Structure of the Myocardium

In *myocardial hypertrophy* all myocardial cells are enlarged. Myofibrils are more numerous but are not thickened and usually appear to be normally branched. Because of the enlargement of cells, the number of mitochondria is increased. At the nuclear poles there are accumulations of rough endoplasmic reticulum and lipofuscin granules as well as newly formed myofibrils. Both nuclei and nuceoli are enlarged (polyploidy). The intercalated disks (cell boundaries) are more folded than normal (increased electrical resistance; altered transmural irritability).

In *cardiac atrophy* the number of myocardial cells is decreased and the number of normal-sized elementary fibrils is reduced. Lipofuscin (= waste pigment) accumulates adjacent to the small-sized nuclei.

In a fresh *myocardial infarct* the sarcomeres are broken (light microscopy shows fragmentation of myocardial cells) and the myofibrillar pattern is erased because of clumping of the filaments. Mitochondria become vacuolated and irreversibly injured. The nuclei show the typical hyperchromatic nuclear walls of necrosis. Contact between cells is lost due to rupture of the intercalated disks.

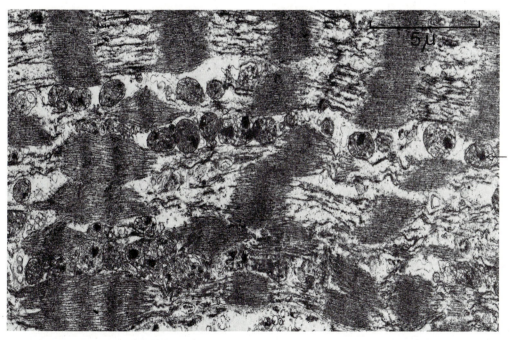

Fig 1–22.—Ultrastructure of fresh infarct 6 hours after ECG confirmation of a myocardial infarct in a 67-year-old man (autopsy material). There is clearly recognizable sarcolysis with beginning clumping of myofilaments. Most mitochondria show dense matrix aggregates (→) (7,500×).

67

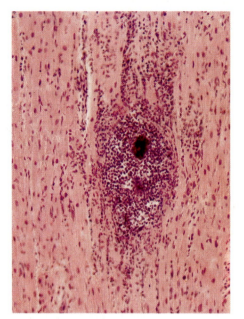

Fig 1–23.—Metastatic (embolic) abscess of heart muscle (hematoxylin-eosin; 141×).

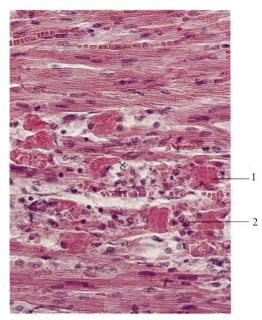

Fig 1–24.—Diphtheritic myocarditis (hematoxylin-eosin; 315×).

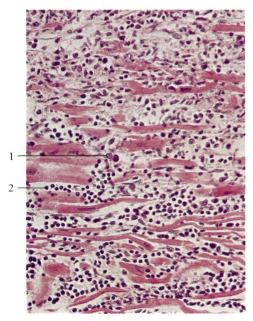

Fig 1–25.—Interstitial myocarditis in scarlet fever (hematoxylin-eosin; 255×).

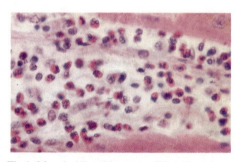

Fig 1–26.—**A,** idiopathic myocarditis with eosinophils (hematoxylin-eosin; 592×).

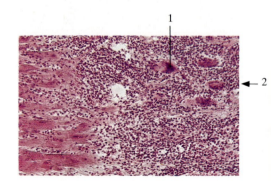

Fig 1–26.—**B,** idiopathic myocarditis with giant cells (hematoxylin-eosin; 110×).

Myocarditis

Inflammations of the heart muscle may be grouped as follows:

1. *Serous myocarditis*
2. *Purulent myocarditis*
3. *Nonpurulent interstitial myocarditis:*
    (a) Degenerative or parenchymatous inflammation *(diphtheria, dysentery)*
    (b) Lymphohistiocytic form *(scarlet fever, infection, hypersensitivity)*
    (c) Granulomatous myocarditis *(idiopathic myocarditis* of Fiedler; active *rheumatic fever* with Aschoff nodules).
4. *Necrotizing myocarditis* (chiefly viral; Coxsackie virus); histologically, focal necrosis and exudate similar to scarlet fever

Serous myocarditis is manifested by inflammatory edema of interstitial tissues (e.g., in thyrotoxicosis, shock, and burn injury, among others).

Purulent myocarditis originates mostly from metastatic colonies of bacteria or from septic arterial emboli (pyemic abscesses, for example, in thromboulcerative endocarditis; see also kidney, Fig 6–38). Figure 1–23 shows a **metastatic abscess of the heart muscle** with centrally situated bacterial colonies (dark blue, round foci), destruction of tissue (abscess), and great infiltration of polymorphonuclear leukocytes. Neighboring tissues are sparsely infiltrated with polymorphs.

Nonpurulent, diphtheritic myocarditis (Fig 1–24) always shows *degenerative changes of the parenchymatous cells,* and the ordinary features of inflammation are not pronounced (parenchymatous or alterative inflammation). In Figure 1–24, different stages of myocardial injury can be recognized: homogenization and clumping of sarcoplasm (→ 1) progressing to sarcolysis, so-called toxic myolysis (see also Fig 1–15). At low magnification, the injured fibers stain intensely red and have irregular shapes. In addition, some myocardial fibers show focal fatty change (see Fig 1–7). Histiocytes have mobilized around degenerated fibers (→ 2), to remove dead and dying debris. In addition, there are occasional polymorphonuclear leukocytes. Healing results in the formation of many small focal scars.

Macroscopic: Dilation of the heart with either small, poorly defined, grayish yellow foci or small scattered scars.

Interstitial myocarditis may occur during the course of scarlet fever. There is *infiltration of lymphocytes and histiocytes* (Fig 1–25) and a less conspicuous degenerative component. Between the widely separated muscle fibers there is a sparse infiltration of histiocytes (→ 1), lymphocytes (→ 2), fibroblasts, and occasional plasma cells and considerable interstitial edema. Some muscle fibers are intact, others are degenerated, and some are necrotic. Develops in the third week of infectious fevers.

In some cases of myocarditis of unknown cause **(idiopathic myocarditis with eosinophils),** the myocardium is either diffusely or focally infiltrated with eosinophils (Fig 1–26,A) (allergic origin?). In addition, granulomatous inflammation **(idiopathic giant cell myocarditis)** (Fig 1–26,B) may occur with a richly cellular infiltration of lymphocytes, histiocytes, fibrocytes, and plasma cells and complete destruction of foci of heart muscle, In such cases, the inflammatory exudate contains giant cells with clumped nuclei, the so-called muscle giant cells (→ 1 and 2). The latter represent aborted muscle cell regeneration. In sarcoidosis, epithelioid cell granulomas develop.

Macroscopic: Dilation of the heart. The cut surface shows numerous small, poorly circumscribed, grayish red or grayish yellow flecklike foci.

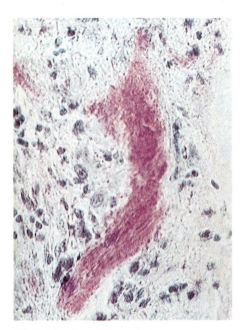

Fig 1–27.—Fresh fibrinoid necrosis (hematoxylin-eosin; 480 ×).

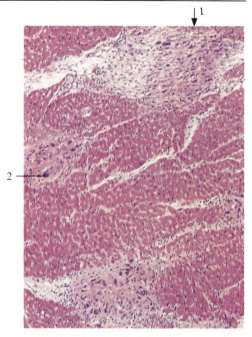

Fig 1–28.—Full-blown Aschoff nodules (hematoxylin-eosin; 120 ×).

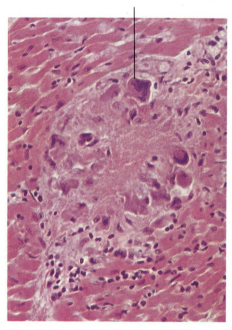

Fig 1–29.—Aschoff nodule (hematoxylin-eosin; 330 ×).

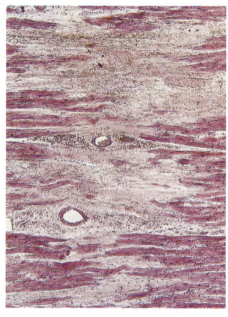

Fig 1–30.—Rheumatic scar (hematoxylin-eosin; 56 ×).

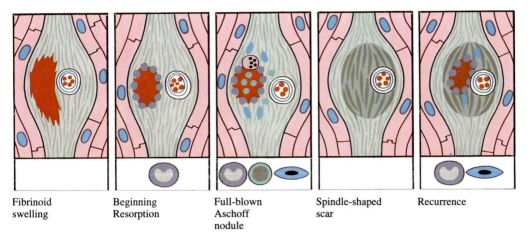

| Fibrinoid swelling | Beginning Resorption | Full-blown Aschoff nodule | Spindle-shaped scar | Recurrence |

Fig 1–31.—Diagram showing time relationships in rheumatic myocarditis.

Figure 1–31 shows the *course of rheumatic myocarditis* in active rheumatic fever. Similar changes take place in the aorta, peritonsillar tissues, heart valves, and joints. *The illness begins with fibrinoid swelling (necrosis) of the perivascular connective tissue* (see also p. 13). *The body reacts by producing a histiocytic granuloma containing giant cells which is called an Aschoff nodule* (Aschoff, 1904). The histiocytes remove the fibrinoid material (phagocytic function of the histiocytes). *The end stage is a perivascular scar of connective tissue* in which histiocytes have been transformed into fibroblasts and have formed collagen fibers. *Recurrences* localize preferentially in old scars.

In examining the tissue microscopically, attention should be directed to the large interstitial spaces. Figure 1–28 was taken at medium magnification and shows many **full-blown Aschoff nodules** (→ 1) with compact accumulations of histiocytes and giant cells (→ 2). High manifestation shows the early change of **fresh fibrinoid necrosis** (Fig 1–27) consisting of bright red, homogeneous material which completely obscures the connective tissues. The host reaction commences immediately with mobilization of histiocytes, which can be recognized by their large, chromatic nuclei, large nucleoli, and poorly demarcated, faintly basophilic cytoplasm. A few lymphocytes are also present. Figure 1–29 shows an **Aschoff nodule** at a somewhat more advanced stage. In the center of this nodule there is fibrinoid material. At the margins there are histiocytes as well as giant cells derived from muscle cells (→), since in this case the inflammation has involved the myocardium.

At the termination of the acute inflammatory phase, the histiocytes become oblong in shape and form collagen fibers. As a result, perivascular **rheumatic scars** develop (Fig 1–30). These scars appear as elongated and pointed bright red areas. In the illustration, a few solitary histiocytes are still embedded in the scar tissue.

Distinguish: Rheumatic fever, rheumatoid arthritis, degenerative arthritis (arthritis deformans), and rheumatoid nodules in soft tissues.

Endocarditis

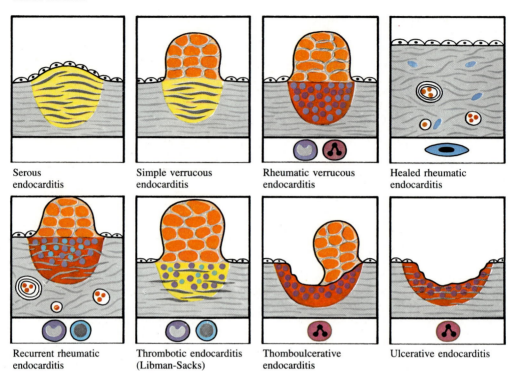

Serous
endocarditis

Simple verrucous
endocarditis

Rheumatic verrucous
endocarditis

Healed rheumatic
endocarditis

Recurrent rheumatic
endocarditis

Thrombotic endocarditis
(Libman-Sacks)

Thomboulcerative
endocarditis

Ulcerative endocarditis

Fig 1–32.—Diagrammatic representations of different sorts of endocarditis.

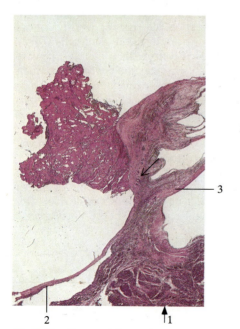

Fig 1–33.—Recurrent rheumatic verrucous endocarditis (hematoxylin-eosin; 10 ×).

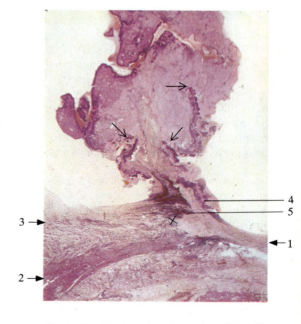

Fig 1–34.—Thromboulcerative endocarditis (subacute bacterial endocarditis) (hematoxylin-eosin; 11 ×).

Endocarditis

Endocarditis is an inflammation of the heart valves and is characterized not only by conspicuous fluid and cellular exudation in the connective tissues of the leaflets or cusps, but also by superimposed thrombosis. The changes occur chiefly at the line of closure of the valve. The aortic cusps and mitral leaflets are preferentially affected.

There are five different sorts of endocarditis. (1) The mildest and most fleeting sort, and perhaps also the precursor of all other forms of endocarditis, is **serous endocarditis** (Fig 1–32), in which blood serum proteins exude into the connective tissue of the valves and cause swelling of the fibers and interstitial edema (macroscopic: slight, glistening swelling). (2) **Simple verrucous endocarditis** (Fig 1–32) is distinguished from rheumatic endocarditis only by the intensity of the edema and cellular reaction. A break develops in the valvular endothelium which is then overlaid by a thrombus consisting almost exclusively of blood platelets, although a small amount of fibrin is also usually present. Frequently seen in shock (deposits of aggregated platelets along the line of closure). (3) **Rheumatic endocarditis** (Fig 1–32) has almost the same microscopic appearance. However, fibrinoid swelling is marked in the valvular connective tissue and correspondingly there is a more pronounced inflammatory reaction of polymorphonuclear leukocytes and histiocytes. Healing (**burned-out rheumatic endocarditis,** Fig 1–32) is accompanied by vascularization and scarification with deformity of the valve. Recurrent attacks of rheumatic endocarditis are frequent (**recurrent rheumatic endocarditis,** Fig 1–33). (4) **Thrombotic endocarditis** (Libman-Sacks) is a nonbacterial endocarditis with soft, coarse thrombi formed of platelets and fibrin. There is marked fibrinoid degeneration of the valvular tissue and a decided inflammatory reaction (Fig 1–32). The lesions are found frequently in *acute disseminated lupus erythematosus* along with renal involvement (wire loop glomerular lesions). (5) **Thromboulcerative and ulcerative endocarditis** (also called endocarditis lenta or subacute bacterial endocarditis, Fig 1–34) are, in contrast to verrucous endocarditis, bacterial infections of the valves, usually *Streptococcus viridans*. Staphylococci and other infectious agents also are common. There is usually marked leukocytic infiltration and destruction of the valves.

Macroscopically, there are valvular deformities and polypoid thrombi. *Complications of endocarditis:* 1. in nonbacterial endocarditis: arterial emboli, valvular defects; 2. in bacterial endocarditis: valvular deformities, metastatic pyemic abscesses, focal embolic glomerulonephritis (Löhlein).

In **recurrent rheumatic endocarditis** (Fig 1–33), low magnification shows thickening of the mitral leaflet due to a superimposed broad layer of red-staining eosinophilic material. Heart muscle (→ 1) is seen at the lower margin of the photograph, and the endocardium of the left atrium at → 2. Medium magnification shows connective tissue thickening of the valve leaflet and numerous capillaries (→). The chordae tendineae show fibrous thickening (→ 3). The thrombus consists of eosinophilic material (blood platelets). From the fact that capillaries are present in the ground substance of the valve, it can be concluded that there was a previous episode of endocarditis.

Thromboulcerative endocarditis (Fig 1–34) *is a form of bacterial endocarditis with destruction of valve leaflets and superimposed, bacteria-laden thrombi.* Both low and medium magnification show aortic media (→ 1), and left ventricular myocardium (→ 2) covered by endocardium (→ 3) that has been thickened by fibrous connective tissue. Remnants of valvular tissue are still plainly seen (→ 4). A thrombus, composed of fibrin and platelets and containing bacterial colonies (→ 5), sits on top of the valve. Calcification of the connective tissue fibers (×) at the base of the leaflet indicates that there had been previous inflammation with subsequent scarring.

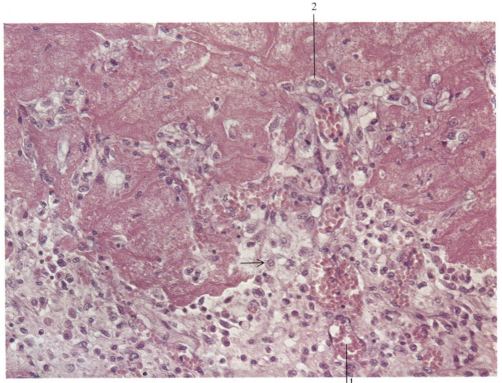

Fig 1–35.—Organizing fibrinous pericarditis (detail) (hematoxylin-eosin; 248 ×).

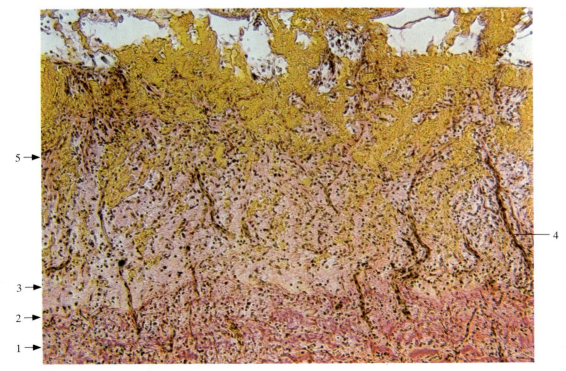

Fig 1–36.—Organizing fibrinous pericarditis (van Gieson's stain; 99 ×).

Pericarditis

Pericarditis is an inflammation of the serous coverings of the heart, including both the visceral or epicardial, and the parietal layers. All variants of the inflammatory reaction may occur (serous, fibrinous, purulent, hemorrhagic, chronic, granulomatous, etc.). *It can arise by metastasis,* for example, in sepsis or infectious diseases; *by direct extension,* for example, from the lung, pleura, or esophagus; or as a *toxic response,* for example, in uremia; or as a result of *myocardial infarction.*

Any inflamed serosal surface (pleura, peritoneum, pericardium) will show the same histologic changes and the same end results.

Figure 1–35 illustrates the **chief changes and the time sequence in fibrinous pericarditis.** The black areas are fibrin.

Figure 1–35 shows **organizing fibrinous pericarditis.** Granulation tissue borders fibrin and has replaced it completely in the lower part of the picture, in which one sees histiocytes (→), lymphocytes, some fibroblasts as well as dilated capillaries containing erythrocytes (→ 1). Inside the forward-thrusting granulation tissue there are histiocytes, surrounded by clear spaces (→ 2).

Organizing fibrinous pericarditis (Fig 1–36). After about 5 days, granulation tissue begins to invade the fibrin. Examination of a microscopic preparation with a hand lens still shows preservation of the three layers (muscle, fat tissue, superficial layer of fibrin), but the subepicardial fat tissue is not clearly demarcated and is densely infiltrated with cells and permeated with collagenous fibrous tissue. With medium magnification and a van Gieson preparation (Fig 1–36), interlacing of the red-stained epicardial fibers can be seen (→ 1) as well as the infiltration of histiocytes, fibroblasts, and lymphocytes (→ 2: original border of epicardium), which originate from the epicardium. This is followed by the appearance of granulation tissue composed of pale red newly formed connective tissue fibers (→ 3). The vascular sprouts in the connective tissue (→ 4) can be seen clearly to have their origin in the pericardium and from there to course perpendicularly to the surface. The granulation tissue shows fibroblast nuclei (cut longitudinally) and occasional lymphocytes. In the upper portion of the section, the remaining strands of fibrin (→ 5) extend in tongue-like projections into granulation tissue. In many places, lacunae of various shapes have formed in the fibrin, where the histiocytes have brought about resorption.

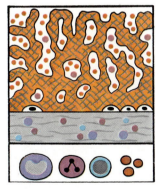

Young fibrinous
pericarditis,
days 1–5

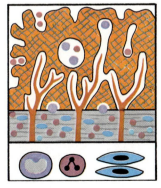

Intermediate
fibrinous pericarditis,
days 5–8

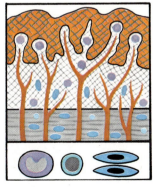

Mature fibrinous
pericarditis,
days 8–20

Fig 1–37.—Schematic representation of the course of pericarditis.

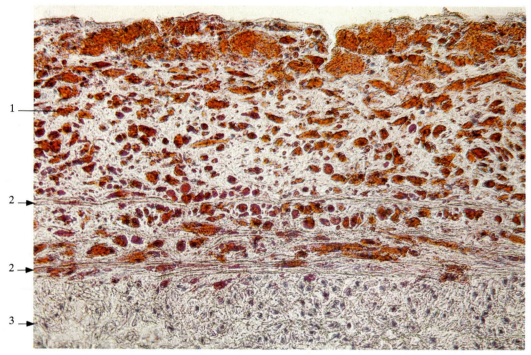

Fig 2–1.—Lipid in intima of aorta (Sudan-hematoxylin).

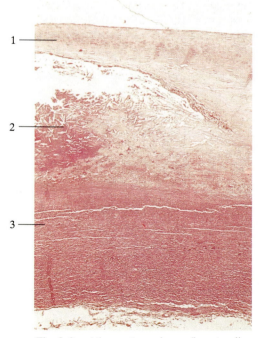

Fig 2–2.—Atheromatous plaque (hematoxylin-eosin; 40×).

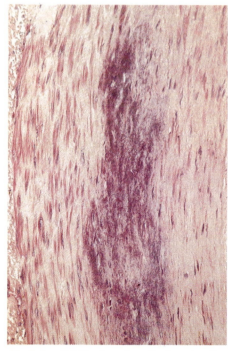

Fig 2–3.—Calcification of media (hematoxylin-eosin; 100×).

2. Blood Vessels

Arteriosclerosis

Fatty streak (lipidosis) of the aorta (Fig 2–1). An early change associated with aortic arteriosclerosis is deposition of lipids, originating from the bloodstream, in the intima. These lipids, however, are not necessarily retained, but may be decomposed and removed (e.g., so-called aortic milk-streaks of children). The process of atherosclerosis is initiated by a reaction of smooth muscle cells in the intima and then becomes progressive.

In frozen sections stained for fat with Sudan stain we see three layers in the aorta: an outer, loose adventitia that contains fat cells and nutrient vessels (vasa vasorum), a middle (media) layer composed of elastic fibers and smooth muscle cells, and an inner layer (intima) which normally is narrow but has become thickened by a fibrous cushion. Examination of the aorta at moderate magnification (Fig 2–1) reveals a broadened intima (top of figure) containing deposits of Sudan-positive lipids, both within cells and between them (→ 1: myointimal cells with phagocytosed lipid). In the lower part of the picture (→ 3) one can see media containing fragmented elastic fibers (→ 2).

In polarizing light the Sudan-positive material can be seen to contain platey or needle-shaped cholesterol crystals with yellow, green, and blue colors (Fig 2–4).

Atheroma of aorta with necrosis (Fig 2–2). Deposition of lipid in the intima is followed by proliferation of intimal myocytes and deposition of collagen (→ 1: cushion of thickened intima with few cells and much collagen). Within this region there is disintegration of collagen, and one can also see deposits of cholesterol which in paraffin sections appear as needle-shaped gaps (→ 2). One may also see dustlike, blue-staining deposits of calcium salts.

Medial calcification (Mönckeberg's sclerosis) (Fig 2–3). In medium-sized arteries (e.g., in the femoral artery) arteriosclerosis may take the form of medial sclerosis. This is recognized by the presence of bands of calcium deposits between well-preserved smooth muscle cells in the media. The picture shows bluish deposits of calcium.

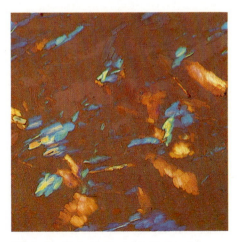

Fig 2–4.—Cholesterol crystals (Sudan stain; polarized light; 250 ×).

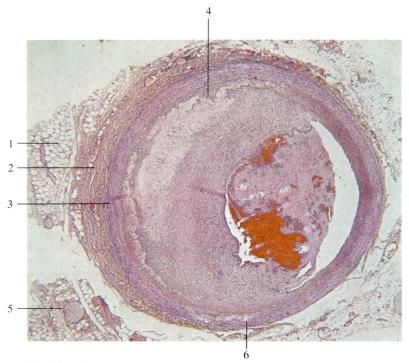

Fig 2–5.—High-grade coronary arteriosclerosis with a recent thrombus (hematoxylin-eosin; 26×).

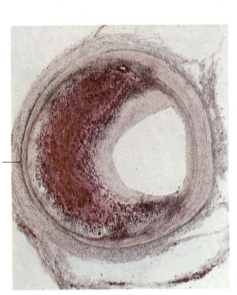

Fig 2–6.—Coronary arteriosclerosis with atheroma (Sudan-hematoxylin; 14×).

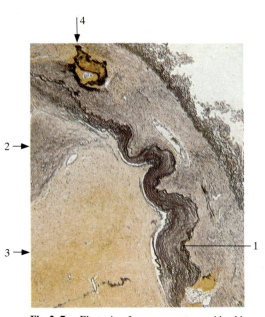

Fig 2–7.—Elastosis of coronary artery with old thrombus (elastica–van Gieson's stain).

78

Coronary Arteriosclerosis

Among the common diseases of the vascular system, coronary arteriosclerosis and its frequent sequel, a myocardial infarct, take the foremost place. It arises like the other forms of arteriosclerosis from fat deposition and is followed by sclerosis. Sometimes, marked edema of the intima develops and the artery is suddenly obstructed (a cause of death in young persons). Complications include secondary thrombosis, bleeding in a sclerotic plaque, or necrosis from excessive swelling, all of which may lead to sudden narrowing of the lumen of the vessel. Today it is generally thought that coronary thrombosis is the primary event. Hyalinization of small intramural (myocardial) branches is also commonly seen. In discussing the pathogenesis of a myocardial infarct, it is necessary not only to consider the state of the coronary arteries, but also the condition of the myocardium. Hypertrophy and increased cardiac function require increased oxygen. For example, if myocardial metabolism is boosted by adrenalin, then a lesser degree of coronary sclerosis can cause necrosis.

High-grade coronary sclerosis with a recent thrombus (Fig 2–5). The changes are well shown by examining a cross section of a coronary artery. The coronary artery is embedded in subepicardial fat tissue (→ 1). The loosely arranged adventitia (→ 2) forms an outer mantle. The media appears as a red ring (→ 3). The intima is thickened by a crescent-shaped layer of fibrous tissue with a lightly stained atheromatous base in which necrosis has occurred as a result of swelling (→ 4). What remains of the lumen is filled with a preformed thrombus consisting chiefly of platelets, fibrin, and erythrocytes (conglutination thrombus, see discussion of thrombosis later this chapter). At → 5, a small nerve can be seen in the fat tissue. Interference with medial nutrition is suggested by a focus of cystic degeneration (→ 6) in the media (medial necrosis). Note that the adventitia adjacent to the crescent-like area of intimal sclerosis shows an increase in collagenous connective tissue. Calcium may be deposited secondarily in both the intima and media.

Coronary arteriosclerosis with atheroma formation (Fig 2–6). Fat stains show clearly the marked deposition of lipid in crescent-shaped areas of intimal thickening. The fatty material is partly within cells resembling histiocytes and partly lying free in the tissues, where it has fused (early atheroma). The inner layer of the sclerotic plaque contains no lipid. Noteworthy is the marked atrophy of the media in the base of the plaque (→), a finding that is almost always present (disturbed medial nutrition caused by the plaque).

Elastosis of a coronary artery filled with an old thrombus (Fig 2–7). Sclerosis is always accompanied by more or less marked elastosis, that is, by splintering and proliferation of the elastic fibers. Figure 2–7 shows such splintering and increase of the elastic fibers (→ 1) together with an old thrombus. The lumen of the artery is partly filled with collagenous connective tissue containing a few blood vessels (cicatrized granulation tissue, → 2). The yellow homogeneous mass (→ 3) is the residue of the old thrombus. In the old scar tissue in the muscle of the media can be seen a few blood vessels (→ 4) that have arisen in the adventitia and growth into the thrombus.

Macroscopic: Lipidosis: yellow, flat deposits. *Sclerosis and atheroma:* lumen narrowed by grayish yellow or yellow plaques which are frequently focal. *New thrombus:* reduction or complete closing of the lumen by gray-red masses. *Old thrombus:* grayish brown to grayish white deposits on the vessel wall, often in a form resembling a rope ladder. Preferred localization of coronary arteriosclerosis: usually 1 cm below the origin of the descending branch of the left coronary artery.

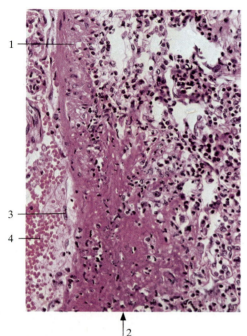

Fig 2–8.—Fresh fibrinoid necrosis in periarteritis nodosa (hematoxylin-eosin).

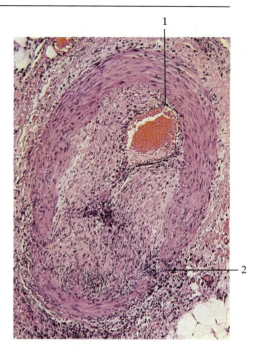

Fig 2–9.—Scar stage (hematoxylin-eosin).

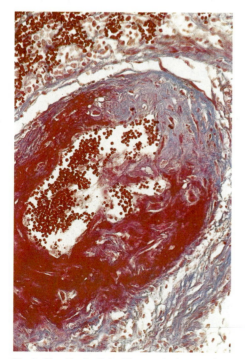

Fig 2–10.—Fresh fibrinoid necrosis (azan stain; 40×).

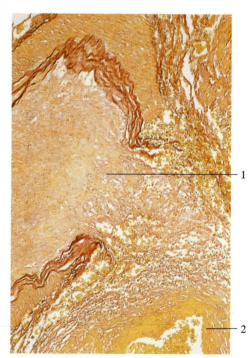

Fig 2–11.—Old and recent periarteritis (recurrence) (elastica–van Gieson's stain; 40×).

Inflammation of Blood Vessels

Periarteritis Nodosa (Polyarteritis Nodosa)

The *earliest stage* is shown in Figure 2–8 (**fresh fibrinoid necrosis in periarteritis nodosa**). *Fresh fibrinoid necrosis* (homogeneous, strongly eosinophilic) has developed in segments of the intima and media (→ 2). In the surrounding tissues there are leukocytes and a beginning granulomatous reaction. At → 1, slightly edematous but otherwise unaffected vascular media can still be seen. The intima is lifted off the area of fibrinoid necrosis (→ 3: endothelial cell) and a loose network of fibrin and erythrocytes lies on the intimal endothelium (→ 4).

The early and late changes of periarteritis nodosa can be demonstrated well with special stains. The azan connective tissue stain shows **fibrinoid necrosis** to be dark red, in contrast to blue-staining connective tissue (Fig 2–10). With van Gieson's stain, fibrinoid necrosis can be identified as homogeneous yellow material (Fig 2–11, → 2). The elastica–van Gieson's stain demonstrates the scar stage to advantage (Fig 2–11): one can recognize necrosis of the vascular wall by the interruption of elastic fibers, especially those of the elastica interna (Fig 2–11, → 1). The necrotic vascular wall is replaced by cellular granulation tissue, which in time becomes hypocellular.

The **scar stage** (Fig 2–13) resembles the appearances seen in Figure 2–12. Fibroblasts and young cellular scar tissue have reduced the lumen to a small channel (→ 1). The place where the artery has been breached by granulation tissue arising from the adventitia can be clearly seen (→ 2), as well as the collagenous scar tissue and occasional lymphocytes.

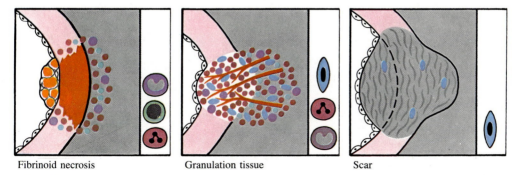

Fibrinoid necrosis   Granulation tissue   Scar

Fig 2–12.—Stages of periarteritis nodosa.

Thromboangiitis Obliterans

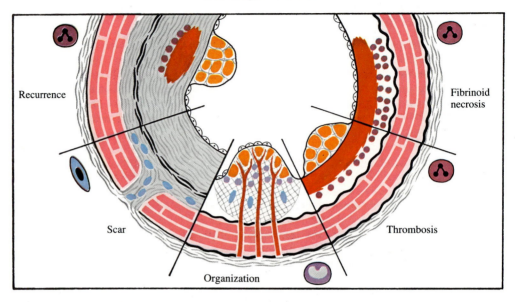

Recurrence

Fibrinoid
necrosis

Scar

Thrombosis

Organization

Fig 2–13.—Diagram of different sorts of vascular inflammations.

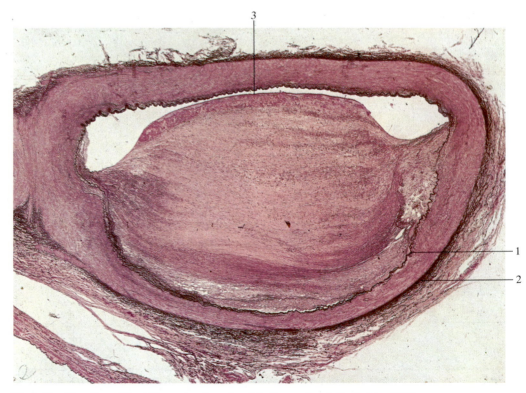

Fig 2–14.—Thromboangiitis obliterans in a leg artery (elastica–nuclear fast red stain; 19×).

Thromboangiitis Obliterans—Endangiitis Obliterans

Thromboangiitis obliterans (Figs 2–13, 2–14) is a chronic disease of arteries and veins that occurs in stages. It encompasses a progressive narrowing of the vascular lumen and leads to gangrene and infarction.

The disease begins with a transient **fibrinoid necrosis of the arterial wall** which in time gives rise to **mural thrombosis** that narrows or closes the lumen (Fig 2–13). Within the thrombus one may see microabscesses that contain granulocytes. The aseptic inflammation may involve neighboring veins, hence the term "angiitis." Necrotic tissue and thrombus material become transformed into **granulation tissue,** which in turn becomes a cushion of **intimal scar** that narrows the lumen.

In the **late stage** (Fig 2–14) there is well-demarcated thickening of the intima that has narrowed or closed the lumen. The picture shows the cross section of an artery with its elastica interna (→ 1) and externa (→ 2). The internal elastica reveals the limit of the original vessel lumen which has been narrowed by collagen-rich, cell-poor scar tissue. One also sees a fresh area of recurrence: the tissue near the luminal surface of the scar shows increased eosinophilia (→ 3: fibrinoid swelling).

The outer layers of affected arteries are also shifted partly or entirely by the intimal proliferation. This is a characteristic finding in thromboangiitis obliterans which serves to differentiate it from arteriosclerosis that is complicated by fresh or organized mural thrombosis.

The disease affects mainly the vessels of the lower extremities, especially in younger men who are chain smokers. However, the disease can also occur in the arteries of various organs (brain, kidneys, heart, and gut). Typical consequences are intermittent claudication, gangrene of extremities, and infarcts of organs. Next to smoking of tobacco, genetic predisposition and hormonal factors may be involved in the pathogenesis of this disease.

Endangiitis obliterans (Fig 2–15). Chronic inflammatory and ulcerating processes can lead to intimal proliferation of neighboring blood vessels, with resulting stenosis or occlusion of the lumen. This is particularly evident at the base of a chronic peptic ulcer. The arterial wall (→) can still be recognized as a dark red band; the lumen has been replaced by cellular and collagenous granulation tissue.

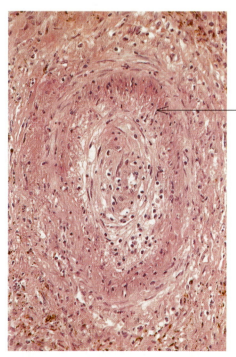

Fig 2–15.—Endangiitis obliterans in a chronic peptic ulcer (hematoxylin-eosin).

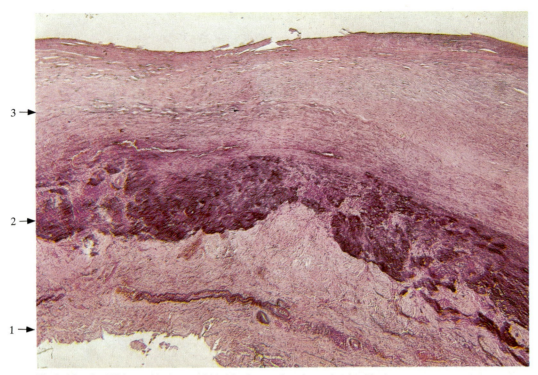

Fig 2–16.—Syphilitic aortitis (mesaortitis) (elastica–nuclear fast red stain; 32×).

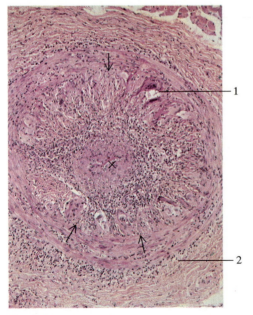

Fig 2–17.—Giant cell arteritis (hematoxylin-eosin).

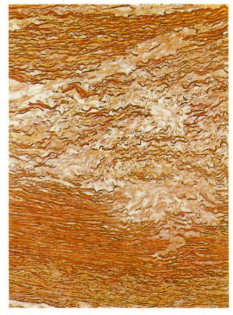

Fig 2–18.—Medial necrosis of aorta (elastica–van Gieson's stain; 100×).

Syphilitic Mesaortitis—Giant Cell Arteritis—Medial Necrosis

Syphilitic Mesaortitis (Fig 2–16). *This in an inflammation of the adventitia and media of the aorta developing in tertiary syphilis.* Figure 2–16, taken at low magnification, shows the typical "moth-eaten" pattern of the destruction of the medial elastica. The adventitia (→ 1) shows an increase in collagenous fibrous tissue (scar formation). The greater part of the media (→ 2) is irregularly replaced by nodular, sparsely cellular scar tissue. The intima (→ 3) is greatly thickened by secondary arteriosclerosis. In the right-hand side of the figure hyalinization of the intima has occurred. The disease process begins with a lymphohistiocytic and plasma cell inflammation around the vasa vasorum of the adventitia and creeps along the vessels into the media. The small medial arteries then show an endarteritis which results in medial ischemia (necrosis), formation of granulation tissue, destruction of elastica, and replacement of the lost tissue by a scar. Since the scar tissue shrinks, the intima is pulled inward over the scar.

From this process results the characteristic *macroscopic* ridges (wrinkles) or tree bark appearance of the intima, especially prominent in the thoracic portion. In addition, the wall of the aorta is thin and the vessel dilated (ectasia). Frequently, the inflammation also encroaches upon the cusps of the aortic valve, causing widening of the commissures and formation of a channel between them. In addition, the cusps contract so that aortic insufficiency develops. Furthermore, the coronary ostia can become obstructed by intimal proliferation, so that death is not infrequently due to a myocardial infarct.

Medium- and small-sized arteries, in particular those at the base of the brain, can also be affected in tertiary syphilis, chiefly in the form of an endarteritis with intimal proliferation.

Giant cell arteritis (Fig 2–17). This relatively benign form of periarteritis nodosa was once thought to affect chiefly the temporal artery of older women. However, more recent statistics indicate that men and women are equally affected. Next to the temporal artery in incidence comes involvement of the ophthalmic artery (blindness), brain, heart, liver, spleen, etc. Fibrinoid necrosis develops locally in the region of the intima, with destruction of the internal elastica. As Figure 2–17 shows, the involvement is preponderantly in the intima and media. In this particular vessel, the intima shows both inflammatory exudate and granulation tissue, and only a small lumen remains (×). The boundary between intima and media is marked by arrows. The internal elastica is broken into fragments that are surrounded by giant cells (→ 1). The media is diffusely infiltrated with lymphocytes and histiocytes. The exudate extends to the adventitia in which collagen is increased (→ 2: adventitia).

Medial necrosis of aorta (cystic medial necrosis). This is a disease of unknown origin involving principally the media of the thoracic aorta. It is thought to result from focal necroses with little tissue reaction or from degenerative changes in the media. Microscopically one sees clefts or cysts in the media which are filled with mucopolysaccharides. Elastica–van Gieson's stain (Fig 2–18) shows fragmented elastic fibers embedded in a slightly basophilic ground substance.

The cause of medial necrosis is unknown (local metabolic changes? hypertension?). It is frequently seen in Marfan's syndrome and is considered the most important factor predisposing to dissecting aneurysm of the aorta, the development of which may be triggered by hypertension or trauma.

Thrombosis—Thrombophlebitis—Organization

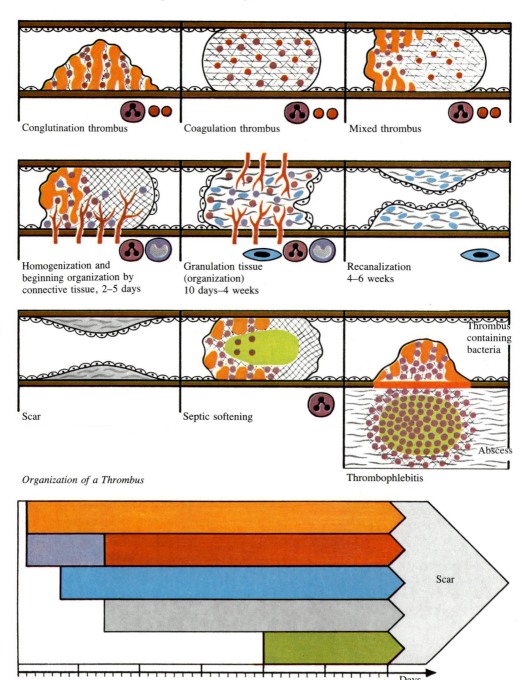

Conglutination thrombus

Coagulation thrombus

Mixed thrombus

Homogenization and beginning organization by connective tissue, 2–5 days

Granulation tissue (organization) 10 days–4 weeks

Recanalization 4–6 weeks

Scar

Septic softening

Thrombus containing bacteria

Abscess

Organization of a Thrombus

Thrombophlebitis

Scar

Days

Fig 2–19.—Diagram of the histologic structure of different sorts of thrombi, the results of secondary changes in a thrombus, and the process of organization. Thrombophlebitis.

Thrombosis—Thrombophlebitis

Thrombosis is the intravascular coagulation of blood during life. Figure 2–19 illustrates in diagrammatic fashion the histologic structure and fate of the different sorts of thrombi and the temporal events in the course of organization.

1. A **conglutination** or **agglutination thrombus,** shown adhering to the vessel wall (a mural or parietal thrombus), has a typical form. Conglutinated blood platelets are built up into a coral-like laminated scaffold. Fibrin surrounds and also lies between the columns of platelets, giving an appearance like that of a reinforced steel building. Leukocytes are enmeshed in the fibrin and accumulate like mantles around the blood platelets. Between the fibrin columns lie masses of erythrocytes (see next page).

Macroscopic: Riblike projections of platelets are seen on the surface of the thrombus, giving it a rippled appearance crosswise to the direction of blood flow like the pattern of a sandbank at the bottom of a river or a wind-swept sand dune. Grayish red in color and friable.

2. A **coagulation thrombus** completely fills the vessel lumen and histologically consists of fibrin lamellae arranged parallel to the vessel wall. Between the lamellae stretches a delicate, irregularly constructed framework of fibrin in the meshes of which erythrocytes have become trapped. Platelets cannot be seen with the light microscope. There is a scanty sprinkling of leukocytes.

Macroscopic: A red, structureless column of coagulated blood.

3. A **mixed thrombus** consists of a headpiece, which has the structure of a *conglutination thrombus,* and a tailpiece, which has the structure of a *coagulation thrombus.* In the femoral vein, both conglutination and coagulation thrombi are frequently intermingled.

Macroscopic: Intermixed red and gray parts. *Postmortem clots,* in contrast to thrombi, have an elastic consistency (clots formed slowly are gray due to the buffy coat; clots formed quickly are red) and show no stratification or other signs of a structure.

4. In **septic thrombophlebitis*** there is a purulent inflammation of the vessel wall of bacterial origin. A thrombus containing bacteria forms at the site of the inflammation and histologically shows irregularly arranged masses of platelets and fibrin and bacterial colonies. If thrombotic material comes loose, then pyemic abscesses develop in the lung or elsewhere (see Inflammation of the Lung, chap. 3). Thrombophlebitic liver abscess in appendicitis!

Macroscopic: Gray to grayish white, cheesy coating of the walls of veins.

5. **Hyaline thrombi** have a red, homogeneous appearance in hematoxylin-eosin–stained sections and are composed of platelets and fibrin. They are found in capillaries and venules, particularly in shock (see Shock Lung, chap. 3).

Fate of Thrombi

1. *Emboli:* parts of a thrombus, or even the whole thrombus, may become detached and circulate with the blood. The danger of embolism is reduced when the thrombus has become organized (10 days). 2. *Alterations in the structure of the thrombus (homogenization):* In the course of disintegration, the contained erythrocytes, granulocytes, and platelets fuse with the fibrin and cell fragments and form a homogeneous mass. This process of homogenization begins in the center of the thrombus as early as the second day and proceeds continuously. The fibrin can be dissolved even after a long time (years), as the results of streptokinase therapy in chronic obstruction of the leg arteries demonstrate. 3. *Dissolution of the thrombus:* (a) *By granulocytes* (softening). When the proteolytic enzymes of the granulocytes are released, they dissolve the fibrin, erythrocytes, and platelets, especially in the center of the thrombus. A puslike fluid results that is flushed away by the bloodstream. (b) *By the fibrinolytic system* (thrombolysis). By the conversion of plasminogen to plasmin, the fibrin in the thrombus can be dissolved by proteolysis (plasmin has a high specificity for fibrin, but does not lyse platelet masses). Plasminogen is present in flowing blood and is absorbed by the fibrin strands in the thrombus. The fibrinolytic system can be activated therapeutically by bacterial products (streptokinase). (c) *By granulation tissue* (organization). One day after it starts to form, monocytes cover the surface of the thrombus and grow into it (transformed to histiocytes and fibroblasts). Sprouts of vascular endothelial cells or subendothelial cells (myocytes?) grow into the base of the thrombus (vascular endothelial cells have fibrinolytic activity).

*Note: in clinical use ''thromboephlebitis'' usually means ''bland,'' i.e., noninfective venous thrombosis associated with the external signs of inflammation (rubor, tumor, dolor, calor).

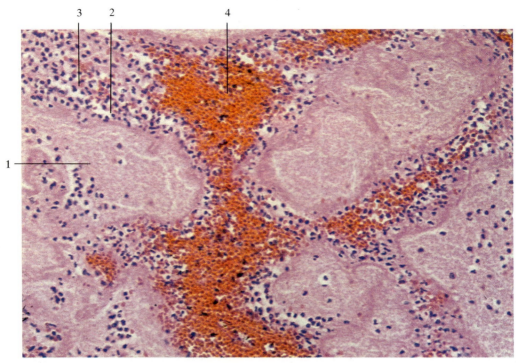

Fig 2–20.—Conglutination (agglutination) thrombus (hematoxylin-eosin; 246×).

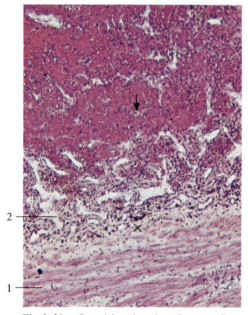

Fig 2–21.—Organizing thrombus (hematoxylin-eosin; 101×).

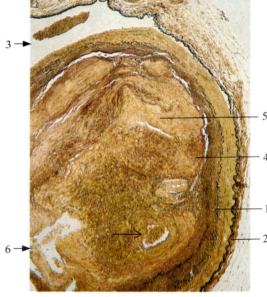

Fig 2–22.—Recanalized arterial thrombus (elastica–van Gieson's stain; 40×).

Capillaries develop from these endothelial cells and grow into the thrombus (about 10 days). About day 5 collagen fibrils, and later some elastic fibers, are laid down. Thus the cellular response of the vessel wall is formation of granulation tissue. Such granulation tissue may release proteolytic enzymes and thus has the ability to dissolve a thrombus, including the homogenized portions, and replace it with connective tissue. In this way a scar may be formed after 4–6 weeks. The new capillaries bring about recanalization of the formerly thrombosed blood vessel.

Special Sorts of Organization: The newly formed connective tissue may become calcified or ossified (phleboliths). The new blood channels in the thrombus can be especially large and numerous (cavernous.) Involvement of the valves of the veins in the process of organization of thrombi in the leg veins may be very important in the development of postthrombotic syndromes (e.g. varicosities, stasis ulcers). 4. *Propagation or "growth" of thrombi:* Simultaneously with the processes of dissolution, a thrombus can also increase in size through the addition of a new thrombus. Such propagation of a thrombus occurs particularly in the veins of the lower extremities (calf veins-femoral, iliac) and always carries a high risk of embolization.

Conglutination (agglutination) thrombus. When a section of such a thrombus is examined under very low magnification, the vessel wall is seen to be covered with a thrombus having a rough, undulating surface. Projecting columns of platelets fill the spaces between erythrocytes. Under medium magnification (Fig 2–20), the coral-like structure of the platelet masses ($\rightarrow$ 1) is easily recognized. Under high magnification, the platelets appear as finely granular material. Fibrin appears as homogeneous bands ($\rightarrow$ 2) which envelop the platelets. Outside the bands of fibrin is a zone of leukocytes ($\rightarrow$ 3). In the spaces between the platelet columns there are thickly massed erythrocytes ($\rightarrow$ 4) and a loose fibrin network. In old thrombi it may be difficult to distinguish between platelets and fibrin. Azan stains are helpful, since platelets stain blue, whereas fibrin stains red.

Organizing thrombus (Fig 2–21). The early stages of resorption and organization begin from the vessel wall and lumen (monocytes!) and are already under way at 2–4 days after the onset of thrombosis. Very low magnification shows red material completely filling the lumen. The wall of the vein ($\rightarrow$ 1) appears as a light red band. Low-power magnification discloses a brighter red, sparsely cellular zone near the vessel wall in the thrombus. Medium magnification (Fig 2–21) shows granulation tissue developing from the vessel wall where markedly dilated capillaries ($\rightarrow$ 2) and erythrocytes are clearly visible. In between lie fibroblasts and histiocytes, and formation of new connective tissue fibers has already started. Vessels are still sparse in the interior of the thrombus. Isolated histiocytes (precursors of granulation tissue) are present, some surrounded by clearings ($\rightarrow$) (compare the organization of a myocardial infarct and pericarditis, Figs 1–17, 1–18, and Fig 1–37). The brownish black granules ($\times$) in the organizing tissue are intracellularly situated products of hemoglobin, i.e., hemosiderin.

Recanalization of an arterial thrombus (Fig 2–22). The microscopic appearance depends on the age and mass of the thrombus and the degree of recanalization. In Figure 2–22, the internal elastic lamina ($\rightarrow$ 1) and external elastic lamina ($\rightarrow$ 2) are present. The former is partly split and fragmented. At $\rightarrow$ 3, the external elastic lamina is lifted off the media and blood fills the breach. The true lumen of the blood vessel is obstructed by connective tissue of different ages (richly cellular young granulation tissue $\rightarrow$ 4; older fibrous connective tissue $\rightarrow$ 5). In the midst of the connective tissue there are spaces lined by endothelium and containing erythrocytes ($\rightarrow$ 6 and arrow). These dilated blood vessels pass through the organized thrombus and terminate in the main lumen of the artery, both before and behind the thrombus.

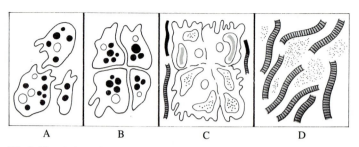

A   B   C   D

Fig 2–23.—Schematic representation of the pathogenesis of thrombosis.

Thrombus formation starts with agglutination of thrombocytes, which is associated with loss of granulation (so-called *viscous metamorphosis*). Later, fibrin accumulates. The results of studies with the electron microscope show that this viscous metamorphosis takes place in four stages (Fig 2–23). Normal thrombocytes (Fig 2–23,A) consist of a *clear* portion (ground substance) and a *granular* portion containing the cellular organelles. In the *first stage* of agglutination (preagglutination), the thrombocytes *swell* (membrane injury?), form *pseudopods,* and stick together (Fig 2–23,B). The existing ATP begins to disintegrate (because of ATPase activity). The integrity of the outer membranes of the thrombocytes is probably preserved through the mediation of ADP and calcium. In the *second stage* of agglutination, the outer membrane of individual thrombocytes is still largely intact (Figs 2–23,B, 2–24). The granular ground substance moves to the center of the platelets. During the *third stage (thrombocytic rhexis),* the outer membranes of the thrombocytes disintegrate (Fig 2–23,C, D). In the center, the various constituents of the granular ground substance deteriorate. At the outer margin, protrusions are formed. Now, for the first time, fibrin is visible at the margins of the aggregates (Fig 2–23,C).

In the last stage, that of *thrombocytolysis* (Fig 2–23,D), the thrombocytes disintegrate completely into granular material and membrane fragments. A large amount of fibrin is intermingled with this remaining wreckage. During the stage of viscous metamorphosis, the thrombocytes give up the following substances: 1, those effecting plasma coagulation [factor 3, thromboplastin (thrombokinase), and factor 4, calcium]: 2, those affecting fibrinolysis—platelet proactivator antiplasmin; 3, those with an effect on the blood vessel wall—adrenalin, noradrenalin, serotonin.

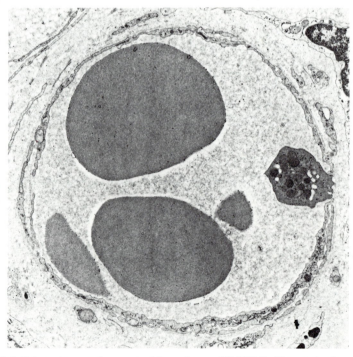

Fig 2–24.—Platelet covers an endothelial gap in a venule as a stand-in or stopgap (13,000×). (Baumgartner)

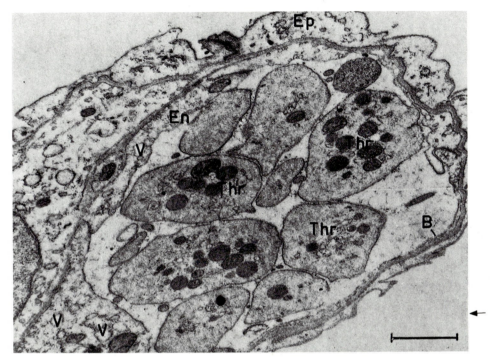

Fig 2–25.—Lung capillary with agglutinated thrombocytes *(Thr)* in the lumen (histamine shock, rabbit). The platelets are heaped on one another, with cytoplasmic organelles mostly located in their centers. The endothelium *(En)* shows numerous vesicles *(V)*, as does the alveolar epithelium *(Ep)* (accumulation of fluid in vacuoles). *B,* basement membrane; → alveolar clearing (20,000 ×). (Nikulin et al.)

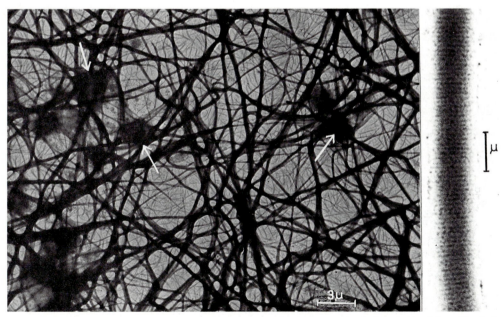

Fig 2–26.—Scaffold of fibrin threads and thrombocytes (→) in spontaneously shed fresh blood (metallic shadowing). Fibrin fibers have formed in both thick bundles and in a fine network (3,000 ×). **Right,** a single fibrin fiber with distinct cross-bands (periodicity of 230 Å) (100,000 ×). (Köppel)

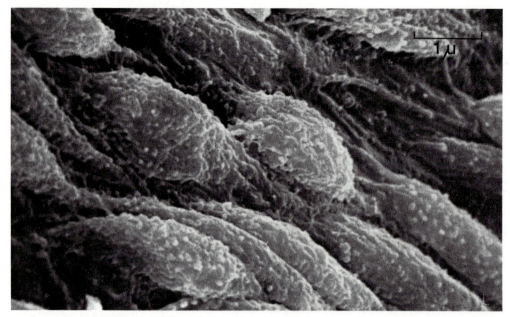

Fig 2–27.—Endothelial cells of normal aorta from a 1-month-old female. The individual endothelial cells are spindle shaped and have a bedlike arrangement. The cells have numerous processes and numerous small out-pouchings of the plasma membranes (scanning electron micrograph; 1,800 ×).

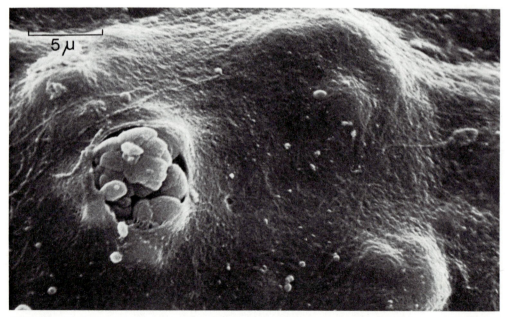

Fig 2–28.—Rupture of an atheromatous lesion in the atherosclerotic aorta of a 67-year-old man. At this particular location in the artery the vascular endothelium is covered by a thick film of fibrin (scanning electron micrograph; 4,500 ×).

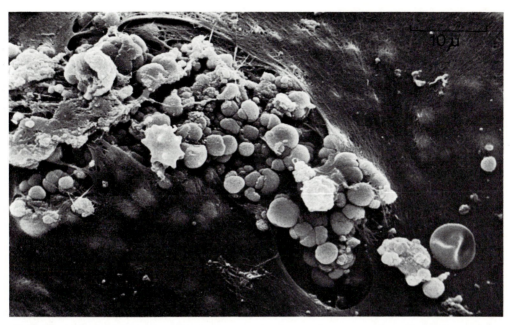

Fig 2–29.—Intimal break in the arteriosclerotic aorta of a 67-year-old man, showing globular particles (lipids) discharged from an atheromatous mass that has broken through several layers of fibrin (scanning electron micrograph; 2,500 ×).

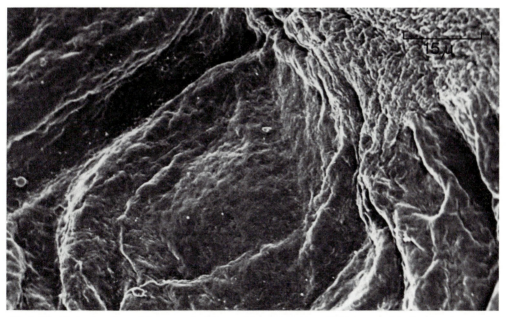

Fig 2–30.—Intimal surface of the aorta of a 76-year-old woman with syphilitic mesaortitis showing circumscribed elevation of endothelium subsequent to injury of elastica with resulting scarring (scanning electron micrograph; 2,000 ×).

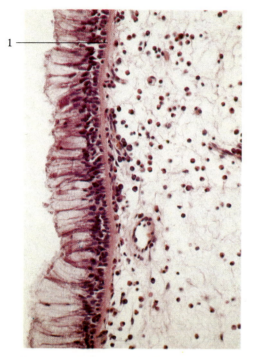

Fig 3–1.—Allergic sinusitis (hematoxylin-eosin; 200×).

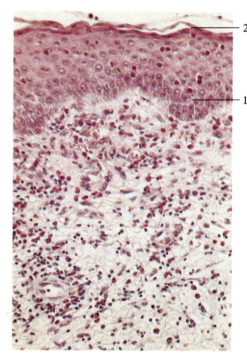

Fig 3–2.—Squamous metaplasia of nasal mucosa in chronic sinusitis (hematoxylin-eosin; 200×).

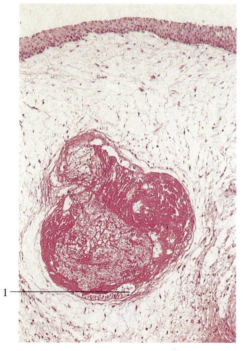

Fig 3–3.—Singer's node (hematoxylin-eosin; 40×).

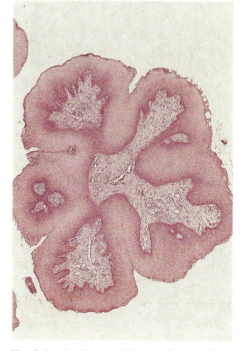

Fig 3–4.—Papilloma of larynx (hematoxylin-eosin; 40×).

3. Upper Respiratory Passages—Lung—Pleura

Sinusitis—Polyps of Vocal Cords—Papilloma of Larynx

Allergic sinusitis (Fig 3–1). The allergic genesis of chronic inflammation of the nasal mucosa (rhinitis) and of the mucosa of the paranasal sinuses (sinusitis) has the following histologic features: the goblet cells of the columnar respiratory epithelium are increased in number, the eosinophilic basal membrane is thickened (→ 1), the stroma is edematous and infiltrated by eosinophilic granulocytes.

Squamous metaplasia in chronic sinusitis (Fig 3–2). If inflammation of the nasal mucosa is persistent the respiratory epithelium may be replaced by stratified squamous epithelium through the process of squamous metaplasia. The microscopic appearance is that of stratified squamous epithelium with indications of basal cell differentiation (→ 1) and superficial keratinization (→ 2). The underlying stroma is heavily infiltrated by lymphocytes and plasma cells (chronic inflammation).

Polyps of vocal cord (singer's node) (Fig 3–3). This is a circumscribed exudative inflammation in the stroma of a vocal cord. Its characteristics are edematous swelling, eosinophilic fibrinous exudate, and cavities that may be lined by endothelium and resemble hemangioma (→ 1). In the later stages these lesions become organized into tissue rich in fibroblasts and collagen ("singer's node"). Vocal cord polyps or nodules occur mainly in consequence of hyperkinetic voice stress in small children and adults, especially singers.

Papilloma of larynx (Fig 3–4) is a benign neoplasm commonly situated on a vocal cord. Histologically it is composed of a framework of collagen covered by multilayered stratified squamous epithelium. The arrangement of cells is regular, and, as a rule, there is no increase in mitoses nor are there signs of infiltrative growth. These papillomas are probably virus-induced tumors. They occur singly or multiply. Although benign, they can spread over the surface of the larynx and can recur after surgical removal. Traumatic local factors occasionally provoke cellular atypia. When this happens it may be difficult to distinguish the lesion from a carcinoma, although malignant transformation is rare in children.

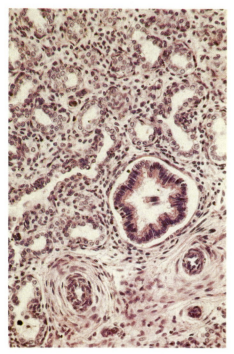

Fig 3–5.—Fetal atelectasis of lung (hematoxylin-eosin; 100×).

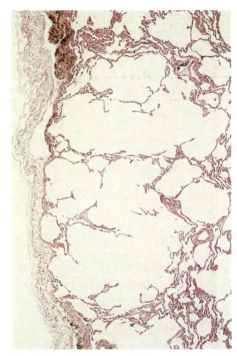

Fig 3–6.—Emphysema of lung (hematoxylin-eosin; 40×).

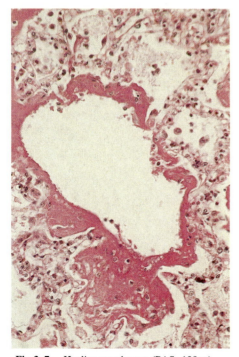

Fig 3–7.—Hyaline membranes (PAS; 100×).

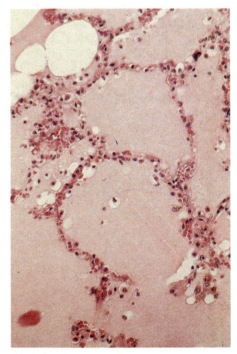

Fig 3–8.—Pulmonary edema (hematoxylin-eosin; 100×).

Lung: Atelectasis—Emphysema—Hyaline Membranes—Edema

Atelectasis of lung (Fig 3–5). This consists of diminished air content of the lung because of insufficient expansion or collapse of alveoli. Microscopically, the alveolar walls are apposed, giving the appearance of increased cellularity. The capillaries are usually dilated. Histologically, the various forms of atelectasis, e.g., compression atelectasis in pneumothorax or pleural effusion, obstructive or reabsorption atelectasis with bronchial tumors, all have the same appearance. Defective maturation and differentiation of lungs should be distinguished from fetal atelectasis.

Emphysema of pulmonary alveoli (Fig 3–6). There is destruction of alveolar septa together with abnormal, persistent enlargement of air spaces distal to terminal bronchioles. There is marked, focal enlargement of alveolar air spaces. The alveolar septa are thin, often torn, and the torn ends project into alveolar spaces. The emphysematous area shown in Figure 3–6 is covered by visceral pleura (left side).

Pulmonary emphysema, chronic bronchitis, bronchial asthma, and bronchiectasis give rise clinically to **chronic obstructive pulmonary disease** (COPD). Pulmonary emphysema is subdivided according to morphological and pathogenetic criteria. An expansion of alveolar spaces that is not accompanied by destruction of tissue is considered to be hyperexpansion (compensatory emphysema). On the basis of the localization of the abnormally expanded terminal air space one can distinguish between centrilobular, panlobular, paraseptal, and irregular emphysema (cf. *Macropathology*).

Hyaline membranes (Fig 3–7). This is the most important morphological finding in respiratory distress syndrome of newborns. It occurs predominantly in premature infants with a weight of less than 2,500 gm. Histologically there is incomplete expansion of alveoli corresponding to the stage of fetal development. The alveoli are lined by an eosinophilic, slightly PAS-positive material consisting of polysaccharides, protein, and lipids.

Similar changes may be seen in adult lungs, for example in chronic shock lung, in pulmonary edema due to toxic agents or uremia, or after prolonged artificial respiration.

Pulmonary edema (Fig 3–8). Fluid exudate has escaped from the bloodstream into the alveoli (intra-alveolar edema). Microscopically the alveoli are seen to be filled with homogeneous eosinophilic cell-free fluid. There are a few solitary, exfoliated alveolar epithelial cells. The capillaries are congested. In some places, alveolar fluid has been lost during preparation of the section, so that empty spaces have resulted (artifacts).

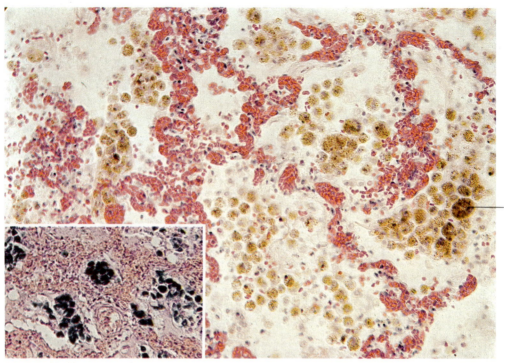

Fig 3–9.—Congestion of the lung (passive hyperemia or stasis) (hematoxylin-eosin; 240×). *Inset,* Prussian blue reaction; 132×).

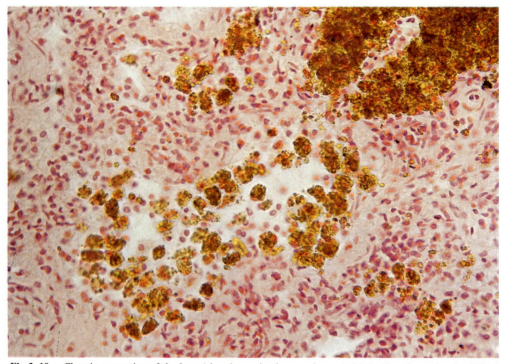

Fig 3–10.—Chronic congestion of the lung (chronic passive hyperemia or stasis) (nuclear fast red stain; 330×).

Congestion of the Lungs

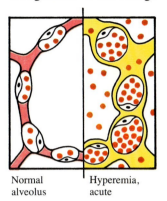 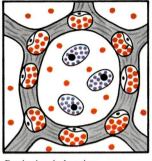 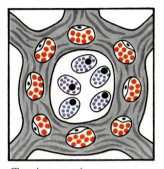

| Normal alveolus | Hyperemia, acute | Beginning induration, subacute | Chronic congestion (stasis) |

Fig 3–11.—Different stages of congestion of the lung.

Passive congestion of the lungs *results from obstruction to the flow of blood from the left side of the heart (e.g., in mitral stenosis). The condition is therefore one of passive hyperemia with morphological alterations corresponding to the severity of the congestion or stasis.* In the **acute stage** (Fig 3–11) there is simple hyperemia, the dilated capillaries projecting into the alveolar spaces in knoblike fashion, and interstitial edema. The capillaries are filled with thickly packed erythrocytes.

Passive congestion of longer duration (subacute to subchronic) (Figs 3–9, 3–11) leads to increased extravasation into the alveoli of erythrocytes which are phagocytosed by alveolar epithelium and the hemoglobin converted into *hemosiderin* (heart failure cells laden with brown intracytoplasmic pigment). An increase in connective tissue and the basement membrane thickens the alveolar walls.

Chronic passive congestion (brown induration) (Figs 3–10, 3–11) is manifested by greatly thickened alveolar septa (collagenous fibrosis), thickening of the basement membrane, and heavy loading of the alveolar epithelium with hemosiderin (heart failure cells may appear in the sputum). Hemosiderin is liberated and may be deposited along with calcium in both the connective and elastic tissue.

Congestion of the lung. Figure 3–9 shows a subacute stage with marked hyperemia of the capillaries so that they project into the alveolar spaces. The alveolar walls are not fibrotic or thickened. The alveolar spaces contain exfoliated alveolar epithelial cells (→), the cytoplasm of which contains finely granular, brown, refractile hemosiderin pigment. The Prussian blue reaction (inset in the lower left-hand corner) shows that the pigment contains Fe^{III}. The iron is probably derived from broken-down hemoglobin.

Chronic passive congestion of lung (Fig 3–10). Inspection under very low magnification shows a thicker lung framework than normal. Alveolar spaces appear narrow because of great thickening of the walls by collagenous tissue. Van Gieson's stain demonstrates an intensely red-staining network of fibers. The cell content, however, is not substantially increased (compare with interstitial pneumonia, later in this chapter). Numerous heart failure cells, with clearly visible brown pigment, are found in the alveolar spaces. In many cases there is also an increase in smooth muscle.

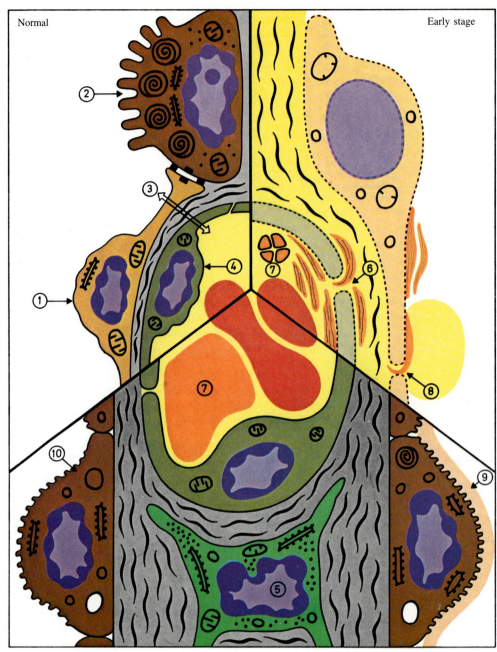

Fig 3–12.—Shock lung. Diagram of ultrastructural changes. **Normal:** *1,* type I alveolar cell; *2,* type II alveolar cell; *3,* attenuated cytoplasm where gas exchange takes place; *4,* capillary endothelial cell. **Acute phase:** loss of contacts between endothelial cells with leakage of edema fluid *(yellow)* and fibrin *(red)* into the interstitium and later *(8)* into the alveolar lumen. In the capillary lumen there are platelet and fibrin thrombi *(7).* **Late phase:** proliferation of type II alveolar cells *(10)* and of fibroblasts *(5)* with deposition of collagen *(gray).* The intra-alveolar exudate leads to the production of hyaline membranes *(9).*

Shock Lung

Shock describes a general failure of peripheral circulation with tissue damage resulting from decreased perfusion of blood. Central to its clinical manifestations are a decrease of the circulating mass of blood platelets (platelet failure—consumption coagulopathy—disseminated intravascular coagulation) and anuria. The respiratory insufficiency of shock patients produces hypoxia due to short-circuiting of blood through arteriovenous anastomoses (up to 67% of the cardiac output), diminished O_2 uptake, and increased blood CO_2 tension. Morphologically and roentgenologically, there is spindle-shaped widening of the blood vessels during the first hours of shock (stage 1) due to perivascular edema. Figure 3–13 shows the **greatly dilated perivascular lymph spaces** that are almost cystic in size (→). Pulmonary lymph flow through these lymph channels is increased. In the following days (3–5 days, stage II) the perivascular edema intensifies and progresses to interstitial edema. X-ray films of the lung now show a cloudy, milk-glass appearance. Grossly, the lung is dusky red and has a spongy, leather-like quality. These changes are shown more clearly in Figure 3–14, where the normal lung tissue in the upper portion is contrasted in the lower portion with the **broad edematous septa** containing an increased number of cells (histiocytes, granulocytes, fibroblasts). Simultaneously (1–2 days), **microthrombi** appear in the lungs. In the third stage of shock, fibroblasts proliferate in alveolar septa, so that roentgenologically there is **reticular striation** (irreversible, progresses to pulmonary fibrosis).

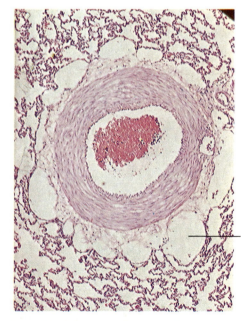

Fig 3–13.—Dilated perivascular lymph spaces in shock lung (hematoxylin-eosin; 60×).

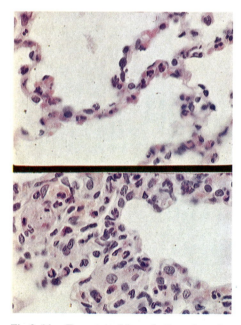

Fig 3–14.—**Top,** normal lung; **bottom,** interstitial edema in shock lung (hematoxylin-eosin; 300×).

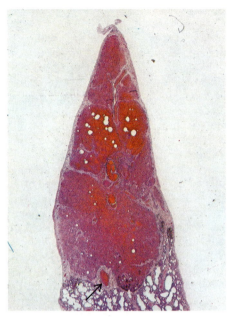

Fig 3–15.—Hemorrhagic infarct of lung (hematoxylin-eosin; 5×).

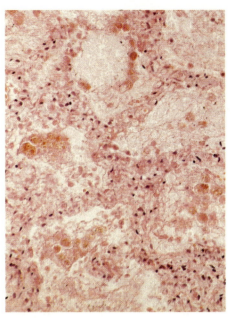

Fig 3–16.—Septal necrosis in a hemorrhagic infarct (hematoxylin-eosin; 150×).

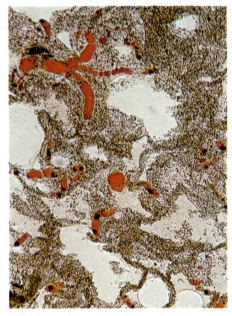

Fig 3–17.—Fat emboli in lung (Sudan stain; 58×).

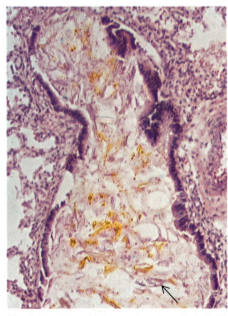

Fig 3–18.—Bronchial aspiration of amniotic fluid (hematoxylin-eosin; 162×).

Hemorrhagic Infarct—Fat Embolism—Aspiration of Amniotic Fluid

Hemorrhagic infarct of lung (Fig 3–15, 3–16). *This denotes focal necrosis and hemorrhage of lung tissue following embolic occlusion of a branch of the pulmonary artery in the presence of passive hyperemia of the bronchial circulation.* Naked eye inspection of a section usually reveals a wedge-shaped, red, homogeneous lesion. The tissue in Figure 3–15 is from the lingula of the lung so that the wedge shape of the infarct is fortuitous. The embolism occlusion (→) of the nutrient branch of the pulmonary artery can be easily seen. Medium and high magnification disclose a monotonous picture: the alveolar spaces are filled with densely packed erythrocytes. In older infarcts, these show only as shadowy forms or are disintegrated into crumbled, eosinophilic, homogeneous, dingy, reddish brown masses. The alveolar septa can scarcely be distinguished from the contents of the alveoli. Septal nuclei have disappeared (evidence of *necrosis,* Fig 3–16).

Infarcts must be *differentiated from aspirated blood,* in which necrosis is lacking, as well as from an embolus.

Fat embolism (Fig 3–17). *Release of fluid fat from bone marrow (also from subcutaneous fat tissue or a fatty liver) after trauma (e.g., burn injury) may cause obstruction of the pulmonary capillaries and eventually escape into the arterial circulation.* In part the fat may also come from nontraumatized fat tissue (adrenalin-caused lipolysis, so-called fat mobilization syndrome). Low magnification reveals small red flecks in the lung parenchyma. Medium magnification shows Sudan-positive material in the capillaries, which have a staghorn or small round disk shape (cross section). There are usually hyperemia and also pulmonary edema. NOTE: Fat embolism is a form of shock. Hyaline thrombi are always present.

Aspiration of amniotic fluid (Fig 3–18) *This occurs during premature respiration in the birth canal.* Microscopically, the signs of aspiration consist of golden brown or greenish amniotic fluid and meconium in small bronchi and in occasional alveoli. Figure 3–18 shows a small bronchus, the lumen of which contains abundant squames (→). These consist of cross-sectioned desquamated squamous epithelium of the vernix caseosa. The masses stained golden brown (bilirubin) consist of meconium. The small round bodies are known as meconium bodies (probably desquamated colonic cells of the fetus). Secondary aspiration pneumonia may develop (infected amniotic fluid) in which maternal leukocytes participate. Aspiration of amniotic fluid occurs chiefly in premature births.

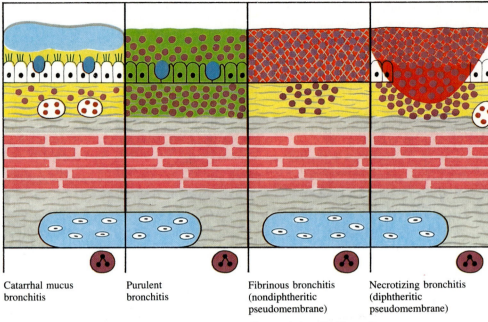

Catarrhal mucus
bronchitis

Purulent
bronchitis

Fibrinous bronchitis
(nondiphtheritic
pseudomembrane)

Necrotizing bronchitis
(diphtheritic
pseudomembrane)

Characteristics of Different Degrees
of Inflammation and Necrosis

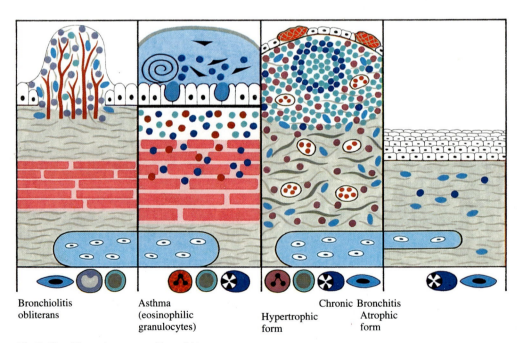

Bronchiolitis
obliterans

Asthma
(eosinophilic
granulocytes)

Chronic Bronchitis

Hypertrophic
form

Atrophic
form

Fig 3–19.—The various sorts of bronchitis.

Etiology of Inflammations in the Lungs (Pneumonia, Bronchitis)

There are two causes of inflammation of the respiratory passages: living agents (infections), and noninfectious noxious agents (radiation, poisons, products of immunologic reactions, i.e., in allergies). Environmental contamination, tobacco smoke, and constitutional factors may facilitate development of infection in the lungs. Normally, bronchi and alveoli are sterile, owing to ventilation and mucociliary function. Pulmonary infection may be facilitated by obstruction of airways, mucociliary insufficiency, retention of mucous secretions, or aspiration.

Classification of pulmonary infections. Four criteria are usually considered:
1. **Anatomical criteria:**
   a. Bronchi: bronchitis
   b. Alveoli: intra-alveolar pneumonia
   c. Interstitial tissue: interstitial pneumonia
2. **Etiologic criteria:**
   a. Nonspecific inflammation (bacteria, such as *Streptococcus pneumoniae, Hemophilus influenzae, Klebsiella pneumoniae,* streptococci, staphylococci, *Pseudomonas,* myxoviruses and adenoviruses)
   b. Specific inflammations
   Bacteria: *Mycobacterium tuberculosis, Actinomyces israeli*
   Fungi: *Candida albicans, Cryptococcus neoformans, Histoplasma capsulatum, Coccidioides immitis, Blastomyces dermatitidis.*
   Viruses: Cytomegalovirus
3. **Clinical course:** Acute or chronic bronchitis/pneumonia.
4. **Histopathologic criteria:** As shown in Figure 3–19, the inflammation may be catarrhal with production of mucus, or purulent, pseudomembranous, pseudomembranous-necrotizing; fibrinous, proliferative, hypertrophic, or atrophic.

Figure 3–19 shows the different forms of bronchitis in diagrammatic form. Acute **seromucous catarrh** shows edema and hyperemia of the tunica propria as well as a layer of mucus containing a few leukocytes. The exudate contains mucus mixed with protein material, occasional leukocytes, and shed epithelium. *Purulent catarrh* is recognized by exudate rich in granulocytes. Erythrocytes predominate in **hemorrhagic inflammation.** In **fibrinous inflammation,** grayish white, cohesive, detachable membranes *(pseudomembrane, croup)* develop which often extend widely (bronchial casts may be formed), whereas *pseudomembranous necrotizing inflammation* (diphtheritic) is distinguished by a patchy, tightly adherent, putty-like layer. In the first case, the fibrin is superficial, replacing the epithelium and the underlying necrotic connective tissue (deeply penetrating fibrinous necrosis). Necrotizing fibrinous inflammation is always followed by proliferation of granulation tissue. When bronchioles are affected in this way, the result is **bronchiolitis obliterans.** In **chronic bronchitis,** all coats are infiltrated by cells and the goblet cells are increased in number. Metaplasia of the epithelium often becomes prominent (see also Fig 3–2).

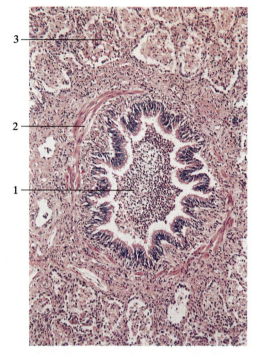

Fig 3–20.—Acute purulent bronchitis (hematoxylin-eosin; 100×).

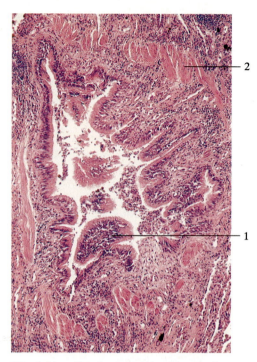

Fig 3–21.—Chronic bronchitis (hematoxylin-eosin; 100×).

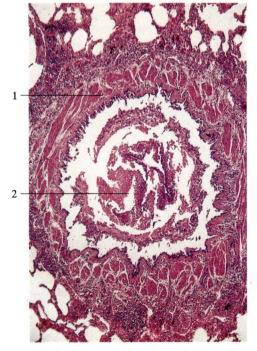

Fig 3–22.—Bronchial asthma (hematoxylin-eosin; 60×).

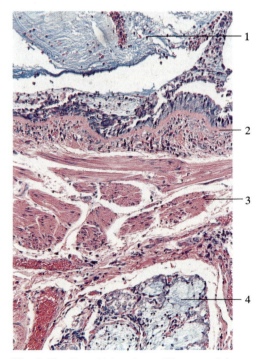

Fig 3–23.—Bronchial asthma (Giemsa stain; 150×).

Bronchitis

Acute purulent bronchitis (Fig 3–20) is characterized by an exudate of pus cells (pyknotic segmented granulocytes) in the bronchial lumen (→ 1). The inflammation may involve the peribronchial stroma with fragmentation of smooth muscle fibers (→ 2). Alveoli (→ 3) become involved only if bronchopneumonia develops.

Acute bronchitis is usually a manifestation of infection of the upper respiratory passages (e.g., tracheobronchitis in influenza) or it may be associated with pneumonia.

Chronic bronchitis (Fig 3–21). In this condition the bronchial mucosa is thrown up into folds that project into the lumen. The stroma shows a dense infiltration by lymphocytes and plasma cells (→ 1). The bronchial muscle layer is thickened owing to an increase in the number of smooth muscle cells (→ 2).

According to WHO, chronic bronchitis is defined as a productive cough persisting for at least 3 months in 2 successive years. Bacterial and viral infections, mucociliary insufficiency, disturbed ventilation of the lungs, environmental pollution, and retained mucous secretions are causative factors.

Bronchial asthma (Figs 3–22, 3–23). This disease is characterized by spells of acute respiratory distress due to contraction of the bronchial muscles associated with increased production of abnormally viscous mucus, with resulting obstruction of bronchi, and is usually due to allergy. Figure 3–22 shows marked hypertrophy of bronchial muscle (→ 1) and inspissated mucus in the lumen (→ 2). The Giemsa stain (Fig 3–23) provides evidence for the allergic pathogenesis: the blue-staining mucus (→ 1), the homogeneously thickened basement membrane of the bronchial mucosa (→ 2), and hypertrophy of the smooth muscle (→ 3) and of the mucous glands (→ 4). The epithelial lining shows changes similar to those described for allergic sinusitis (see Fig 3–1).

Bronchiolitis obliterans (pseudomembranous necrotizing bronchiolitis, Fig 3–24). In this condition necrotic and inflammatory exudate and fibrin are replaced by granulation tissue. Thus the lumen of bronchi or bronchioles may be completely plugged. A similar process may occur in proliferative bronchiolitis. Low magnification reveals closure of bronchioles by highly cellular granulation tissue. Intermediate magnification reveals partial absence of ciliated columnar epithelium (× in Fig 3–24). The plug of granulation tissue that fills the lumen is composed of fibroblasts, collagen fibers, capillaries, and lymphocytes. The walls of bronchioles contain chronic inflammatory cells. → 1 indicates bronchial smooth muscle; → 2, ciliated columnar epithelium.

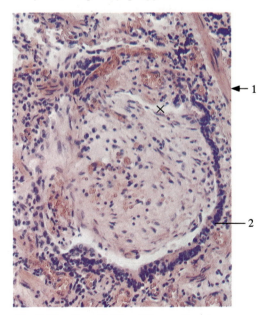

Fig 3–24.—Bronchiolitis obliterans (hematoxylin-eosin).

Inflammation of the Lung

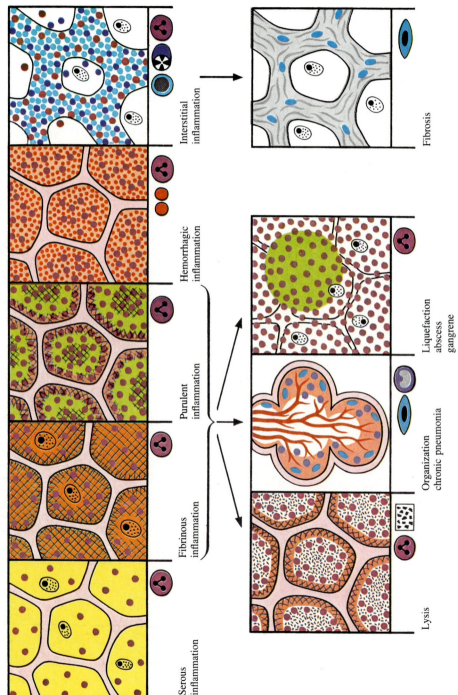

Focal Pneumonitis—Lobar Pneumonia—Interstitial Pneumonia

Serous inflammation

Fibrinous inflammation

Purulent inflammation

Hemorrhagic inflammation

Interstitial inflammation

Fibrosis

Liquefaction abscess gangrene

Organization chronic pneumonia

Lysis

Fig 3-25.—Summary of the various sorts of inflammation of the lung, the results of healing, and the complications that may develop.

Inflammation of the Lung—Pneumonia, Pneumonitis

Two large categories of inflammation of the lung can be distinguished and further subdivided:

1. **Pneumonias characterized by an intra-alveolar exudate.**
   a. **Focal pneumonias,** also called **lobular pneumonias,** and **bronchopneumonias.** These may involve parts of one or several lobes. The process can spread along bronchi and secondarily to surrounding alveoli. It may also originate from a septic embolus (Fig 3–26) and give rise to a septic lung abscess. In Figure 3–26 a cross-sectioned pulmonary artery is plugged by an embolus (→ 1). This embolus is composed of fibrin and platelets (eosinophilic) and bacteria (blue). The lumens of neighboring capillaries are filled with bacteria (→ 2).
   b. **Lobar pneumonias** are characterized by more or less simultaneous involvement of entire lobes.

2. **Interstitial pneumonias** show predominantly accumulations of lymphocytes, plasma cells, or histiocytes in alveolar walls.

With respect to clinical course as well as the microscopic picture of the lungs, one distinguishes acute from chronic pneumonia as well as serous, fibrinous, purulent, abscess-forming, gangrenous, and organized (fibrous) pneumonias (Fig 3–25).

Results of pulmonary inflammations (Fig 3–25). Under favorable conditions, the inflammatory exudate undergoes lysis through enzymatic action and is resorbed. The lung is then restored to normal. Severe inflammation (highly virulent bacteria and/or reduced resistance of the host) may lead to tissue necrosis (abscess). This may be followed by organization of the inflammatory exudate, leaving a scar, or may continue as chronic pneumonia. Interstitial pneumonitis may result in septal fibrosis.

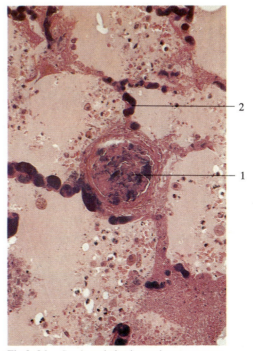

Fig 3–26.—Septic embolus in a pulmonary artery (hematoxylin-eosin; 150×).

109

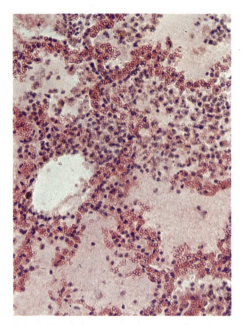

Fig 3–27.—Lobar pneumonia: stage of engorgement (hematoxylin-eosin).

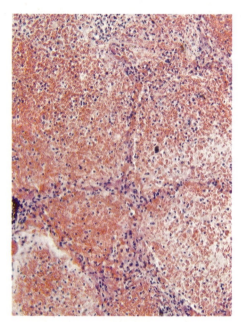

Fig 3–28.—Lobar pneumonia: stage of red hepatization (hematoxylin-eosin).

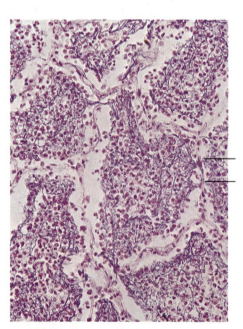

Fig 3–29.—Lobar pneumonia: stage of gray hepatization (Weigert's fibrin stain).

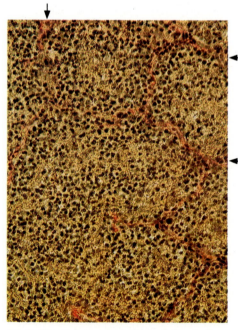

Fig 3–30.—Lobar pneumonia: resolution (yellow hepatization) (van Gieson's stain).

Lobar Pneumonia

The term lobar pneumonia refers to that type of pneumonia in which there is sudden involvement of an entire lobe by an inflammatory process caused by *Streptococcus pneumoniae* (95% of cases) or, much less frequently, by *Klebsiella* or other bacteria. The natural course of the disease runs in stages. These are shown in Figures 3–27 through 3–30.

Stage of engorgement (Fig 3–27). On the first day of the illness pulmonary hyperemia predominates. The septal capillaries are packed with erythrocytes. Soon thereafter, serous fluid streams into the alveolar spaces. The exudate becomes progressively richer in protein. It is seen as eosinophilic material containing desquamated alveolar epithelial cells and granulocytes.

Stage of red hepatization (Fig 3–28). On the second and third day of the illness there is marked leakage of erythrocytes and fibrinogen into the alveolar lumens, in addition to continued pronounced hyperemia of the capillaries. The intra-alveolar exudate is now characterized by predominance of erythrocytes, embedded in a network of fibrin.

Stage of gray hepatization (Fig 3–29). The fibrinous component of the inflammatory exudate is most prominent between the fourth and sixth day of the illness. Weigert's fibrin stain reveals a dense network of fibrin (when stained by hematoxylin-eosin, the threads of fibrin are best seen when the condenser of the microscope is lowered). The fibrin mesh network now contains segmented granulocytes. The arrows in Figure 3–29 indicate alveolar septa.

Stage of resolution (yellow hepatization, Fig 3–30). On the seventh and eighth days of the illness fibrinolysis is evident, owing to the action of proteolytic enzymes. Microscopically, the exudate is dominated by pyknotic segmented leukocytes. The alveolar septa can be demonstrated with van Gieson's stain (pink in Fig 3–30).

The further course of lobar pneumonia may be characterized by complete liquefaction of the intra-alveolar exudate (within 4 weeks of onset). The liquefied exudate is coughed up. This **lysis** is accompanied by gradual expansion of alveoli with air. If fibrin is not enzymatically decomposed, the exudate becomes organized into granulation tissue (see also Organized Pneumonia, later in this chapter). In unfavorable circumstances (e.g., chronic alcoholism or severe diabetes mellitus), lobar pneumonia may be followed by formation of abscesses.

The term **hepatization** refers to the liver-like consistency of an affected lobe. In this stage of gray hepatization the cut surface is gray and dry.

Differential diagnosis: Lobular pneumonias (bronchopneumonias) may become confluent and thus resemble lobar pneumonia. However, histologically the picture is more varied. Lobular bronchopneumonias also run through stages, but these are not synchronous. Thus, in confluent lobular pneumonia several of the stages described for lobar pneumonia may be present concurrently.

Apart from the complications already mentioned (organization, abscess formation), pleuritis (pleurisy) must be mentioned. The latter is a fibrinous inflammation involving the visceral pleura, which are covered by fibrinous exudate.

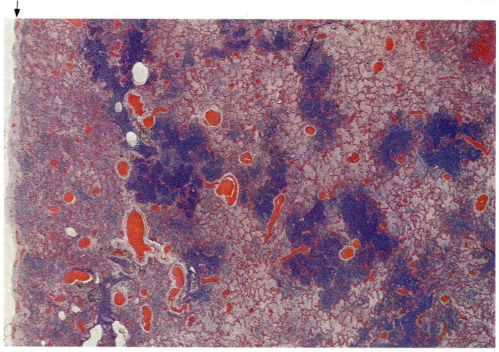

Fig 3–31.—Bronchopneumonia (hematoxylin-eosin; 12.5×).

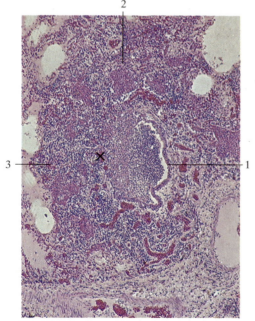

Fig 3–32.—Peribronchial focal pneumonia (hematoxylin-eosin; 64×).

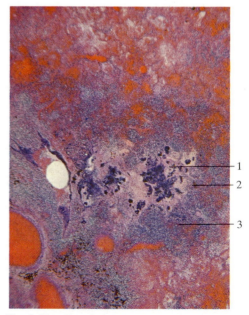

Fig 3–33.—Hemorrhagic necrotizing bronchopneumonia (hematoxylin-eosin; 36×).

Focal (Patchy, Lobular) Pneumonia

Focal pneumonias may have a variety of causes and their pathogenesis may be different (endobronchial, peribronchial, hematogenous). Common to all forms is the spread from multiple small foci to the rest of the lung tissue.

Bronchopneumonia (Fig 3–31). *There is patchy inflammation of lung tissue with involvement of single groups of alveoli and not sharply limited to the anatomical units (lobules).* With low magnification, irregular, poorly defined, blue-staining foci are seen in the lung (→ pleura). The alveoli between these foci contain palely stained red exudate. If the center of one of the nodules is examined with higher magnification, the alveoli will be seen to be thickly packed with polymorphonuclear cells. Alveolar walls are preserved and the capillaries are hyperemic. The further one looks toward the periphery, the fewer the number of leukocytes and fibrin threads that can be seen. Adjacent alveoli are filled with inflammatory edema, shed alveolar epithelium, and a few polymorphonuclear leukocytes (*focal inflammatory edema*). The bronchi contain purulent exudate and shed ciliated epithelial cells.

Peribronchial focal pneumonia (Fig 3–32). *In this type, the inflammation extends from the bronchial wall into adjacent lung tissue so that mantle-like peribronchial lesions develop.* Low-power magnification shows blue-stained lesions, in the center of which lies a small bronchus. With medium magnification, the bronchus can be recognized by its ciliated epithelium (→ 1), which is missing in one place (×) in the illustration. Reddish fibrinous membranes can be seen in the bronchi (pseudomembranous inflammation). During the healing process, such an area may develop into bronchiolitis obliterans (see Fig 3–24). The lumen of the bronchus is filled with granulocytes and the wall is densely infiltrated with them. The blood vessels are hyperemic. The adjacent alveoli contain fibrin (→ 2) and granulocytes (→ 3). More distant alveoli are filled with inflammatory edema fluid.

Hemorrhagic necrotizing bronchopneumonia (Fig 3–33). *Lobular or focal peribronchial pneumonia with hemorrhagic exudate occurs chiefly in infectious diseases (e.g., in influenza) caused by a mixture of etiologic agents (a virus plus influenza bacilli or various cocci).* The microscopic picture is variegated. Low magnification shows large, irregularly shaped, red and blue focal lesions. Bacterial colonies (→ 1) are seen in the center of the lesion. The surrounding lung tissue is necrotic (→ 2). Outside of this lies a zone of granulocytes (→ 3) mixed with exuded erythrocytes. Farther toward the periphery, the exudate is entirely hemorrhagic.

In very acute and toxic cases of influenza there is only hemorrhagic edema with hemorrhagic infarction and hyaline vascular thrombi (shock).

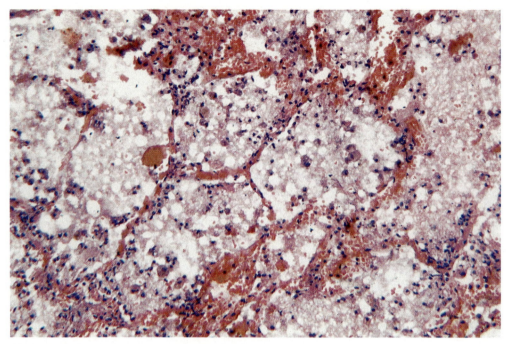

Fig 3–34.—Pneumonia due to *Klebsiella pneumoniae* (hematoxylin-eosin, 150×).

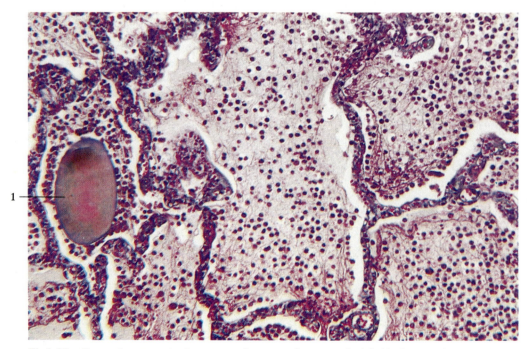

1 —

Fig 3–35.—Hypostatic pneumonia. A corpus amylaceum can be seen on the left side (hematoxylin-eosin; 150×).

114

Pneumonia due to *Klebsiella* and Hypostatic Pneumonia

Klebsiella pneumonia ("Friedländer bacillus pneumonia," Fig 3–34). Pneumonia due to *Klebsiella pneumoniae* is usually secondary to other disease and can involve one or more lobes of the lung (either confluent lobular or lobar pneumonia). The causative organism, *Klebsiella pneumoniae,* is a gram-negative bacillus with a polysaccharide capsule. Microscopically there is marked hyperemia of the septal capillaries (orange-red network in Fig 3–34). Within the alveoli there is a mucoid, slightly basophilic exudate in which there are scattered leukocytes (granulocytes and macrophages).

The infection may be nosocomial but is often a complication of serious disease elsewhere in the body, associated with lowered resistance, prolonged artificial respiration or bed rest, or aspiration. Grossly, the stringy exudate and the confluent lobular to lobar involvement are characteristic. The stringy mucoid nature of the exudate is mainly due to the capsular carbohydrate of the causative bacteria.

Hypostatic pneumonia (Fig 3–35). This condition is seen as a terminal complication in bedridden patients. Inflammation develops predominantly in the dependent (dorsal) parts of the lungs and is microscopically characterized by rather discrete intra-alveolar exudates. Figure 3–35 shows a serofibrinous exudate (eosinophilic material containing delicate fibrin strands) in which there are scattered segmented granulocytes. Commonly one also finds signs of chronic passive hyperemia, usually due to cardiac insufficiency. Associated with this may be **corpora amylacea** (→ 1). These are round or oval laminated bodies that are situated within alveoli and superficially resemble amyloid.

Hypostatic pneumonias are also secondary to other diseases that are particularly common among older bedridden patients who have suffered from prolonged cardiac insufficiency and diminished pulmonary ventilation. Causative organisms are various gram-positive and gram-negative bacteria, e.g., staphylococci, *Proteus, E. coli, Klebsiella.*

Special forms of pneumonia:

1. **Hemorrhagic pneumonia.** This is usually a complication of viral infections, e.g., influenza. Hemorrhagic pulmonary exudates also occur in plague, smallpox, and anthrax and are thought to reflect highly virulent etiologic agents.
2. **Eosinophilic pneumonia.** Eosinophilic infiltrates in the perihilar regions of the lungs are seen occasionally and are accompanied by increased numbers of eosinophils in liver and bone marrow. The infiltrates may be due to allergic reactions or passage of intestinal parasites through the lungs. A separate category of eosinophilic pneumonia is **Loeffler's syndrome.** This is a bronchopneumonia with a granulomatous reaction, necrotizing angiitis, and infiltration of eosinophiles. These exudates often become organized and may be due to immune hypersensitivity.
3. **Aspiration pneumonia.** Food, stomach contents, or inhaled medications may reach the lower respiratory passages and there cause localized inflammation with foreign body reactions. Aspiration pneumonia is frequently seen in infants who have difficulty in swallowing (e.g., in congenital malformations); also, after instillation of oily nose drops; and in gravely ill adults. Patients who are unconscious and vomit are in particular danger of developing aspiration pneumonia.

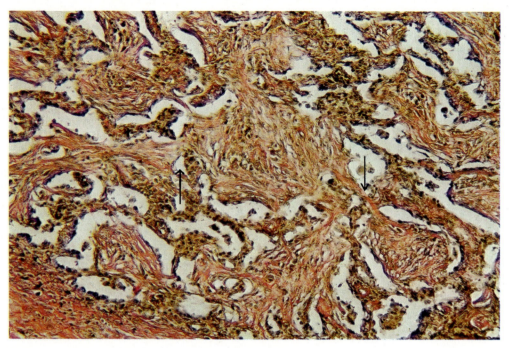

Fig 3–36.—Organized pneumonia (elastica–van Gieson's stain).

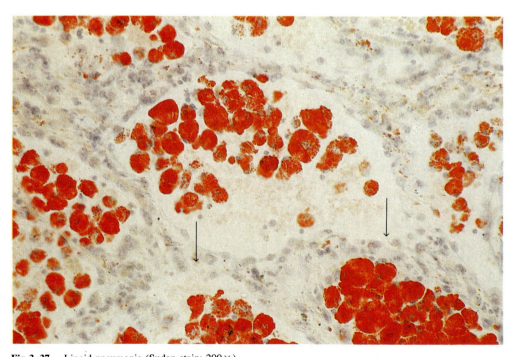

Fig 3–37.—Lipoid pneumonia (Sudan stain; 200 ×).

Organized Pneumonia—Lipoid Pneumonia—Cytomegalovirus Pneumonia

Organized pneumonia (Fig 3–36). Fibrinous intra-alveolar exudates that are not re-sorbed via lysis become organized by ingrowth of granulation tissue originating from the region of the respiratory bronchioles. Van Gieson's stain reveals red to yellow plugs that fill the alveoli. At higher magnification these are seen to be composed of young, yellow-staining and old, red-staining collagen fibers, between which there are angioblasts, newly formed capillaries, fibroblasts, and histiocytes. This granulation tissue replaces fibrin, as is especially evident by its growth through the pores of Kohn, so that granulation tissue in neighboring alveoli is bridged (→). Lymphocytes and histiocytes infiltrate the alveolar septa. The granulation and fibrous tissue in the alveoli retracts, so that there are gaps between it and the alveolar walls. These may be lined secondarily by alveolar epithelial cells, typically by cuboidal epithelium.

Lipoid pneumonia (Fig 3–37). In this condition collections of macrophages, filled with aspirated fatty material, are situated focally or diffusely in pulmonary alveoli and produce consolidation of the lung. Sudan stain (Fig 3–37) reveals a faintly outlined alveolar frame-work (→). In the alveolar lumens large phagocytic cells can be seen, whose cytoplasm is occupied by Sudan-positive fat droplets. These may represent vegetable or mineral oil or animal fats (cod liver oil), oily nose drops, milk, and x-ray contrast media.

The intrapulmonary response to aspirated material is quite varied. Unsaturated lipids provoke intra-alveolar phagocytosis and foreign body reactions. Lipoid pneumonia is to be distinguished from xanthomatous pneumonia that may follow chronic suppurative inflam-mation in the lung (e.g., in pulmonary actinomycosis).

Cytomegalovirus pneumonia (Fig 3–38). This disease is caused by a virus of the herpes group and affects mainly infants and adults with diminished immune competence. Typically, one sees enlarged cells (diameter > 40 μm) in which the nucleus contains a basophilic inclusion body (→). The inclusion body contains DNA. The inflammatory re-sponse is varied and often quite focal. Parenchymal cells in salivary glands, liver, kidney tubules, pancreas, and gut may be infected and enlarged. In the lungs, cytomegalic disease occurs mainly in adults. The inclusion bodies in alveolar cells are composed of DNA and nonhistone proteins.

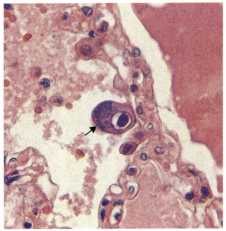

Fig 3–38.—Alveolar cell (→) with intranuclear cytomegalovirus inclusion body (hematoxylin-eosin; 250×).

Tuberculosis

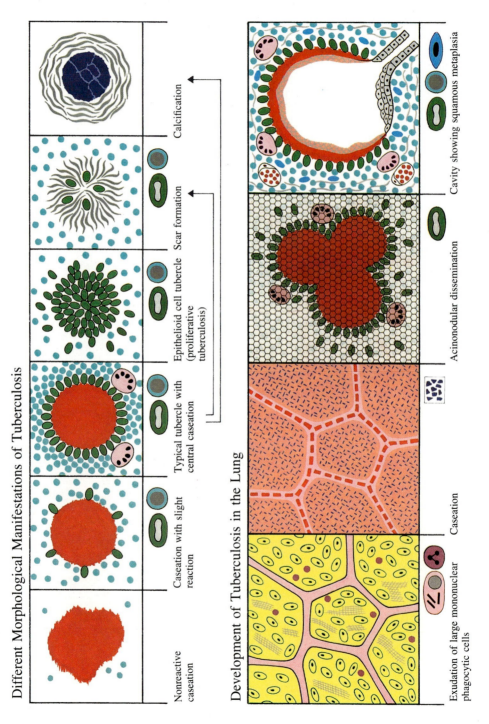

Different Morphological Manifestations of Tuberculosis

Nonreactive caseation

Caseation with slight reaction

Typical tubercle with central caseation

Epithelioid cell tubercle (proliferative tuberculosis)

Scar formation

Calcification

Development of Tuberculosis in the Lung

Exudation of large mononuclear phagocytic cells

Caseation

Acinonodular dissemination

Cavity showing squamous metaplasia

Fig 3-39.—Various histologic manifestations of the tubercle. Development of primary tuberculosis.

Tuberculosis

Figure 3–39 illustrates the **various histologic appearances of a tubercle.** The *"typical"* *tubercle* consists of a *necrotic center (caseation),* a zone of *epitheloid cells* (modified histiocytes), *Langhans' giant cells* and *granulation tissue,* and a more or less well-marked outer margin of *lymphocytes.* In lymph nodes and in certain diseases *(Boeck's sarcoid),** the principal manifestation of tuberculosis may be proliferative, i.e., the formation of a *tubercle composed of epithelioid cells* and few giant cells and showing no central caseation. Caseation occurs as a secondary manifestation (see Figs 3–39 and 3–41 through 3–44).

All the manifestations of the tubercle shown to the *right* in the diagram (Fig 3–39) indicate a *defense reaction* by the host (productive tuberculosis). Epithelioid cell tubercles as well as caseous tubercles heal by removal of the necrotic material and increased production of collagen fibers and scar formation (e.g., hyaline scars in lymph nodes, indurated slate-colored nodules in the lung). The caseous material may calcify secondarily *(calcified nodules).*

The manifestations of the *left* in Figure 3–39 arise when there is reduced host resistance (exudative tuberculosis). In these cases, the caseation is progressive. Epithelioid cells are always scanty and the chief host reaction is necrosis. Finally, acute bacteremia and sepsis develop with nonreactive necrosis (fulminant tuberculous sepsis).

In the **development of tuberculosis in the lung** (Fig 3–39), there is an exudative preliminary stage consisting of an acute serous inflammatory exudate containing many large mononuclear phagocytic cells (3–40). Macrophages with ingested tubercle bacilli fill the alveoli. Necrosis then ensues very rapidly *(caseation).* *Cavities* develop as a consequence of the tissue destruction (i.e., softening of the caseous necrosis) and may lead to bronchial spread with development of *acinonodular tuberculosis* characterized by cockadeshaped areas of necrosis and typical tuberculous granulation tissue.

---

*NOTE: Epithelioid cell tubercles are a special sort of tissue reaction which occurs in several conditions—Boeck's sarcoid, regional enteritis, etc.

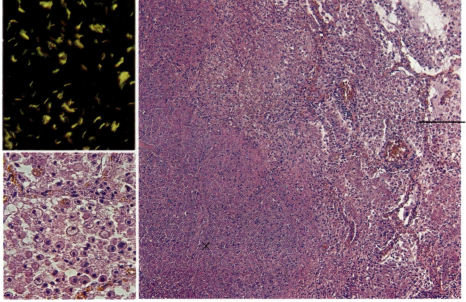

Fig 3–40.—Pulmonary tuberculosis, showing fresh caseation necrosis and exudation of large mononuclear phagocytic cells (hematoxylin-eosin; 82×). **Top left,** phagocytized tubercle bacilli (Auramin stain, fluorescence microscopy; 1,000×). **Bottom left,** exudate with numerous mononuclear macrophages (hematoxylin-eosin; 195×).

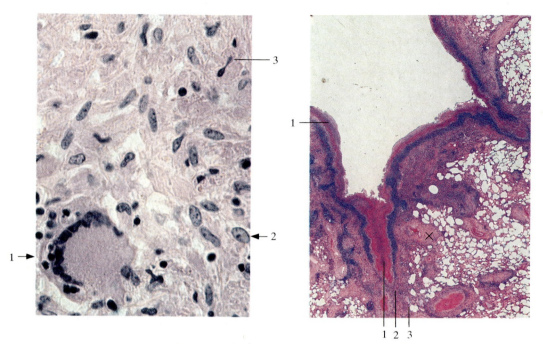

Fig 3–41.—Langhans' giant cell and epithelioid cells (hematoxylin-eosin).

Fig 3–42.—Tuberculous cavity (hematoxylin-eosin).

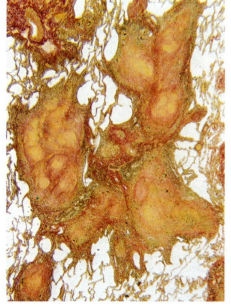

Fig 3–43.—Acinonodular tuberculosis of lung (van Gieson's stain).

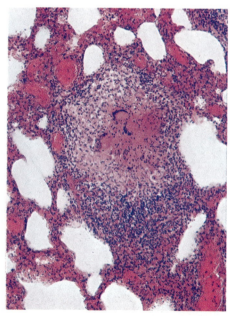

Fig 3–44.—Miliary tubercle in lung (hematoxylin-eosin).

Tuberculous granuloma (Fig 3–41). Microscopically, productive tuberculosis is characterized by the presence of ''specific granulomas'' with or without central caseous necrosis. The cellular component of the granulomas consists of epithelioid cells, lymphocytes, and multinuclear Langhans' giant cells. The latter (→ 1) possess multiple nuclei in horseshoe or semicircular arrangement. The nuclei of epithelioid cells are oval or elongated (→ 3), with a hazy basophilic aspect. The cytoplasmic margins of the epithelioid cells are indistinct.

Tuberculous cavity (Fig 3–42). *As a result of enzymatic digestion of the caseous material (leukocytic enzymes) and removal of the liquefied material by way of a draining bronchus, a cavity may develop in the wall of which three layers can be recognized histologically* (Fig 3–42). The innermost layer (→ 1) consists of a narrow band of homogeneous, eosinophilic, *necrotic tissue* (yellow in van Gieson's stain). Next comes a dark blue layer in which *cellular granulation tissue* and epithelioid cells (→ 2) can be seen under high magnification. Finally, the third and outside layer consists of *cicatrized granulation tissue* (→ 3) infiltrated with nodular collections of lymphocytes. Notice that the blood vessels in the region of the cavity (×) are nearly completely obstructed by intimal proliferation. At a distance from the cavity there are small and large caseous nodules.

Bronchial spread in pulmonary tuberculosis (acinonodular tuberculosis) (Fig 3–43). *The lesions give a characteristic appearance as they cluster around the bronchial passages.* The tubercle bacilli either lodge in the territory served by a terminal bronchus (in the pulmonary acinus) or cause peribronchial inflammation, a focal peribronchial pneumonia. As a result, many closely grouped caseous nodules are found, some of which have fused, while others are completely enveloped by fibrous tissue. Higher magnification shows all the typical features of a tubercle (necrosis, a collar of epithelioid cells, Langhans giant cells, and granulation tissue). Figure 3–43, which is stained with van Gieson's method, shows the yellow central area of necrosis, surrounded by red collagenous connective tissue and peripheral lymphocytes. Numerous giant cells are seen. Notice the emphysema next to the nodules.

Miliary tubercle (Fig 3–44). *These are millet seed-sized tubercles of lymphogenous or hematogenous origin (miliary tuberculosis).* In miliary tuberculosis, low magnification shows numerous small, richly cellular nodules scattered throughout the lung tissue. Higher magnification shows a small central eosinophilic zone of necrosis surrounded by epithelioid cells and lymphocytes. In the illustration, many Langhans' giant cells can be seen at the edge of the necrotic zone.

Acute (fulminant) tuberculosis with extensive caseous necrosis (Fig 3–45). *Acute tuberculosis results from marked reduction of host resistance (or increased virulence of the infectious agent). It is sometimes seen as a terminal stage in the treatment of tumors with cytotoxic drugs or in advanced cachexia.* Histologically, there are eosinophilic, maplike areas of necrosis without significant cellular boundary. The illustration shows necrotic pulmonary lesions with serofibrinous exudate and occasional lymphocytes. The alveolar septa are destroyed or indistinct.

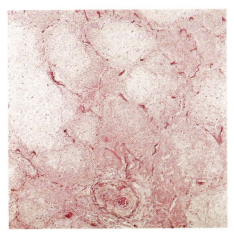

Fig · **3–45.**—Caseous tuberculous pneumonia (elastica–nuclear fast red stain; 60×).

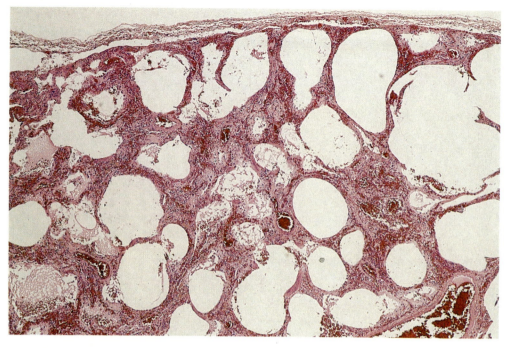

Fig 3–46.—Interstitial pulmonary fibrosis (hematoxylin-eosin; 40×).

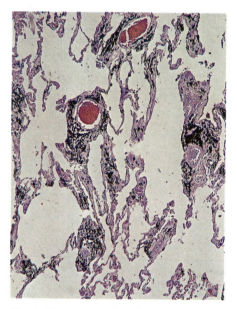

Fig 3–47.—Anthracosis of lung (hematoxylin-eosin).

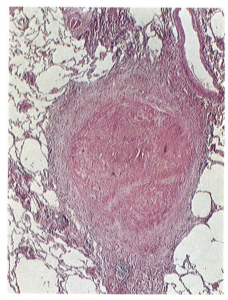

Fig 3–48.—Silicosis of lung (hematoxylin-eosin).

Interstitial Fibrosis—Anthracosis—Silicosis—Asbestosis

Interstitial pulmonary fibrosis (Hamman-Rich, Fig 3–46). This is a nonspecific inflammation of the lung of unknown etiology which runs its course in the interalveolar septa and leads to diffuse fibrosis of the lung. In the early phase the septa become infiltrated with lymphocytes, plasma cells, and histiocytes. This is followed by proliferation of connective tissue (chiefly fibroblasts) and leads to disturbance of pulmonary gas exchange. Figure 3–46 shows this later stage. There is proliferation of interstitial connective and granulation tissue (→ 1) which has arisen in the alveolar septa. Alveoli are replaced by cystic spaces, and these are lined with cuboidal epithelium (→ 2). In isolated places, cystic spaces are filled with protein-containing material (→ 3).

Causes: Antigens such as bird excrement (pigeon handler's disease), moldy dust (farmer's lung), virus infections, irradiation, busulfan, bleomycin, and other cytostatic drugs. Unknown (Hamman-Rich). Autoimmunity? Also seen in prolonged shock.

Anthracosis of the lung (Fig 3–47). In this condition, coal pigment is deposited in the interstitial tissues. Coal dust reaching the alveoli is phagocytosed by type I pneumocytes or macrophages. The coal dust is insoluble, and phagocytic cells carry it into the lymphatic vessels, where it accumulates. The host reaction consists of slight fibrosis of the perilymphatic connective tissue. Figure 3–47 shows the black pigment (the differential diagnosis of various pigments is given in Table 2, section on General Pathology) and the slight perivascular fibrosis and lack of cellular infiltration. Occasionally the deposits fuse into nodules.

Silicosis of the lung (Fig 3–48). Particles of quartz dust (1–5 μ in size) entering the lung are phagocytized and deposited in the lymphatics. The liberated silicates induce accumulation of histiocytes and proliferation of fibroblasts, and deposition of reticular fibers, which later hyalinize, resulting in acellular fibrous nodules. In Figure 3–48 a fibrous nodule with concentric layers of collagen has replaced normal lung tissue. Histiocytes containing coal pigment can be seen at the periphery of the silicotic nodule. The quartz particles can be detected readily in histologic preparations mounted in water and examined with polarized light. Emphysema is present in the areas adjacent to the silicotic nodules. Similar changes are observed in the hilar lymph nodes of the lungs.

Asbestosis of the lung (Fig 3–49). Asbestos is a collective term for several kinds of mineral fibers or spicules composed of silicone, magnesium, and calcium (chrysotile amosite, crocidolite). The asbestos elicits diffuse pulmonary fibrosis. Dumbbell- or club-shaped asbestos needles encrusted with protein and iron (brown color) are situated in the fibrous tissue. In Figure 3–49, typical asbestos bodies are seen in scar tissue.

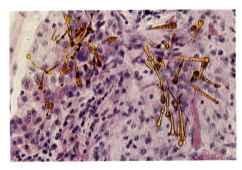

Fig 3–49.—Asbestosis (hematoxylin-eosin; 255×).

123

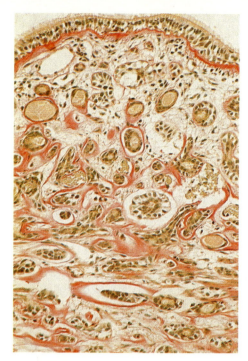

Fig 3–50.—Bronchial adenoma: cyclindroma (van Gieson's stain; 100×).

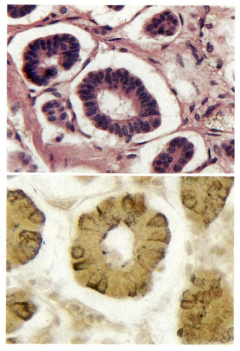

Fig 3–51.—Bronchial adenoma: carcinoid (**top,** hematoxylin-eosin; **bottom,** Bodian silver stain 250×).

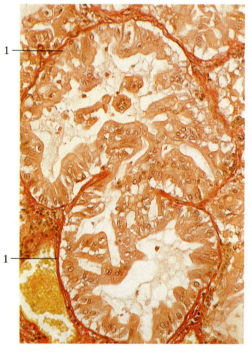

Fig 3–52.—Bronchioloaveolar carcinoma (terminal bronchiolar carcinoma) (elastica–van Gieson's stain; 150×).

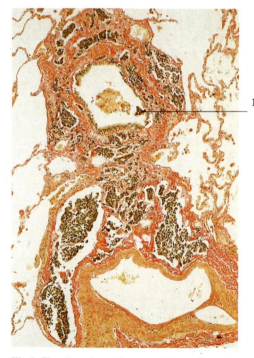

Fig 3–53.—Lymphangiolar spread of carcinoma in lung (elastica–van Gieson's stain; 60×):

Lung Tumors: Adenoma—Carcinoma—Lymphangiolar Dissemination of Carcinoma

Neoplasms in the lungs can be primary or secondary (metastatic), benign or malignant, and of either epithelial or nonepithelial ("mesenchymal") origin.

Bronchial adenomas are primary lung tumors that arise from bronchial epithelium, generally in the large bronchi. Although they appear to be histologically benign, their biologic behavior is that of slow-growing infiltrative new growths that tend to recur after surgical excision and sometimes metastasize. For this reason, they are nowadays considered to be low-grade malignancies (or potentially malignant neoplasms) and terms such as *cylindroma of bronchus* and *carcinoid of bronchus* are applied to them.

a. Cylindroma of bronchus (Fig 3–50). This tumor is composed of cords, nests, and glandlike structures that resemble cylindromas of sweat glands. The groups of tumor cells are embedded in a loose stroma and are often demarcated by a basement membrane. In Figure 3–50 the respiratory epithelium lining a bronchus can be seen near the top. The intact respiratory epithelium and its basement membrane cover the cylindroma, as is usually the case.

Bronchial cylindroma arises mainly in primary bronchi. It occurs as polypoid growths that infiltrate the bronchial wall and can attain a diameter of 3 cm. This sort of bronchial adenoma metastasizes three times as often as bronchial carcinoid.

b. **Carcinoid of bronchus** (Fig 3–51). This tumor is composed of glandlike structures that are lined by cuboidal cells with compact nuclear chromatin. Individual neoplastic glands are surrounded by connective tissue and have central lumens. The Bodian silver stain reveals black cytoplasmic granules in the cuboidal carcinoid cells in 90% of cases. The granules correspond to neurosecretory granules of APUD tumor cells, as demonstrated by electron microscopy. This neoplasm is probably derived from Kulchitsky cells in the bronchial mucosa.

The common **primary carcinomas of the lung** are the squamous cell carcinoma, the adenocarcinoma, the anaplastic small cell carcinoma, and the bronchioloalveolar carcinoma (terminal bronchiolar carcinoma).

Bronchioloalveolar carcinoma (Fig 3–52) arises from the terminal bronchioles, from where it spreads into nearby alveoli, where the tumor cells replace the normal alveolar living cells. The irregularly arrayed new growths show nuclear and cytoplasmic polymorphism. The original pulmonary framework of collagen and elastic fibers can be demonstrated with the elastica–van Gieson's stain. Thus, connective tissue elements of the alveolar septa are preserved and are important diagnostic criteria.

This tumor (accounting for 1%–5% of all primary lung tumors) was formerly known as **alveolar cell carcinima** or **adenomatosis of the lung.** Morphologically it resembles the infectious pulmonary adenomatosis of sheep, known as "Jagziekte" in South Africa. Grossly, bronchioloalveolar carcinomas may mimic pneumonia. Metastases (mainly in the lymph nodes) occur in 45% of cases.

Lymphangiolar dissemination of carcinomas in the lungs (Fig 3–53). Primary as well as metastatic lung tumors (usually carcinomas) can spread through the intrapulmonary lymphatics. On microscopic examination one sees dilated lymphangioles filled with compact collections of tumor cells and situated along the major pulmonary arteries and bronchi (→ 1).

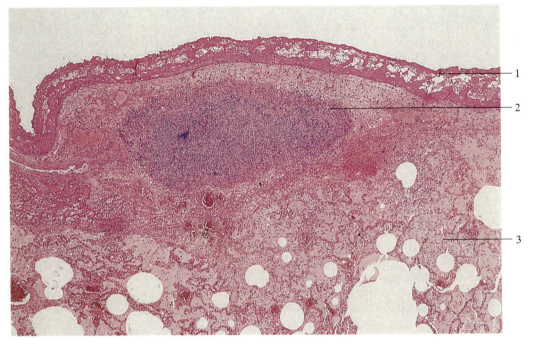

Fig 3–54.—Fibrinous pleuritis with subpleural lung abscess (hematoxylin-eosin; 40×).

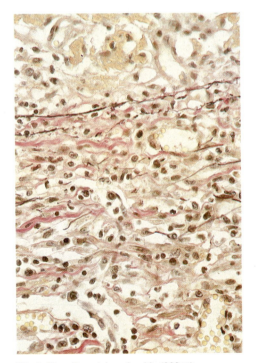

Fig 3–55.—Organizing pleuritis (200×).

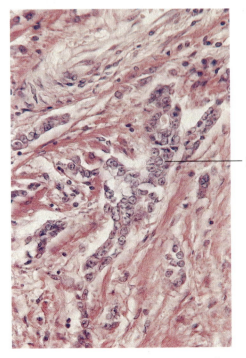

Fig 3–56.—Pleural mesothelioma (hematoxylin-eosin; 200×).

Pleura: Pleuritis—Mesothelioma

Acute fibrinous pleuritis (Fig 3–54). The surface of the visceral pleura is covered by an eosinophilic pseudomembrane that is composed of fibrin and scattered leukocytes. During its formation such an exudate is at first tufted but later it becomes a rough-surfaced sheet with hollows (→ 1). Beneath this exudate is the pleural surface. The underlying lung parenchyma surrounds a pyemic abscess, seen as a collection of pus with necrosis of lung tissue (→ 2). There is also some pulmonary edema (→ 3).

Fibrinous pleuritis (pleurisy) is usually a secondary phenomenon or complication of disease. For example, the pleura over a hemorrhagic infarct in the lung may be covered by a thin fibrinous exudate. Pneumonias are associated with more marked fibrinous pleuritis. Fibrinous or hemorrhagic fibrinous pleuritis may complicate pulmonary tuberculosis. One can also distinguish between fibrinous and serofibrinous pleuritis. When there is a massive granulocytic exudate, pus forming in the pleural space gives rise to an **empyema.**

Organizing pleuritis (Fig 3–55). In this condition fibrinous exudate is replaced by granulation tissue consisting of capillaries and chronic inflammatory cells. The capillaries grow into the exudate through the pleural elastic and collagen fiber zone and into the fibrinous sheet that covers the visceral pleura.

Extensive inflammation of both visceral and parietal pleura can lead to obliteration of the pleural space, at first by fibrinous adhesions, later by fibrous tissue (adhesive pleuritis). Most frequently one sees localized strandlike fibrous adhesions that indicate healed pleuritis.

Malignant Neoplasms Involving the Pleura are most frequently metastases of pulmonary or extrapulmonary carcinomas. **Mesotheliomas** are primary tumors of the pleura. They may be localized benign tumors or diffusely spreading malignant tumors. Figure 3–56 shows a diffusely growing malignant mesothelioma of pleura that contains a collagen-rich stroma and neoplastic cells resembling epithelium, with pseudoglandular structures (→ 1). The combination of mesenchymal and epithelial elements has been called "biphasic growth." When the mesenchymal elements predominate, the tumor resembles sarcomas. In other instances it may be impossible to differentiate it histologically from carcinomas. The "epithelial" tumor cells contain acid mucopolysaccharides that take the alcian blue stain and can be removed by treatment with hyaluronidase.

Localized (benign) pleural mesotheliomas are composed of collagen-rich tissue and usually have the appearance of *fibromas*. Large pleural fibromas may produce paraneoplastic hypoglycemia.

Malignant pleural mesotheliomas occur most frequently in persons that have been occupationally exposed to asbestos. However, in such patients typical asbestos bodies are situated in lung parenchyma, not in the tumor (see Fig 3–49).

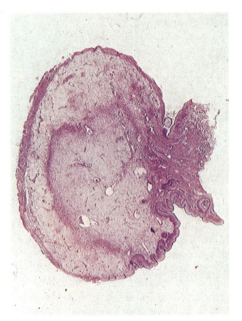

Fig 4–1.—Hemangiomatous epulis (granuloma pyogenicum) (hematoxylin-eosin; 20×).

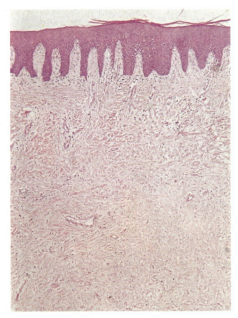

Fig 4–2.—Fibroma (hematoxylin-eosin; 60×).

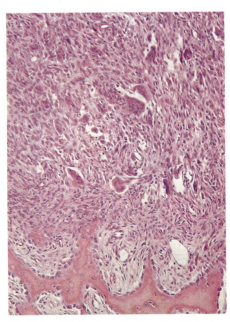

Fig 4–3.—Giant cell epulis (hematoxylin-eosin; 60×).

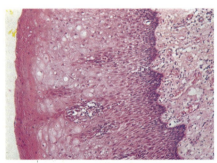

Fig 4–4.—Pachydermia (hematoxylin-eosin; 40×).

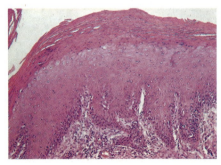

Fig 4–5.—Leukaplakia (hematoxylin-eosin; 40×).

4. Oral Cavity—Gastrointestinal Tract—Pancreas

From ancient times the **oral cavity** has been considered a *mirror of disease,* since many diseases manifest themselves there (e.g., leukemia, agranulocytosis, infectious diseases, etc.). Only a few examples have been selected for consideration here, chiefly because they occur frequently or have special diagnostic or therapeutic significance.

Hemangiomatous epulis ("granuloma pyogenicum") (Fig 4–1). This is a rather common condition of the lower lip or tongue. Macroscopically there is a bright red nodule, about 0.5 cm in size, partly covered with squamous epithelium (Fig 4–1). On the right-hand side of the figure the oral mucous membrane is unaltered. The spongy structure of the lesion is clearly shown in the illustration. Proliferation of capillaries occurs just as it does in a capillary hemangioma (see Hemangioma, chap. 9). In addition there is a sparse infiltration of granulocytes. The lesion usually results from trauma; infrequently it is a true tumor. Women are preferentially affected.

Fibroma (Fig 4–2) is the most frequent "tumor" of the oral cavity. This *true fibroma* is rich in fibrocytes (occurring especially in the cheeks near the line of closure of the teeth) and is different from a fibroma due to irritation which is a fibrous hyperplasia resulting from chronic pressure, e.g., a prosthesis or tooth crown. Figure 4–2 shows a fibroma due to irritation that is covered with noncornified squamous epithelium and composed of broad tongues and bands of collagen fibers and a few fibroblasts.

A **giant cell epulis** (Fig 4–3) occurs on the gingiva or alveolar process as a nodular bluish or gray tumor (chiefly near front teeth, the mandible; in young women). It always shows a relation to periodontal tissue. Histologically there is a rich proliferation of capillaries and foreign body–type giant cells derived from vascular endothelium. Frequent microhemorrhages lead to hemosiderin-laden macrophages. Later plasma cells may appear *(granulomatous epulis)* and even bony deposits (osteoplastic epulis). A giant cell epulis is a reactive granulomatous lesion caused by minor trauma, for example in chronic reactive processes in the periodontium.

Pachydermia (Fig 4–4): White flecks on the mucous membranes of the cheeks or lips (chiefly in men) that cannot be distinguished grossly from leukoplakia. Histologically there is orderly hyperplasia of the squamous epithelium with hyperkeratosis (rarely parakeratosis). Transition to leukoplakia?

This is a harmless change, in contrast to **leukoplakia,** which is regarded as a precancerous lesion and frequently develops on alveolar processes of the lower jaw or on the mucosa in the cheek folds. Histologically (Fig 4–5) there are *hyperkeratosis, parakeratosis* (nuclei are present in the horny layer), *acanthosis,* and *dysplasia* (mitosis present in all layers, loss of polarity in the epithelial layer, hyperchromasia of nuclei) *as well as dyskeratosis* (cornification of single cells). Additionally, the submucous layer is infiltrated by *inflammatory cells.* Transition to carcinoma occurs in 5%–10% within 5–20 years. Men are chiefly affected. Causes: tobacco abuse. Either carcinoma in situ or frank carcinoma may hide beneath a lesion that grossly appears to be leukoplakia.

Ameloblastoma (adamantinoma, Fig 4–6). A benign, cystic tumor arising in the region of the molar teeth of the lower jaw. Histologically there are islands of teeth corresponding to the ameloblasts of developing teeth. The cells have a palisade arrangement and surround reticulum-like cells (→). Hollow spaces lined with pavement epithelium that sometimes has a horny layer may develop.

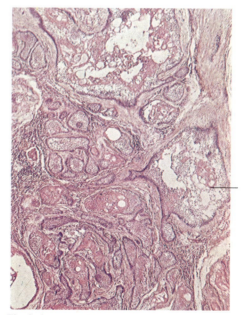

Fig 4–6.—Ameloblastoma (adamantinoma) (hematoxylin-eosin; $60 \times$).

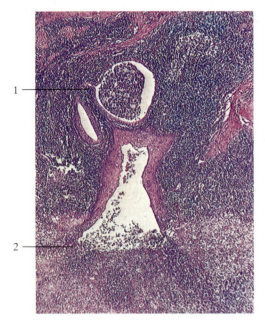

Fig 4–7.—Tonsilitis (hematoxylin-eosin; 100×).

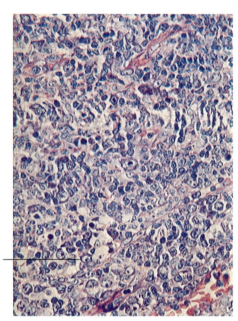

Fig 4–8.—Tonsil: infectious mononucleosis (Giemsa stain; 380×).

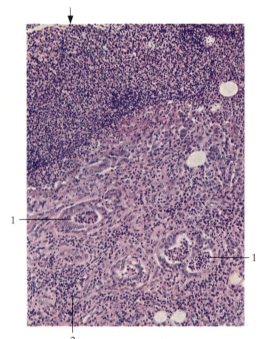

Fig 4–9.—Purulent sialadenitis with abscess (hematoxylin-eosin; 120×).

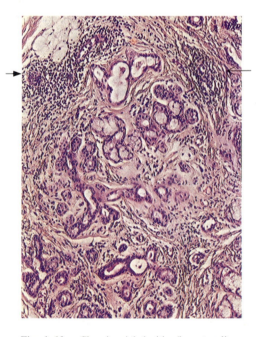

Fig 4–10.—Chronic sialadenitis (hematoxylin-eosin; 100×).

Tonsils and Salivary Glands

Tonsillitis (Fig 4–7) is chiefly due to streptococcal infection of the faucial tonsils. The term *angina* is used when all the lymphoid tissues of the pharynx are affected. The tonsillar crypts may be filled with plugs of pus (→ cross section of a crypt filled with granulocytes). The lower end of a longitudinally sectioned crypt (→ 2) has been destroyed by an abscess (necrotic tissue and granulocytes). In the upper part of the figure there is scar tissue indicating previous inflammation.

Necrotizing tonsillitis occurs in scarlet fever (hemolytic streptococci), diphtheria, and Vincent's angina (fusiform bacteria and spirochetes). In chronic recurrent tonsillitis the crypts contain cellular detritus, fibrin, granulocytes, and colonies of fungi or bacteria.

Angina of infectious mononucleosis (glandular fever, Fig 4–8). In this condition there may be a superficial necrotizing tonsillitis as an expression of generalized infection with Epstein-Barr virus (DNA virus of the herpes group) accompanied by enlargement of liver, spleen, and lymph nodes. Smears of peripheral blood contain up to 90% lymphoid cells (normal lymphocytes plus abnormal lymphocytes or glandular fever cells) which are derived from lymphatic tissue. Lymph nodes and tonsils contain many of these abnormal basophilic lymphoid cells (immunoblasts →), lymphoblasts, and plasma cells so that the normal structure of the nodes is unclear. The reaction centers of secondary lymphoid follicles may be preserved.

Age: 15–25 years, chiefly males. Diagnosis: heterophil agglutination (Paul-Bunnell) test. *Epstein-Barr virus* is also thought to be the cause of *Burkitt lymphoma* (see Fig 40, section on General Pathology), *nasopharyngeal carcinoma,* occurring in the south Chinese, and perhaps other malignant lymphomas.

Inflammation of salivary glands may be caused by bacteria, viruses, fungi, irradiation, or an immunologic agent. Virus infections like mumps (epidemic parotitis) cause bilateral swelling of the parotid glands (interstitial serous inflammation with lymphocytic infiltrate). Testes, pancreas, and meninges may also be affected (viremia). *Cytomegalic inclusion disease* is seen in newborn infants or adults (see Fig 37, section on General Pathology) with lowered resistance or undergoing cytostatic therapy. Typical findings include large, round, DNA-rich nuclear inclusions in the epithelium of parotid ducts. All organs may be affected. *Sjögren's syndrome* is an autoimmune disease (antibodies against parotid duct extract) that affects postmenopausal women and leads to atrophy of the parotid and tear glands (sicca syndrome: xerostomia, keratoconjunctivitis sicca) and sometimes may be associated with chronic rheumatoid arthritis.

Purulent sialadenitis with abscess (Fig 4–9), usually bilateral, occurs in debilitated patients with poor resistance, frequently following an operation. Calculi may trigger an ascending infection, mostly in the submandibular gland and chiefly in men. Histologically, dilated excretory ducts and their branches contain granulocytes (→ 1). The gland itself is edematous and packed with polymorphonuclear leukocytes and lymphocytes (→ 2). Often there is tissue destruction and abscess formation (→).

Chronic sialadenitis of the submandibular gland (Fig 4–10) presents as a hard, tumorlike lesion. Cause: duct calculi. Men are mainly affected. Histologically there are scanty infiltration of lymphocytes (→) and collagenous connective tissue surrounding excretory ducts. The glandular acini are destroyed by chronic inflammation. The result is sclerotic scarring of the gland similar to that seen in cirrhosis of the liver.

Granulomatous inflammation with many epithelioid cells may occur in sarcoidosis (see Specific Inflammation of Lymph Nodes, chap. 11).

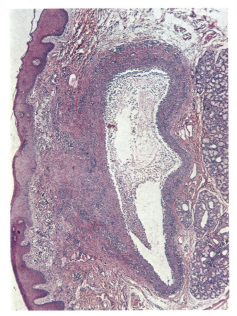

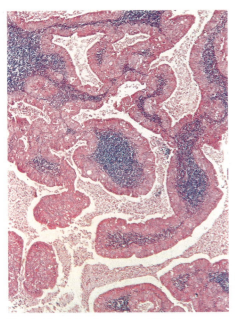

Fig **4–11.**—Mucocele (hematoxylin-eosin; 20×).

Fig **4–12.**—Adenolymphoma (Warthin tumor) (hematoxylin-eosin; 60×).

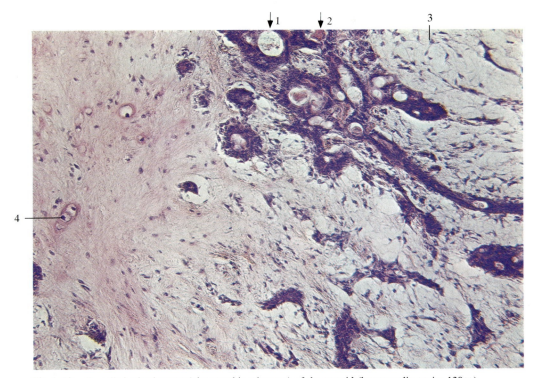

Fig 4–13.—So-called mixed tumor (pleomorphic adenoma) of the parotid (hematoxylin-eosin; 130×).

Salivary Gland Tumors

Mucocele (retention cyst of salivary gland, salivary gland granuloma, Fig 4–11) occurs chiefly in the lower lip as a result of injury of the salivary excretory duct from biting. They are pseudocysts without epithelial linging (true cysts have an epithelial lining). Secretion accumulates in the tissues as a result of the trauma (or of chronic inflammation), leading to a granulomatous tissue reaction which walls off viscid secretion. On the left-hand side of the illustration, there is surface epithelium; on the right, salivary gland. A large true cyst is called a *ranula* (submaxillary or sublingual gland).

Adenolymphoma (Warthin tumor, Fig 4–12). A benign tumor, almost exclusively of the parotid glands, mostly unilateral, virtually restricted to elderly men. Macroscopically the cut surface is finely cystic. Histologically there are cystic spaces lined by a double layer of epithelium with eosinophilic cytoplasm. Characteristically, lymphoid tissue lies between the cysts.

Mixed tumor of the parotid (pleomorphic adenoma, Fig 4–13). Mixed tumors may arise in any of the salivary glands of the oral cavity but are most frequent in the parotid gland. The current opinion is that the tumor is a *true adenoma* showing pseudomesenchymal differentiation. Foci of mucus, hyalin, and cartilage are thought to be derived either from cells of the glands or from myoepithelium. Examination of the tumor with a scanning lens reveals foci of several different sorts of tissue: solid strands of cuboidal and cylindrical epithelium that may form glands (→ 1). Masses of homogeneous hyaline fill the lumina of the glands (→ 2). The solid strands border homogeneous tissue containing abundant blue-staining ground substance and branched cells having stellate processes (mucoid portion → 3) or cells with halos that resemble cartilage cells (→ 4). The epithelial formations are derived from salivary gland ducts.

Macroscopic: Well-defined grayish white tumors often with a glistening cut surface. Prone to recur. In older people, about 5% show malignancy (adeno- or squamous carcinomas).

Adenoidcystic carcinoma (cylindroma, Fig 4–14). This is a locally malignant epithelial tumor which grows by local infiltration, frequently recurs after removal, but metastasizes only rarely (lungs). It shows a Swiss cheese pattern histologically, with adenoid cellular structures having both small and large cystic spaces filled with mucus. The cysts are formed by accumulation of the mucus secreted by epithelial cells that are embedded in hyaline stroma. Typically there is a thickened PAS-positive basement membrane.

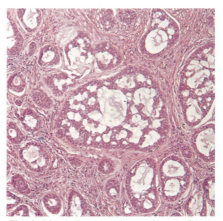

Fig 4–14.—Adenoidcystic carcinoma (hematoxylin-eosin; 60 ×).

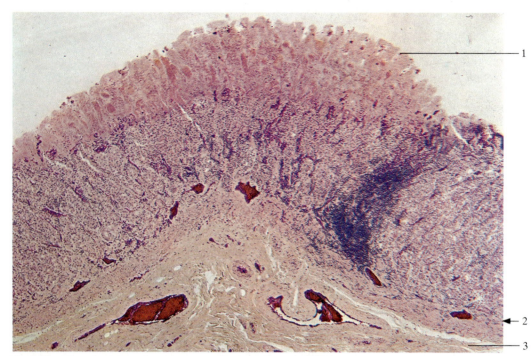

Fig 4–15.—Corrosive injury of gastric mucosa (hematoxylin-eosin; 50×).

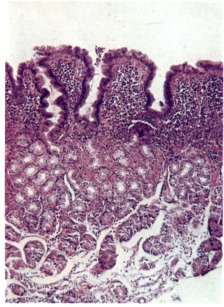

Fig 4–16.—Chronic superficial gastritis (hematoxylin-eosin; 90×).

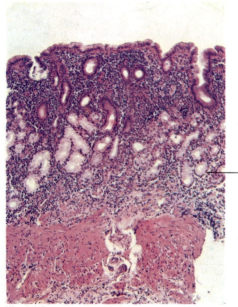

Fig 4–17.—Chronic gastritis with early mucosal atrophy (hematoxylin-eosin; 90×).

Gastrointestinal Tract

The normal architecture of the gastrointestinal tract should be recalled in interpreting histopathologic appearances (mucosa: squamous epithelium—cylindrical epithelium—glands; character of the villi; tunica propria, muscularis mucosa, submucosa, muscularis propria, and subserosa). It is important to note the cellular constituents of the individual coats and any defects in the mucosa or atypical proliferation of the glands.

Corrosive injury of the gastric mucosa (Fig 4–15). Corrosive acids cause coagulation necrosis of the gastric mucosa, while lye causes liquefaction necrosis. Figure 4–15 shows an area of fresh corrosion of the gastric mucosa due to HC1. The necrosis (coagulation necrosis → 1) can be seen on the surface. The cytoplasm of the necrotic cells in the glands is stained more strongly with eosin than the cells that lie deeper. The cells in the necrotic area lack nuclei. The necrotic zone is bordered by a narrow rim of granulocytes, scant numbers of which are also present in the submucosal stroma. With the passage of time, the necrotic mucosa sloughs off and an ulcer results. → 2 muscularis mucosae, → 3 submucosa.

Macroscopic: In the early stage of scab formation, there are different colors, depending on the kind of corrosive: sublimate (HgCl₂)—grayish white, HNO₃—yellowish, H₂SO₄ and HCl—dark brown. The following sequelae may develop: perforation, cicatricial stricture (e.g., in the esophagus).

Gastritis

Gastritis. Normally there is slight inflammation of the entire gastrointestinal tract with infiltration of small numbers of granulocytes (‘‘physiologic’’ inflammation). For the diagnosis of gastritis, histologically there should be necrosis of epithelium with a tissue defect and a more marked inflammatory reaction. Histologic gastritis may not have a clinical counterpart.

1. Acute gastritis: Catarrhal inflammation, edema, and a small epithelial defect. Recovery in a few days (alcohol abuse!).

2. Chronic superficial gastritis (Fig 4–16): Chiefly confined to the antrum but also encroaching on other regions of the stomach. Figure 4–16 shows no alterations in mucous glands in the antrum. The tips of the villi are widened by inflammatory exudate (lymphocytes, plasma cells, granulocytes) and appear plump. Small defects in the superficial epithelium are visible. Epithelium with dark nuclei and basophilic cytoplasm has replaced the normal mucus-secreting superficial epithelium.

3. Chronic gastritis with early atrophy of mucosa (Fig 4–17). Figure 4–22 illustrates the reduction of mucosa compared to normal and the extension of inflammatory exudate to the mucosa muscularis. The inflammatory process extends from the surface to involve the entire mucosa. In contrast to superficial gastritis, the mucosa is reduced in width and has bulky borders and flat foveolae. The inflammatory exudate consists of granulocytes, plasma cells, and many lymphocytes. Typical lymph follicles may be present. Both chief cells (pepsinogen production) and parietal cells (HCl production) are reduced in number. Likewise the mucous glands (→) in the antrum are decreased.

4. Chronic atrophic gastritis (Fig 4–18). The mucosa is markedly atrophied (Fig 4–18, 4–22). Both chief cells and parietal cells have vanished, as have antral mucous glands. The entire mucosa consists only of the surface epithelial layer and broad gastric pits with elongated marginal tips. The inflammatory infiltrate may be as in **3** above or may consist only of lymphocytes. Frequently the lymphoid tissue is hyperplastic (lymph follicles). Clinically: achlorhydria, achylia gastrica.

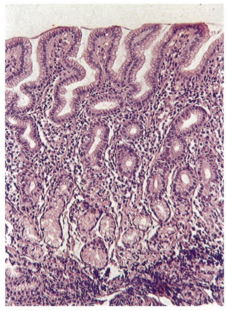

Fig 4–18.—Chronic atrophic gastritis (hematoxylin-eosin; 100 ×).

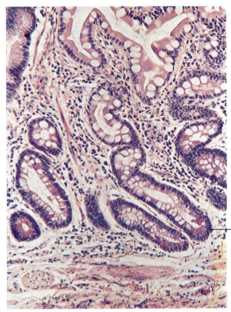

Fig 4–19.—Atrophy and intestinal metaplasia of gastric mucosa (hematoxylin-eosin; 200 ×).

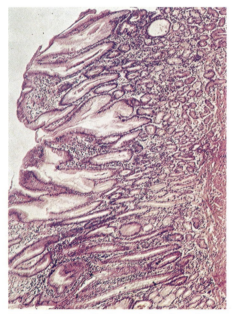

Fig 4–20.—Foveolar hyperplasia of gastric mucosa (hematoxylin-eosin; 100 ×).

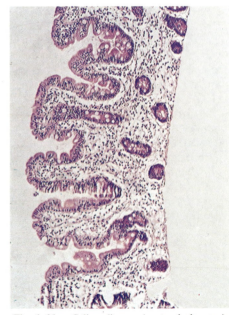

Fig 4–21.—Celiac disease (nontropical sprue): jejunum (hematoxylin-eosin; 100 ×).

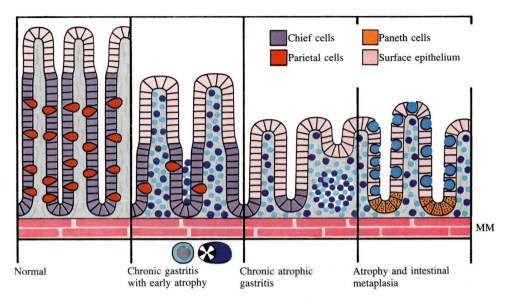

Chief cells
Parietal cells
Paneth cells
Surface epithelium

Normal | Chronic gastritis with early atrophy | Chronic atrophic gastritis | Atrophy and intestinal metaplasia

MM

Fig 4–22.—Diagram of different sorts of chronic gastritis (redrawn from Oehlert). *MM*, muscularis mucosae.

5. Atrophy of gastric mucosa with intestinal metaplasia (Fig 4–19). The mucosa is atrophied just as in chronic atrophic gastritis. The foveolae extend to the muscularis mucosae and resemble the crypts of the jejunal mucosa. Goblet cells are abundant and there are granular Paneth cells (→). For the most part the epithelium is basophilic (dark red cytoplasm, no pale secreting epithelium). Occurs in the end-stage of chronic atrophic gastritis, pernicious anemia, senile atrophy, and in the margins of chronic gastric ulcers. It is regarded as precancerous lesion and may result in early cancer (see Early Carcinoma of the Stomach, later this chapter).

6. Atrophy of gastric mucosa. Occurs in the aged, in chronic atrophic gastritis, and in pernicious anemia. Normally extrinsic factor (vitamin B_{12}) is bound to intrinsic factor of the parietal cells and thus protected from destruction. Loss of parietal cells (**atrophy, chronic gastritis, after gastrectomy**) may lead to a deficiency of B_{12}. A genetic defect may also operate.

Causes of gastritis: Chronic alcohol abuse, age-determined disturbance of regenerative capacity (after 60 years 50%–80% of persons have superficial chronic atrophic gastritis), autoaggression.

Hyperplasia of gastric mucosa (Fig 4–20). In the *Zollinger-Ellison syndrome* there is glandular hyperplasia of the mucosa, whose rugae have increased prominence macroscopically. The mucosa is thickened because of hyperplasia of the glands and of both chief cells and parietal cells. The usual cause is a gastrin-producing tumor of the pancreas. *Result:* multiple gastric and duodenal ulcers. *Giant hypertrophic gastropathy* (Ménétrier's disease): gigantic mucosal folds and increase in thickness of mucosal epithelium. Increased mucous production → protein loss → hypoproteinemia.

Foveolar hyperplasia in chronic gastritis (Fig 4–20). Mucosal epithelium is widened with loss of chief and parietal cells.

Celiac disease (nontropical sprue, gluten enteropathy, Fig 4–21). The malabsorption syndrome occurs after resection of the small intestine, in Whipple's disease (discussed later this chapter) exudative enteropathy, and sprue. In **nontropical sprue** (Fig 4–21) there is sensitivity to gluten (enzyme defect?). There are villous atrophy (flattening and broadening with increase of parietal cells) and a lymphoplasmacytic infiltrate. *Clinical:* Large, fatty stools.

137

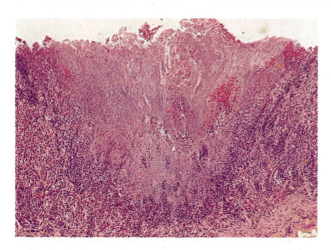

Fig 4–23.—Hemorrhagic infarct of the gastric mucosa (hematoxylin-eosin; 72×).

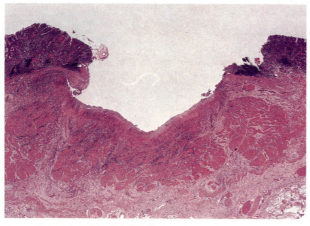

Fig 4–24.—Fresh gastric ulcer (hematoxylin-eosin; 14×).

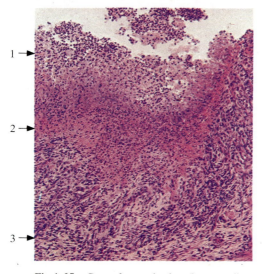

Fig 4–25.—Base of a gastric ulcer (hematoxylin-eosin; 102×).

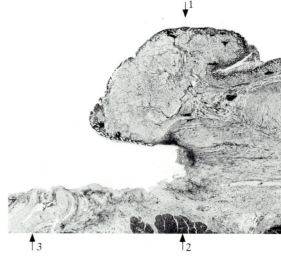

Fig 4–26.—Chronic penetrating gastric ulcer (hematoxylin-eosin; 6×).

Gastric Ulcer

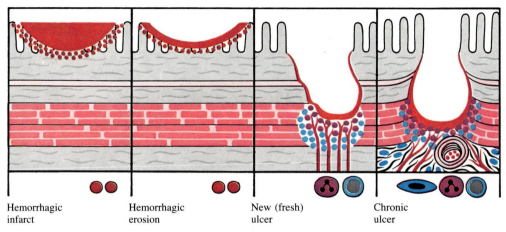

| Hemorrhagic infarct | Hemorrhagic erosion | New (fresh) ulcer | Chronic ulcer |

Fig 4–27.—Probable pathogenesis of a gastric ulcer.

First stage: *hemorrhagic infarction of the mucosa* (see Fig 4–23). The necrotic material is being excavated from the lumen *(hemorrhagic erosion)*. The erosion can either heal or progress to ulceration. A *new ulcer* (Fig 4–24) frequently is steplike on the oral edge, while on the aboral edge it rises steeply. A *chronic ulcer* (Fig 4–26), in contrast, is flask shaped with a margin of dense scar tissue.

NOTE: Erosion: defect limited to mucosa. Ulcer: defect involves additional layers of stomach wall.

Hemorrhagic infarct (Fig 4–23). A wedge-shaped area lacking stained nuclei is seen in the mucosa. Medium magnification shows faintly staining erythrocytes lying in anuclear necrotic tissue. The villi of the surface mucosa have disappeared (slight erosion).

Macroscopic: Irregularly shaped black focus with shallow mucosal defect.

Fresh gastric ulcer (Fig 4–24). Under low magnification, the defect in the wall can be seen extending to the muscularis and showing the usual mucosal overhang (on the aboral edge to the left of the illustration). In the base of the ulcer, there is a pale grayish red zone (fibrin) and a darker zone (necrosis and granulation tissue). Under higher magnification, it is easier to analyze these layers. **Base of a gastric ulcer** (Fig 4–25): At the top, there is a loose layer of fibrin and polymorphonuclear leukocytes (→ 1) lying on an intensely eosinophilic bandlike zone of fibrinoid necrosis (→ 2): necrotic material composed of fibrin and nuclear fragments. Granulation tissue (→ 3) surrounds the necrotic layer and invades it. The capillaries in the granulation tissue run perpendicularly to the surface. Fibroblasts, lymphocytes, histiocytes, and mature connective tissue make up the lower third of this zone.

Macroscopic: A steplike or flat, round or oval defect in the wall. The base is gray.

Chronic penetrating ulcer (Fig 4–26). In this figure, the mucous membrane has been elevated (→ 1) and contains hyperplastic pyloric glands. In the neighborhood of the ulcer, there is an increased amount of connective tissue. The defect in this instance extends to the pancreas (→ 2). The necrosis has eroded a large artery → 3 (clinically: fatal hemorrhage).

Macroscopic: A round defect with firm margins and a smooth base. Pancreatic lobules can often be seen in the base of the ulcer.

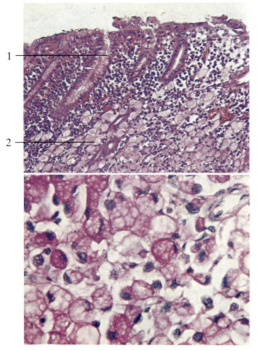

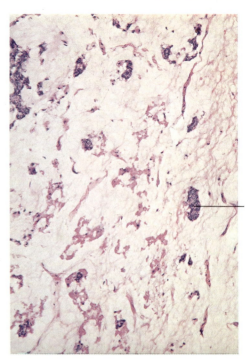

Fig 4–28.—Top, early infiltrating carcinoma of stomach (hematoxylin-eosin). **Bottom,** mucinous carcinoma of stomach with signet ring cells (PAS; 320×).

Fig 4–29.—Mucinous carcinoma of stomach (hematoxylin-eosin; 100×).

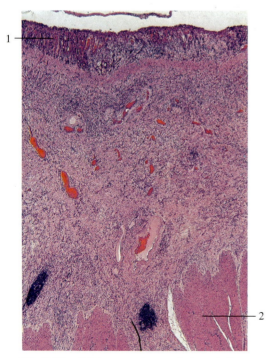

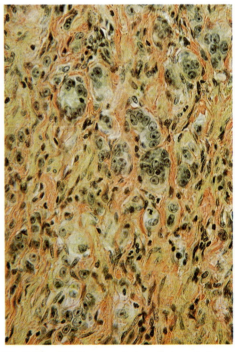

Fig 4–30.—Scirrhous carcinoma of stomach (hematoxylin-eosin; 30×).

Fig 4–31.—Scirrhous carcinoma of stomach (van Gieson's stain; 320×).

Stomach: Early, Mucinous, and Scirrhous Carcinomas

Early carcinoma of the stomach ("early cancer," Fig 4–28). This is an infiltrating epithelial cancer that is limited to the mucosa and is frequently composed of signet ring cells. The mucosal lining is preserved, so that one might easily overlook the infiltrating neoplasm. Figure 4–28, top, shows the epithelial lining with gastric pits (→ 1), but in the stroma underneath there are groups of paler cells (→ 2) that can be recognized as signet ring cancer cells at higher magnification (Fig 4–32), especially after staining with PAS (Fig 4–28, bottom).

Use of gastroscopy and gastric biopsies has led to the recognition of this early stage of gastric carcinoma. Proper therapy yields a 5-year survival rate of over 90%. Histologically, one can distinguish between an M type (tumor limited to mucosa) and an SM type (invasion of muscularis mucosae, but relatively good prognosis). Note, however, that signet ring carcinoma and early carcinoma (or cancer) are not synonymous: signet ring carcinomas can be aggressively infiltrating growths, with distant metastases. Also, some early carcinomas are gland-forming adenocarcinomas.

Mucinous carcinoma (Fig 4–29) is associated with massive production of mucinous material. Masses of pale-staining, slightly basophilic, and finely stranded mucin might be mistaken for edema fluid. These mucinous deposits are interspersed with small nests of carcinoma cells (→), only some of which have the appearance of signet ring cells (intracellular mucin).

Mucinous carcinomas occur along the gastrointestinal tract, in the ovaries, and frequently in mammary glands. Mucinous carcinomas of the mammary gland have a better prognosis than other infiltrating mammary gland carcinomas although they can become quite large.

Scirrhous carcinoma (Figs 4–30, 4–31) contains abundant collagenous stroma in which tumor cells or rests of tumor cells are scattered. At low magnification one sees marked thickening of the stomach wall (Fig 4–30). Near the top of the illustration the intact mucosa can be seen as a more darkly staining band (→ 1), and near the bottom are parts of the muscularis, which has been infiltrated by tumor (→ 2). The submucosa (between → 1 and → 2) has been markedly broadened by infiltrating tumor. At high magnification (Fig 4–31) one sees small groups of carcinoma cells with relatively large nuclei and prominent nucleoli. These cells are embedded in a stroma that consists of collagen (red in Fig 4–31) and fibroblasts with thin, fusiform nuclei.

Highly collagenous scirrhous carcinomas of the stomach may be difficult to diagnose. Sometimes these tumors are associated with a considerable inflammatory reaction and proliferation of capillaries. This form of cancer has been called granulomatous carcinoma and has been misinterpreted as granulation tissue.

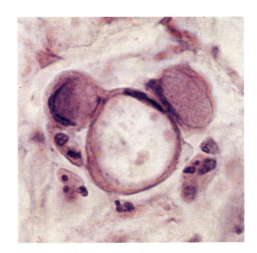

Fig 4–32.—Signet ring cell (hematoxylin-eosin; 900 ×).

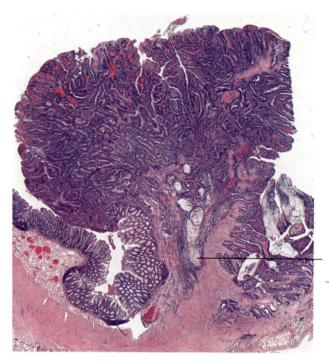

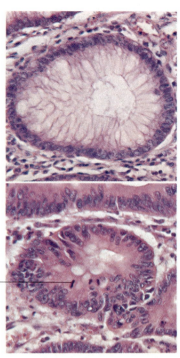

Fig 4–33.—Villous adenoma of rectum with malignant change (hematoxylin-eosin; 8×).

Fig 4–34.—**Top,** normal colonic crypt. **Bottom,** glandular adenocarcinoma (hematoxylin-eosin) (200×).

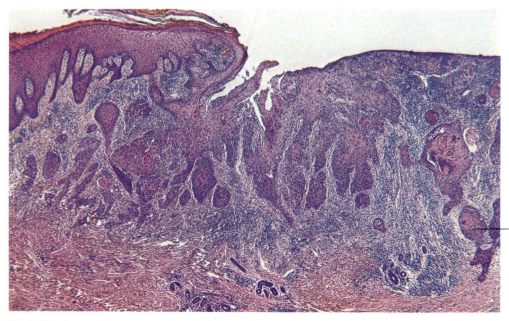

Fig 4–35.—Squamous cell carcinoma of anus (hematoxylin-eosin; 30×).

Carcinoma of the Colon and of the Anus

Malignant change in villous adenoma (Figs 4–33, 4–34). Carcinoma of the colon often arises in a villous adenoma. Figure 4–33 shows a broad-based adenoma with papilliform growth. The neoplastic cells appear more basophilic than the adjacent mucosa. Invasion of the muscularis mucosae and infiltration of the submucosa are histologic criteria of malignant change. In Figure 4–33 one can see infiltration down into the base of the adenoma (i.e., into the wall of the colon, →). Figure 4–34 contrasts a normal colonic crypt with a glandlike formation of carcinoma cells. The picture at the top of Figure 4–34 shows a normal crypt with a distinct lumen. The globlet cells have basal nuclei and an orderly arrangement. The glandlike formation of carcinoma cells (Fig 4–34, bottom) has an irregular lumen, and the lining cells possess larger nuclei that vary in size, are hyperchromatic, and are no longer strictly basal. There is little mucin in the cytoplasm, and mitoses are relatively frequent (→).

Squamous cell carcinoma of anal mucosa (Figs 4–35, 4–36). This is a multilayered, infiltrating, malignant tumor in which there may be prickle cells with intercellular bridges and other signs of keratinization. Low magnification (Fig 4–35) reveals the markedly infiltrative growth. Pegs of epithelium have infiltrated the corium. Smaller nests of carcinoma cells are visible in the deeper layers (→); these are surrounded by stroma in which there are many chronic inflammatory cells (mainly lymphocytes). In the left half of Figure 4–35 one can see noncancerous but hyperplastic epidermis. Higher magnification (Fig 4–36) reveals the more lightly stained prickle cells (→ 1). Peripheral to the latter and next to the stroma are carcinoma cells that resemble normal basal cells. Formation of keratin pearls typifies squamous cell carcinoma (→ 2). A stratum granulosum corresponding to that of normal skin is usually absent.

Squamous cell carcinomas frequently occur in skin that has been previously compromised (e.g., by overexposure to sunlight). They also occur on the lips, in the oral cavity (especially the tongue), in the larynx and esophagus, as well as in the bronchial and cervical mucosa (after squamous metaplasia). These cancers must be distinguished from pseudoepitheliomatous hyperplasia and leukoplakia (see Benign Epithelial Tumors, section on General Pathology) and from other changes that are associated with proliferation of prickle cells, for example keratoacanthoma.

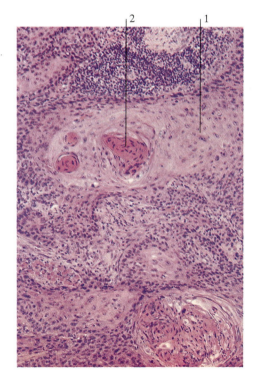

Fig 4–36.—Squamous cell carcinoma, higher magnification (hematoxylin-eosin; 100 ×).

143

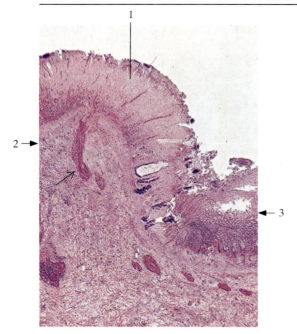

Fig 4–37.—Dysentery (hematoxylin-eosin; 28 ×).

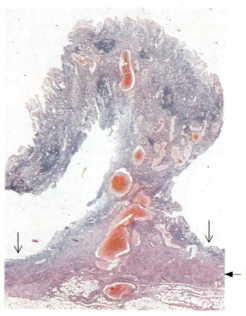

Fig 4–38.—Chronic ulcerative colitis (hematoxylin-eosin; 11 ×).

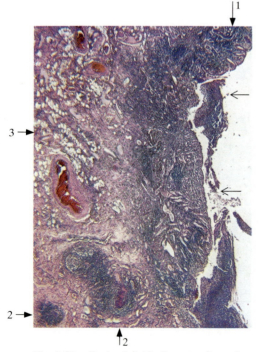

Fig 4–39.—Regional ileitis (hematoxylin-eosin; 20 ×).

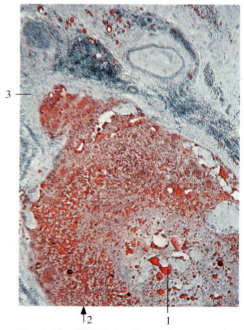

Fig 4–40.—Whipple's disease in mesenteric lymph node (Sudan-hematoxylin; 64 ×).

Dysentery (Fig 4–37). *Intestinal infestation by Shigella organisms or amebae. The colon is most frequently affected, the distal ileum less frequently.* In the early stages, there is edema and hyperemia of the mucosa, which is followed by hemorrhagic inflammation, necrosis, and a fibrinous exudate on the surface of the mucosa (pseudomembranous, necrotizing inflammation). The terminal stages show ulceration. Figure 4–37 shows an area of expanding necrosis of the colonic mucosa (→ 1) and considerable edematous loosening of the submucosa (→ 2) in shigellosis. The blood vessels are widely dilated and partly filled with erythrocytes and fibrin thrombi (→). There is a longitudinal pseudomembranous layer of fibrin (→ 3).

Macroscopic: Redness and edema of the intestinal wall. Mucosal necrosis is forming a dirty yellowish brown, mushy covering. Sharply circumscribed ulcers with undermined margins. The colon contains blood mucus.

Chronic ulcerative colitis (Fig 4–38). *This is a chronic relapsing, noninfectious inflammation of the mucosa of the colon (an autoimmune disease with mucosal ulceration and granulation tissue → clinical bleeding, scarring, polypoid mucosal regeneration, and, in about 7% of cases, carcinoma; usually 0.3%. Seen chiefly in neurotic young persons, but may occur at any age.)* In the fully developed disease, there are extensive ulcers (→) extending to the muscularis propria (→ 1), together with islands of preserved colonic mucosa. These islands of colonic mucosa are polypoid and have stalks containing connective tissue (the elevation of the mucosa to the left in the illustration is an artifact).

Macroscopic: Extensive, irregular, longitudinal mucosal defects with polypoid overgrowth of mucosal islands. The wall is stiff and the lumen narrowed. The muscularis shows cross rippling.

Regional ileitis (terminal ileitis, regional enteritis, Crohn's disease, Fig 4–39). *This is a chronic, recurring disease of the ileum or colon involving all intestinal coats. Etiology is unknown. Age: 15–35 years. Frequently familial.* After the edema, hyperemia, and hemorrhage of the acute stage, the chronic stage is characterized by extensive ulceration (→) with thickened mucosa (→ 1) and accompanied by a chronic inflammatory infiltrate and epithelioid cell granulomas (→ 2) with Langhans'-type giant cells (this is not tuberculosis, but rather a nonspecific granuloma). In Figure 4–39 the ulcer extends to the subserosa (→ 3). Beneath this, there is an increased amount of collagenous connective tissue (scarring) and hypertrophy of the muscularis.

Macroscopic: In the chronic stage, the intestinal wall is thick and rigid, the surrounding tissues are adherent, and there are irregular mucosal defects.
Complications: Perforation, hemorrhage, stenosis, fistulas, extension, frequent recurrence.
NOTE: Often multiple segments are involved with frequent recurrences.

Whipple's disease (intestinal lipodystrophy, Fig 4–40). *This is a progressive disease of the small intestine and mesenteric lymph nodes in which there is stasis of chyle, fat storage, and granulomatous inflammation. It is probably caused by a bacterial infection (Corynebacteria?, Hemophilus?).* Histologically, the intestinal lymph vessels are dilated and filled with fat. The sinuses of enlarged mesenteric lymph nodes are also dilated, cystic, and crammed with phagocytosed fat (partially dissolved out → 1). Histiocytic granulation tissue is also present (→ 2) with large foam cells containing lipid droplets (also glycoproteins). It is in these cells that the above-mentioned bacteria have been demonstrated. In the later stages, scarring may result from the chronic inflammation (→ 3).

Macroscopic: Chylous ascites, dilated, yellow lymphatic channels in the intestinal serosa, enlarged cystic lymph nodes with yellow contents.
Pathogenesis: Bacterial infection.
Clinical: Chiefly rheumatic complaints, endocarditis, steatorrhea, anemia, cachexia. Obstruction of the thoracic duct (stasis?).

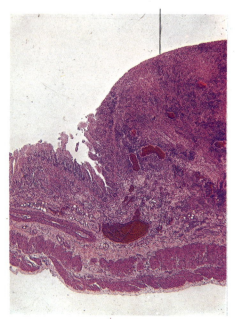

Fig 4–41.—Typhoid fever: marked inflammatory swelling (hematoxylin-eosin; 26×).

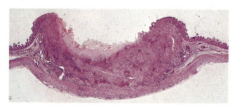

Fig 4–42.—A, typhoid fever: ulceration and scab formation (hematoxylin-eosin; 6×).

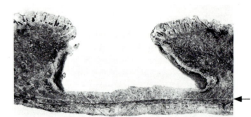

Fig 4–42.—B, typhoid fever: ulcer (hematoxylin-eosin; 8×).

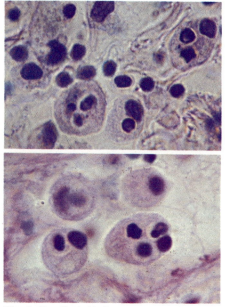

Fig 4–43.—Typhoid fever: large macrophages (hematoxylin-eosin; 640×).

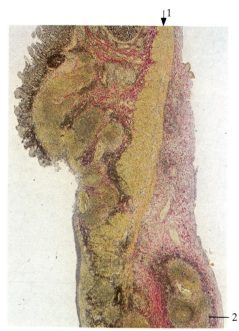

Fig 4–44.—Tuberculous ulcer of intestine (van Gieson's stain; 12×).

Typhoid Fever

The typhoid bacillis (Salmonella typhi) *causes an inflammatory disease of the lower ileum and occasionally the colon that runs a characteristic course. The inflammation starts in the region of Peyer's patches and progresses to necrosis and ulceration. Four stages are recognized, each lasting approximately 1 week. Both the intensity of the inflammation and the duration of the disease vary greatly.*

1st stage (1 week); **marked inflammatory swelling** (Fig 4–41), with either diffuse or focal enlargement of the lymphoid follicles which is characterized by infiltration of swollen macrophages and palely stained lymphocytes (architecture erased). Figure 4–41 shows the dense cellular infiltration of a swollen follicle (bluish red), with beginning necrosis of the surface mucosa (→). **Higher magnification** (Fig 4–43) reveals an increased number of large round macrophages with abundant cytoplasm that contains pyknotic nuclei, nuclear fragments, erythrocytes, and bacteria within phagosomes.

Macroscopic: Pea-sized, grayish red nodules or gray plaques.

2nd stage (2 weeks); a **scab** (Fig 4–42,A) can be seen in the necrotic portion of the markedly swollen and superficially ulcerated tissue (area devoid of nuclei). The necrotic area is surrounded by granulocytes.

Macroscopic: Yellowish green necrosis stained with bile.

In the third week the necrotic tissue sloughs, and this results in the *3rd stage; ulceration* (Fig 4–42,B). The ulcer extends to the muscularis (→). A narrow strip of necrotic tissue can still be recognized in the edges at each side.

In the *4th stage* (4 weeks) *the ulcer is cleaned up finally* by granulation tissue, which is then converted to a *scar* and finally epithelialized from the adjacent mucosa. The scars are smooth and thin because of the absence of lymph follicles. After about 4 months, only a thin zone in the intestinal wall marks the previously diseased area. Typhoid scars never cause stenosis.

Clinical: Temperature rises during the first week to 39°–40° C and continues to week 4, then falls; florid diarrhea (pea soup stools), skin rash (rose spots), splenomegaly.
Complications: Perforation with peritonitis in the ulcer stage (3 weeks), fatal intestinal hemorrhage, typhoid pneumonia, waxy hyalin, degeneration of the abdominal muscles.

Intestinal Tuberculosis

Intestinal tuberculosis (Fig 4–44). *Tubercle bacilli may colonize the lymph follicles of Peyer's patches and cause caseous tuberculosis.* Under low magnification, a defect is seen which extends to the muscularis (→ 1). The base is formed by a narrow zone of necrosis (caseation) containing many polymorphonuclear leukocytes (secondary infection). At the margins, there are round nodules that can be identified as typical tubercles under higher magnification. The tubercles extend through the entire wall at the base of the ulcer and into the serosa (→ 2). There is an increase in connective tissue.

Macroscopic: Flat ulcers with tattered margins, often surrounded by a circle of small white nodules on the serosa. Tuberculous lymphangiitis develops. The nearest lymph nodes draining the area are also always involved. Intestinal tuberculosis appears either as a result of ingestion of tubercle bacilli (primary intestinal tuberculosis with a primary complex) or, more frequently, as a secondary tuberculous process in association with active pulmonary tuberculosis.
Complications: Scarring of the ulcers with resultant intestinal stenosis, rarely perforation into the peritoneal cavity or into neighboring hollow organs. Bleeding may occur from a tuberculous ulcer; or generalized tuberculous peritonitis may develop.

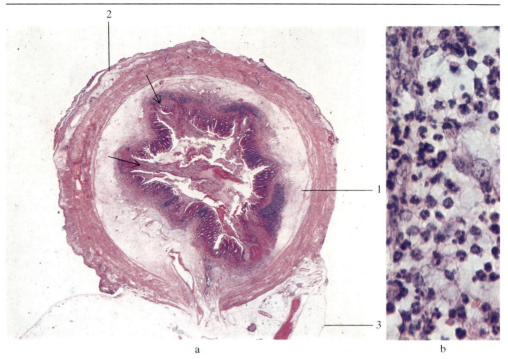

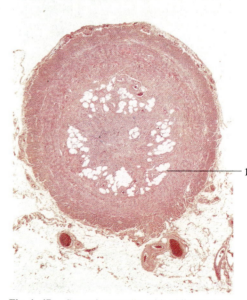

a

b

Fig 4–45.—**A,** phlegmonous appendicitis (hematoxylin-eosin; 10×). **B,** higher magnification of the submucosa (600×).

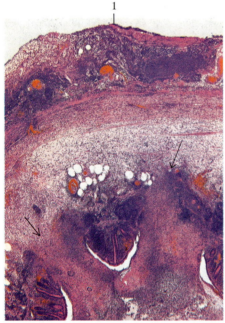

Fig 4–46.—Acute appendicitis with a so-called focus of primary infection (hematoxylin-eosin; 23×).

Fig 4–47.—Scarred appendix with obliterated lumen (hematoxylin-eosin; 40×).

Appendicitis

Inflammation of the vermiform appendix usually has an intestinal origin (invasion of obstructed glands by intestinal bacterial flora or streptococci: or obstruction from a fecalith). Only rarely is appendicitis hematogenous, although it may follow an acute viral infection such as influenza, chickenpox, or measles.

The *inflammation* starts in a small focus in the mucosa *(primary infection)* and then spreads like a *phlegmon* through all coats of the wall. Intraumural abscesses, secondary ulceration, empyema, necrosis, and gangrene of the wall frequently occur as a result of the development of arteritis and hemorrhagic infarction.

Figure 4–45,A shows an example of **acute phlegmonous appendicitis** at low magnification. Fibrin and leukocytes fill the lumen. Several primary sites of infection are seen with mucosal necrosis covered with fibrin and leukocytes. The markedly increased thickness of the submucosa (edema → 1) and sparsity of granulocytic infiltration are remarkable (higher magnification, Fig 4–45,B). Fibrin covers the peritoneum (→ 2). The inflammation also commonly extends into the mesoappendix (→3).

In Figure 4–46, two **primary foci of infection** can be seen under higher magnification (2 arrows in the picture). The inflammation has originated in a crypt and the granulocytic exudation has involved the tunica propria. Following this, the epithelium is breached and the mucosa destroyed by focal inflammatory exudation of fibrin and granulocytes. Later the necrotic tissue may slough and an ulcer form (acute ulcerative appendicitis). In Figure 4–46, the whole wall is infiltrated with granulocytes (→ 1: peritoneum covered with fibrin and granulocytes).

Acute appendicitis is usually a rapidly progressive illness that requires prompt surgical intervention. The urgency of the intervention becomes clear when the number of serious complications of untreated appendicitis is compared with the rapidity of recovery after appendectomy.

In chronic appendicitis there is infiltration of the appendix by lymphocytes and plasma cells, but lymph follicles may be preserved. The lumen of the appendix may become obliterated by scar tissue (Fig 4–47). This is thought to be due to replacement of necrotic mucosa after acute appendicitis. There is marked fibrosis of the submucosa, which may also contain foci of adipose tissue (→ 1). Chronic appendicitis occurs rarely (2%–6% of surgically removed appendices).

Complications of appendicitis: Perforation, pertonitis, pericecal abscess, spreading retroperitoneal inflammation (phlegmonous), subphrenic abscess, pyelophlebitic liver abscess, chiefly in the left lobe, hydrops, mucocele.

Oxyuriasis (Fig 4–48). The picture shows cross sections of oxyuris vermicularis in the lumen of the appendix. Frequently this is an incidental finding. The cross section of the parasite shows typical septation as well as a centrally located digestive tubule. The lowest part of the picture shows intact appendiceal mucosa.

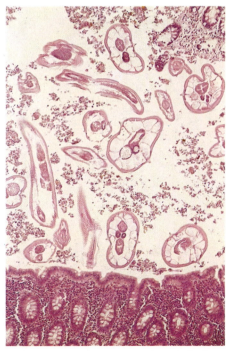

Fig 4–48.—Oxyuris in lumen of appendix (hematoxylin-eosin; 150×).

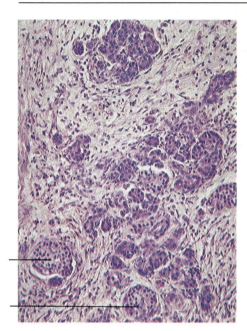

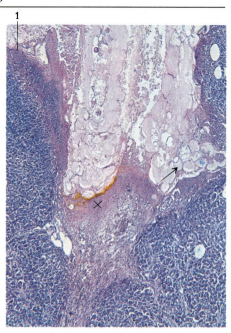

Fig **4–49.**—Chronic pancreatitis (hematoxylin-eosin; 120×).

Fig **4–50.**—Parenchymatous and fat necrosis of the pancreas (hematoxylin-eosin; 43×).

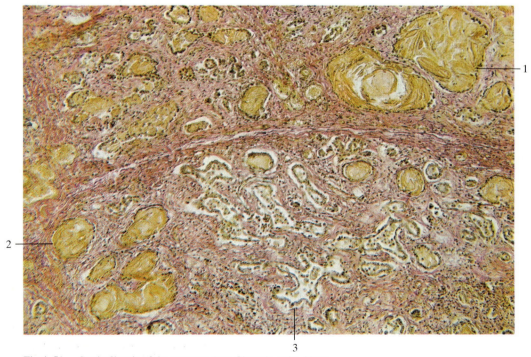

Fig **4–51.**—Cystic fibrosis of the pancreas (van Gieson's stain; 80×).

Pancreas

Chronic pancreatitis (Fig 4–49). This is a chronic recurrent inflammation with destruction, reconstruction, and replacement of the exocrine parenchyma of the pancreas by connective tissue. The etiology is varied: primary infection metabolic (alcohol), enzymatic autodigestion, idiopathic.

Histologically there is marked fibrosis with foci of chronic inflammatory infiltrates rich in lymphocytes, plasma cells, and histiocytes. The fibrous tissue infiltrates the acini, splitting and finally completely destroying them. Small fresh areas of pancreatic necrosis are frequently seen (enzymatic pancreatitis). Mostly the disease has a slow course, often with acute exacerbations. There may be large areas of acute necrosis that later become cystic. It is remarkable that the islets of Langerhans (→) remain intact for a considerable time. In the final stages (the burned-out pancreas), however, they also are destroyed and diabetes mellitus develops. Excretory ducts may proliferate and ectasia of ducts containing pancreatic calculi may develop (x-ray!).

Clinical: Pancreatic insufficiency (fatty stools, diarrhea). A past history of alcohol abuse is frequent. In 50% of cases there is latent hyperparathyroidism. Persons with pancreatic carcinoma often have had chronic pancreatitis previously.

Fat necrosis of the pancreas (Fig 4–50). Necrosis of the parenchyma and fat tissue of the pancreas is initiated by autodigestion (trypsin, lipase) resulting from previous disturbance of the local circulation. The pathogenesis of this very complex process is still under dispute. Microscopically, there is necrosis of the parenchyma and of islands of fat tissue in the pancreas, frequently accompanied by hemorrhage (hemorrhagic pancreatic necrosis). Under intermediate magnification, the ghostlike outlines of the fat cells can be recognized in many of the necrotic areas (→). In other areas, the fat is replaced by homogeneous, pale pink or blue material. Often crystals of fatty acids are precipitated. Hematoidin is deposited at the edge of the area of fat necrosis (×) in Figure 4–50. The necrosis also extends into the parenchyma (→ 1), which appears eosinophilic and shows loss of nuclei. In the acute stages of the necrosis, granulocytes accumulate at the margins, while in later stages a collar of granulation tissue or mature connective tissue containing foam cells may be found. Fat necrosis developing after death lacks any evidence of tissue reaction such as exudation of leukocytes.

Macroscopic: In the initial stages, there is edema and focal parenchymatous necrosis (large, dirty gray pancreas): in hemorrhagic necrosis, the pancreas is dark red and bloody; secondary liquefaction with cyst formation may develop. Fat necrosis appears as chalky white, freckle-sized nodules. The disease is more common in men than in women, but obese women are especially prone to it and there is often alcohol abuse with fatty cirrhosis of the liver.

Cystic fibrosis of the pancreas (Fig 4–51). Not only is the pancreas involved in this recessively heritable disease, but so also are the mucous glands of the intestine, bile ducts, lungs, and salivary glands (mucoviscidosis). It affects chiefly infants who have meconium ileus. Marked inflammatory changes are present in the lungs of affected children (bronchiectasis) and, finally, chronic deficiency of pancreatic enzymes leads to the development of stasis of secretions of high viscosity, except in sweat glands, where the defect involves abnormal electrolyte transport and resorption. Microscopically, the normal lobular structures are surrounded by strands of connective tissue. Both the ducts (→ 1) and acini (→ 2, 3) are widely dilated and cystic. The contents of the cysts consist of homogeneous or laminated secretions. An increased amount of interstitial tissue is distributed randomly through the lobules (red connective tissue in van Gieson's stain). In addition, there is scanty infiltration of lymphocytes and plasma cells. In general, the organ is reconstructed in a way similar to hepatic cirrhosis.

Macroscopic: The pancreas is firm and grayish white. In the late stages there are numerous small cysts and the surface is granular.

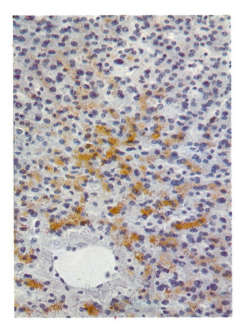

Fig 5–1.—Brown atrophy of the liver (111×).

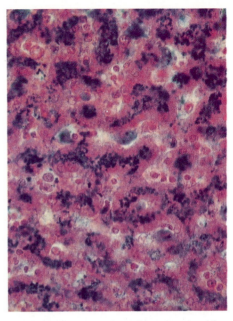

Fig 5–2.—Siderosis of the liver (Prussian blue reaction; 456×).

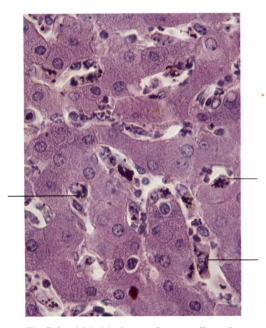

Fig 5–3.—Malarial pigment (hematoxylin-eosin; 480×).

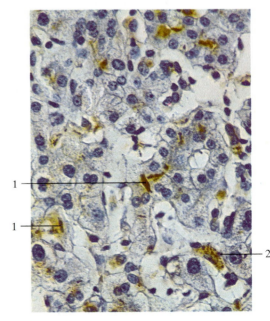

Fig 5–4.—Icterus of the liver (hematoxylin-eosin; 310×).

5. Liver—Gallbladder

Familiarity with the normal microscopic anatomy of the liver is an essential prerequisite for interpretation of the microscopic appearances of abnormal liver. The traditional morphohistologic unit of the liver is the "liver lobule." A modern point of view subdivides the liver into acini or acinar units, but for the sake of simplicity we shall refer to liver lobules. For purposes of orientation, the *periportal field* will serve as a good starting point [Glisson's triad of bile ducts (cylindrical epithelium), artery (heavy muscular wall), and branches of the portal vein]. The periportal field is enveloped by a sheath of liver cells, known as the *limiting plate*. Plates of liver cells accompanied by sinusoids course toward the central vein. When trying to understand pathologic changes in the liver lobules, it should be borne in mind that different parts of the liver lobule can be affected separately (e.g., either the central or peripheral zones). This depends on peculiarities of the circulation and of the cellular complement of enzymes. Concepts about the fundamental functional unit of the liver are still not well established. For example, instead of the "classic" liver lobule centered around the central vein *(central vein unit),* a so-called *portal vein unit* has been proposed. In this scheme, the periportal zone lies at the center and the central vein marks the peripheral boundary of the liver lobule. Many pathologic alterations can be well correlated with the functional findings with this concept (e.g., the pattern of stasis). *Attention should be paid to the following features in pathologic material:* the cell constituents of the periportal field, the integrity of the liver cell cords (i.e., liver cell plates as seen in cross section) and of the liver cells themselves, particularly in the limiting plate, Kupffer cells, and any deposits of pigments or other substances (e.g., fat, amyloid).

Brown atrophy of the liver (Fig 5–1). *In brown atrophy, which may affect any internal organ and especially the heart and liver, there is an increase in lipofuscin.* The pigment is best seen in histologic sections stained with hematoxylin without a counterstain. Low magnification shows a prominent brownish cast in the region of the central portion of the lobule. Under higher magnification, brown cytoplasmic granules can be seen. Figure 5–1 shows the central vein and surrounding cords of liver cells, which contain less and less pigment the farther they are situated from the center of the lobule. In addition, the liver cells are also atrophic and have compactly arranged nuclei.

Macroscopic: Brown, shrunken organ with a wrinkled capsule.

Siderosis of the liver (Fig 5–2). *In this condition, iron-containing pigment, often derived from hemoglobin, is deposited in the cytoplasm of both the liver and the Kupffer cells.* In contrast to lipofuscin pigment, siderin is found chiefly in hepatocytes at the periphery of the liver lobule, especially in the cytoplasm near the bile canaliculus (see Table 2, section on General Pathology). In this way, the midline between two rows of cells becomes intensified. The pigment appears yellowish brown in sections stained with hematoxylin-eosin, but the Prussian blue reaction colors the pigment a deep blue. The stellate Kupffer cells also contain deposits of iron pigment.

Macroscopic: A brown liver of normal size, often associated with siderosis of other organs (pancreas, spleen, salivary glands), especially in hemochromatosis (see Hepatic Cirrhosis, later this chapter).

Malarial pigment (Fig 5–3). *Brownish black pigment originating from destruction of blood cells in malaria is deposited in the reticuloendothelial cells.* Accordingly, it is found in the Kupffer cells of the liver. Figure 5–3 shows the black granules in the swollen Kupffer cells (→) and is a good demonstration of the phagocytic capacities of these lining cells of the sinusoids.

Macroscopic: Smoky gray discoloration of liver and spleen.

Icterus of the liver (Fig 5–4). *In jaundice, granules of bile pigment appear in the cytoplasm of the liver cells and bile casts form in the ductules or larger bile ducts.* Under intermediate magnification, greenish, sausage-shaped secretions (bile casts, incorrectly called bile thrombi → 1, see also Table 10) can be seen. Isolated, fine droplets of bile are also seen in the cytoplasm of the liver cells. In obstructive jaundice and extrahepatic jaundice, the central zone of the liver lobule is particularly affected, whereas in hepatocellular jaundice all parts of the lobule are involved.* The Kupffer cells may also contain bile pigment (→ 2) or phagocytosed necrotic liver cells.

Macroscopic: The liver has either a green (biliverdin) or a golden brown color (bilirubin).

---

*Drug-induced jaundice has become very important (sex hormones, ovulation arresting drugs, psychotherapeutic drugs such as chlorpromazine).

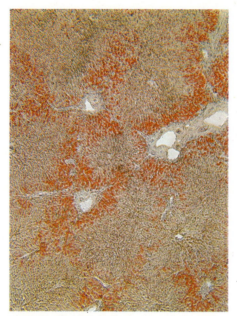

Fig 5–5.—Peripheral fatty metamorphosis of the liver (Sudan stain; 22×).

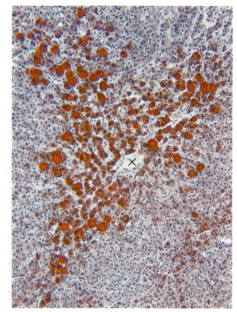

Fig 5–6.—Central fatty metamorphosis of the liver (Sudan stain; 84×).

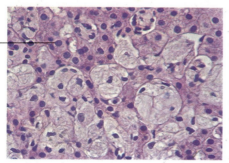

Fig 5–7.—Gaucher's disease (hematoxylin-eosin; 300×).

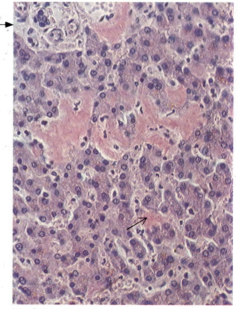

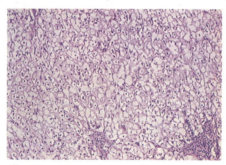

Fig 5–8.—Glycogen storage disease (hematoxylin-eosin; 300×).

Fig 5–9.—Amyloidosis of the liver (Congo red stain; 155×).

Fatty Metamorphosis of the Liver—Storage Diseases—Amyloidosis

The lipids of the liver cells are bound to cell components and are not normally seen. When fat appears in the form of droplets in the cytoplasm of the liver cells, the condition is known as *fatty metamorphosis*. Three forms of fatty metamorphosis occur in the liver: *peripheral fatty metamorphosis* (e.g., alimentary fatty metamorphosis), *central fatty metamorphosis* (e.g., metabolic or toxic), and *diffuse fatty metamorphosis,* particularly in chronic alcohol abuse (see fatty liver). Diffuse fatty metamorphosis occurs with excess accumulation of fats or carbohydrates in diabetes and with the use of antibiotics, cytostatic drugs, or cortisone.

Peripheral fatty metamorphosis (Fig 5–5) is manifested by the occurrence of large droplets of fat in the cytoplasm of liver cells at the periphery of the lobules. Low-power examination of preparations stained with Sudan shows a red ring surrounding a pale central zone. Higher magnification shows that the liver cells are filled with large droplets of fat; frequently, a single large fat globule fills the cytoplasm. The nucleus is displaced to the periphery of the cells.

Macroscopic: Yellow network with brownish red centers.

Central fatty metamorphosis (Fig 5–6) shows the reverse picture. With the scanning lens, the central zones of the lobules appear as red areas surrounded by a blue halo. Low magnification reveals the position of the fat deposits. The central vein ($\times$) lies in the middle of the fatty area. A further point of distinction from peripheral fatty metamorphosis is that most of the fat droplets are very fine and distributed diffusely through the cytoplasm.

Macroscopic: Small yellow pointlike lesions scattered on a brown background.

Storage diseases (Figs 5–7, 5–8). Excessive storage of various substances in cells results from certain genetically determined metabolic defects in which specific lysosomal enzymes are lacking, so that degradation of these substances does not occur and they accumulate within cells. In *Gaucher's disease* cerebrosides (kerasin) accumulate because of a deficiency of glucocerebrosidase and α-galactosidase in lysosomes. Thus, erythrocytic membranes are only partially destroyed by cells in the reticuloendothelial system, and cytoplasmic accumulation of the lipids occurs in the spleen, liver, and bone marrow. Figure 5–7 shows large cells of the reticuloendothelial system with finely granular cytoplasm which have compressed liver cells and even caused pressure atrophy ($\rightarrow$). In *glycogen storage diseases* there is a lack of enzymes, with the result that lysosomal glycogen is not metabolized. Nine different sorts of enzyme defects are known. *Von Gierke's disease* (lack of glucose-6-phosphatase) involves liver and kidney, *Pompe's disease* (absence of lysosomal maltase) chiefly the heart (frequency, $1:100,000$ births). Figure 5–8 shows the typical appearance of the liver, with large cells having clear cytoplasm. The glycogen, being water soluble, dissolves out of the cells in Formalin-fixed tissue. In tissue fixed in alcohol, the glycogen is preserved and can be demonstrated by special stains.

Amyloidosis of the liver (Fig 5–9). The amyloid, which is a pathologic protein, is deposited in the space between the walls of sinusoids and liver cells (Disse's space); periportal field ($\rightarrow$). At first only a narrow strip of homogeneous red material (positive for Congo red) is seen next to the capillaries ($\rightarrow$ inside picture). If the deposits are marked, they may cause pressure atrophy of the liver cords, which may disappear completely. The lumina of the sinusoids may be greatly reduced as a consequence of the infiltration. Amyloid can be stained with either Congo red or methyl violet (red metachromasia, see Tables 1 and 3, section on General Pathology). Amyloid stained with Congo red shows color birefringence (green color when viewed with polarized light).

155

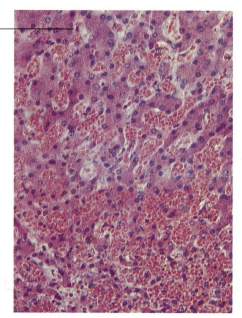

Fig 5–10.—Mild congestion (stasis) of liver (hematoxylin-eosin; 250×).

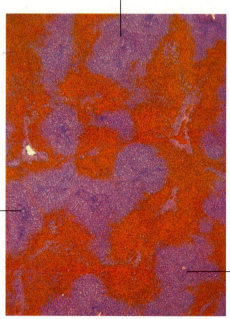

Fig 5–11.—Marked congestion of liver (hematoxylin-eosin; 29×).

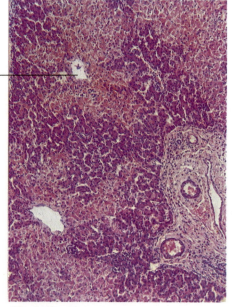

Fig 5–12.—Hypoxemic (ischemic) necrosis of liver (hematoxylin-eosin; 60×).

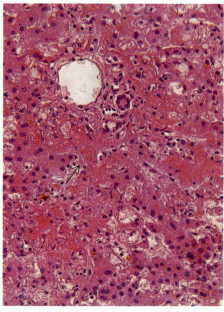

Fig 5–13.—Liver necrosis in eclampsia (hematoxylin-eosin; 200×).

156

Congestion of the liver (Fig 5–10). Stasis due to obstruction of the venous return to the right heart (right heart insufficiency) manifests itself first in the *central zone of the liver lobules*. At a later stage, lakelike vascular channels develop by fusion of the congested central zones of adjacent liver lobules. In the early stages, low-power magnification reveals red zones in the central regions of the lobules; higher magnification discloses the greatly dilated sinusoids. Figure 5–10 shows a section of a central zone (the central vein lies below and outside the picture), with the sinusoids greatly distended by numerous erythrocytes. If the liver cells in the uncongested upper portion of the illustration are compared with those in the congested areas, it can be clearly seen that the liver cells in the latter are atrophic because of compression by dilated sinuses. This often leads to deficient oxygenation of the cells so that they also show fatty change (→: unaltered Kupffer cell).

Macroscopic: Enlarged, firm liver. The cut surfaces show dark red central areas surrounded by pale brown peripheral zones. Often, fatty change is also present and imparts a yellow appearance.

Marked congestion of the liver (Fig 5–11). When congestion has been present for some time, it also involves the intermediate zones of the lobules, but the peripheral zones only where lobules adjoin each other. In this manner, congested channels are formed which connect one liver lobule with another and lead to a *reversal of the normal liver pattern* so that the periportal field (→) is in the middle of a red ring of hyperemia (see notes on histology at beginning of this chapter). The red ring and the broad channels can be seen even with the scanning lens. With low-power magnification, the periportal fields are seen to be at the center. Higher magnification of the congested area shows the greatly dilated sinusoids. In these areas, the liver cells have disappeared. Frequently, the walls of the sinusoids cannot be recognized. Lakes of blood have formed. Most of the intact parenchyma shows fatty change.

Macroscopic: The liver is large and dark red. The cut surfaces show a dark red network on a yellow background (fatty metamorphosis), the so-called nutmeg liver.

Hypoxic (Ischemic) **liver necrosis** (Fig 5–12). *Necrosis of the liver can affect either single cells (see Viral Hepatitis, later this chapter) or groups of cells in either the intermediate zones of the lobules or without any particular localization.* Focal necrosis can be caused by *toxins* (e.g., diphtheria) or it may be dependent on *acute oxygen lack*. Figure 5–12 shows geographical areas of necrosis in the centers of the liver lobules (→: central vein). The areas of necrotic liver cells are apparent from the pale red stain. Nuclei are decreased in number. Kupffer cells, for the most part, are preserved. The condition is also seen in shock.

Liver necrosis in eclampsia (Fig 5–13). *Eclampsia usually develops toward the end of pregnancy, especially during labor. The pathogenesis is now considered to be either a direct action of a toxin formed in the placenta on the parenchymatous cells or a secondary outcome of a disturbance of the circulation (shock?). Liver, kidney, and brain are preferentially affected.* In contrast to hypoxic liver necrosis, which develops in the area of greatest oxygen deficiency, the necrosis of eclampsia is distributed at random throughout the lobule. Examination with a scanning lens discloses irregularly scattered, eosinophilic, maplike lesions. Intermediate magnification shows that the liver cell cords and sinusoids in the homogeneous red areas are no longer arranged next to one another. Cell nuclei have disappeared. The cytoplasm of the liver cells has become homogeneous and structureless. The blood in the sinusoids is coagulated into solid masses (→) as a result of stasis or the formation of fibrin and platelet thrombi (hyaline thrombi → evidence of shock).

Macroscopic: Gray or grayish yellow, maplike lesions.

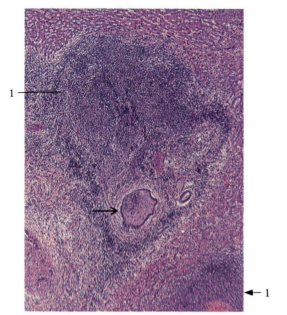

Fig 5–14.—Ascending suppurative cholangitis (hematoxylin-eosin; 50×).

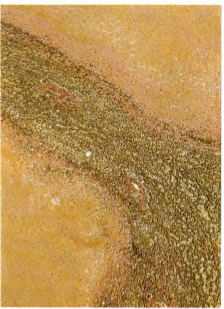

Fig 5–15.—Gumma of the liver (van Gieson's stain; 40×).

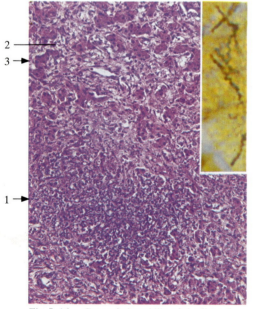

Fig 5–16.—Congenital syphilis of the liver (hematoxylin-eosin; 120×). *Inset:* spirochetes (Levaditi stain; 2,350×).

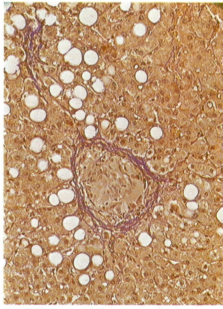

Fig 5–17.—Sarcoid granuloma in the liver (hematoxylin-eosin; 330×).

Ascending suppurative cholangitis (Fig 5–14). *This is caused by ascending bacterial infection (mostly* Escherichia coli) *of the bile ducts and is often associated with bile stasis (stones, tumors).* The bile ducts in the periportal spaces are dilated and contain exudate rich in polymorphonuclear leukocytes (→). The entire periportal field is infiltrated with polymorphonuclear leukocytes, which also are found in the adjacent parenchyma where there is tissue necrosis *(cholangiolytic abscess → 1).* In Figure 5–14 there is an increase in the periportal fibrous tissue, which forms a concentric, collar-like arrangement around the bile ducts (→). This is often an indication of previous cholangitic disease (see Primary Cholangitis, later this chapter).

Macroscopic: The liver is bile-stained, with widening and proliferation of the periportal fields and foci of greenish necrosis (abscesses).

Gumma of the liver (Fig 5–15). *In the third stage of syphilis, granulomas (gummas) with a rubbery consistency appear in affected organs.* These are sharply demarcated, round or maplike foci of necrosis which, as can be easily seen with elastica and van Gieson's stains, contain connective tissue or elastic fibers which arise in the surrounding tissues and penetrate the necrotic areas. Figure 5–15 shows the necrotic areas (yellow with van Gieson's stain and lacking nuclei) surrounded by a narrow band of granulation tissue. Epithelioid cells resembling those of tuberculosis (see Tuberculosis, chap. 3) are seen in the granulation tissue. These, however, are present in smaller numbers than in tuberculosis. Next to this layer there is a layer of connective tissue vascularized with capillaries and containing fibroblasts and lymphocytes. In the outermost zone, scar tissue has formed (red in van Gieson's stain). Langhans'-type giant cells are occasionally present. However, in contrast to tuberculosis, numbers of plasma cells are present in the granulation tissue of a gumma and the neighboring blood vessels show endarteritis.

Macroscopic: Yellow, maplike areas of necrosis having a rubbery consistency.

Congenital syphilis of the liver (Fig 5–16). Under low magnification, the normal architecture of the liver can be scarcely recognized. There are small, richly cellular, blue-staining focal lesions *(syphilomas).* The liver cords are widely separated by an interstitial cellular infiltrate and have been segregated as groups of liver cells. Medium magnification reveals miliary granulomas (→ 1) showing areas of fresh necrosis, nuclear fragments, polymorphonuclear leukocytes, and lymphocytes. In these areas, the liver cells are completely destroyed. In the surrounding tissue, a chronic interstitial hepatitis has developed in which the interstitial tissue is markedly distended with histiocytes (→ 2), fibroblasts, lymphocytes, and fibrous tissue. Remnants of liver cords lie in between (→ 3). Numerous *spirochetes* can be demonstrated with special stains (Levaditi silver stain, inset, Fig 5–16).

Macroscopic: The liver is of firm consistency and the cut surfaces show grayish brown flecks.

Congenital syphilis localizes principally in the skeletal system *(syphilitic osteochrondritis, syphilitic saddle nose, syphilitic periosteitis),* in the skin *(syphilitic pemphigus),* lungs *(pneumonia alba),* and brain. In addition, the victims may show the so-called *Hutchinson triad* (keratitis, inner ear deafness, and malformed teeth).

Sarcoid granuloma of the liver (Fig 5–17). Sarcoidosis *(Boeck's sarcoid)* may spread via lymphatics from pulmonary hilar lymph nodes or by the bloodstream and can affect all organs. The liver is affected in 60% of cases and consequently a liver biopsy may be diagnostically helpful, as may a lymph node biopsy. Figure 5–17 shows an epithelioid cell granuloma with a typical collagenous ring in the outer zone (beginning scar ring). Peripheral to this zone there is fatty change in hepatocytes, with large droplets of fat.

Viral Hepatitis

Massive Liver Necrosis

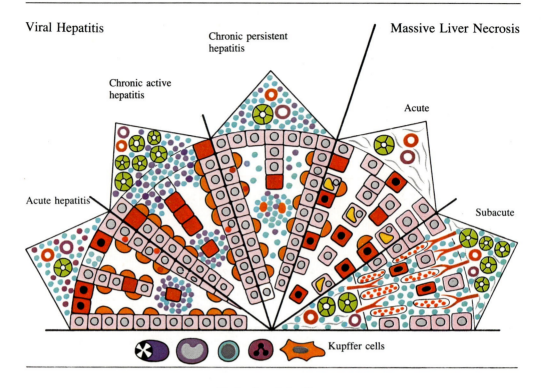

Chronic persistent
hepatitis

Chronic active
hepatitis

Acute

Acute hepatitis

Subacute

Kupffer cells

Cirrhosis of the liver

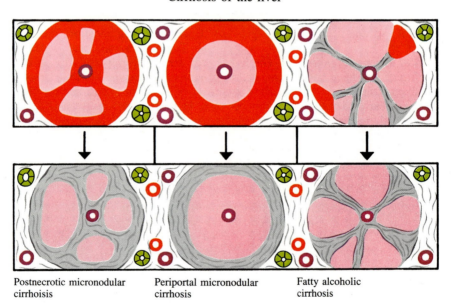

Postnecrotic micronodular
cirrhoisis

Periportal micronodular
cirrhosis

Fatty alcoholic
cirrhosis

Fig 5–18.—Diagram of the histologic changes in viral hepatitis, massive liver necrosis, and cirrhosis of the liver. In the lower half of the figure red indicates necrosis; gray, fibrous scars.

Viral Hepatitis—Massive Liver Cell Necrosis—Cirrhosis

Figure 5–18 shows in schematic form the histologic appearances of these three diseases, which will be considered together because of certain similarities. *In essence, all three show destruction of liver cells (necrosis) accompanied by resorption and a secondary mesenchymal reaction that takes the form of granulation tissue. There is, in addition, reorganization of the structure of the liver and parenchymal regeneration.* In many cases of cirrhosis, *primary proliferation of granulation tissue (inflammation) with simultaneous or subsequent destruction of parenchyma* occupies a prominent place.

Viral hepatitis (see also Figs 5–19 through 5–21 and accompanying text) is initiated by *necrosis of single cells* (acidophilic necrotic cytoplasm). These are resorbed by histiocytes. The periportal zones show an infiltrate of lymphocytes and histiocytes which break through the limiting plate and extend farther into the parenchyma. *Chronic hepatitis* develops in about 5% of cases, either as *chronic active hepatitis,* which shows a patchy inflammatory exudate extending from the periportal field into the parenchyma, or as *chronic persistent hepatitis,* which runs a course of many years and does not show extension of the periportal inflammatory exudate into the liver parenchyma.

In massive liver cell necrosis (see also Figs 5–30 through 5–32 and accompanying text), the necrosis involves either the entire liver or a part of it. In the majority of cases, it is now thought to be a *fulminant form of viral hepatitis.* The acute stage (*massive cytolytic necrosis,* formerly *acute yellow atrophy*) is manifested by dissociation of the liver cell cords, necrosis of cells, and pyknosis of nuclei. In the *subacute stages,* a large part of the parenchyma is demolished and the periportal zones collapse and are infiltrated with chronic inflammatory cells.

Cirrhosis of the liver (see also Hepatic Cirrhosis, later this chapter) is a disease in which there is *destruction of parenchyma* with *progressive reconstruction* of the entire liver and formation of nodules of parenchyma.

Two essentially different types of cirrhosis are recognized: 1. *macronodular postnecrotic cirrhosis,* 2. *micronodular cirrhosis (including biliary cirrhosis).*

In **postnecrotic cirrhosis** there is massive parenchymal necrosis which either involves isolated segments of the liver lobule or more commonly embraces several liver lobules or large areas of the parenchyma. As a result large irregular zones of fibrosis develop and surround the remaining parenchymal tissue in an irregular fashion. In addition, regeneration of the parenchyma takes place by division of spared hepatocytes, but this, too, occurs in irregular ways. The entire liver displays a pattern of nodularity, with some nodules measuring several centimeters in diameter while others have diameters near 1 cm. In some cases, the postnecrotic process results in a more uniform, diffuse nodularity of the liver, with nodules measuring between approximately 0.5 and 1.5 cm.

If many liver lobules are destroyed, large scars develop in which the periportal fields are packed closely. Eventually only small islands of parenchyma remain (see Fig 5–33).

Periportal, posthepatitic cirrhosis is due to chronic inflammation starting in the periportal field with secondary periportal necrosis resulting in the formation of large uniform islands of parenchyma bounded by a ring of fibrous tissue. The central vein may lie in the center but often is displaced to the periphery of the islands of parenchyma (see Figs 5–34, 5–35). The cirrhosis is micronodular and regeneration of parenchyma is irregular.

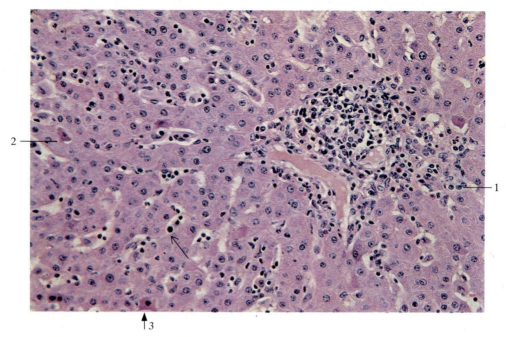

Fig 5–19.—Acute viral hepatitis (hematoxylin-eosin; 60 ×).

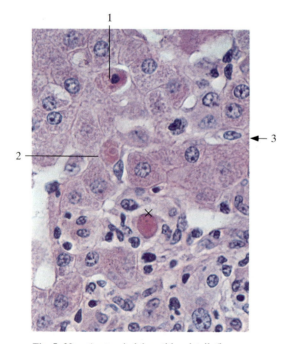

Fig 5–20.—Acute viral hepatitis, detail (hematoxylin-eosin; 500 ×).

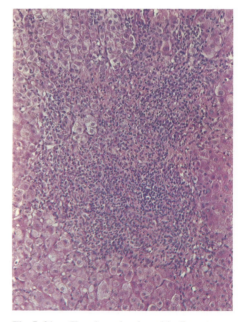

Fig 5–21.—Chronic active hepatitis (hematoxylin-eosin; 100 ×).

162

Viral Hepatitis

Acute and chronic viral hepatitis shows a *characteristic histologic picture* so that, in most cases, it is possible to diagnose the sort of hepatitis and the prognosis. Study of needle biopsy specimens has aided in unraveling the course of the disease.

Clinically **acute viral hepatitis** begins with malaise, loss of appetite, nausea, and mild jaundice. SGOT is slightly elevated. The disease lasts about 6 weeks. It is transferred orally in epidemics of virus A (infectious hepatitis). The virus has been successfully transmitted to monkeys. Incubation period 15–20 days. **Serum hepatitis** (homologous serum hepatitis, virus B) is transmitted orally or parenterally (blood transfusion, injections, "hippie" hepatitis). Incubation period 45–160 days. Viral antigens can be detected in blood [so-called Australia antigen, HB surface antigen$_{(HBsAg)}$, other antigens]. HBsAg can also be detected by immunofluorescence techniques in the cytoplasm of liver cells. With the light microscope the cytoplasm has a ground-glass appearance. The disease is more severe and persists longer than does hepatitis A. Both forms of hepatitis have the same histologic features, the necrosis of individual cells eliciting a secondary inflammatory reaction of the Kupffer cells and in the periportal fields. Since the framework of supporting fibers is preserved, it is possible for regeneration to occur without destruction of liver parenchyma. Hepatitis B can progress to chronic hepatitis.

Other forms of hepatitis are now of major importance because of their marked tendency to become chronic. The term "non-A, non-B" hepatitis is used in relation to these forms. Electron microscopy has revealed several possible etiologic agents. The disease has the attributes of viral hepatitis and is now the most common form of "serum hepatitis" in the United States.

Acute viral hepatitis (Fig 5–19, 5–20). Low magnification reveals widening and cellular infiltration of the periportal fields, but with preservation of architecture and scanty cellular infiltration of the parenchyma. Somewhat higher magnification (Fig 5–19) shows the periportal infiltrate to consist of lymphocytes and a few polymorphonuclear leukocytes which have breached the limiting plate of the lobule and invaded the parenchyma (→ 1). Between the liver cell cords there are *swollen Kupffer cells* (stellate shaped) and round cells with a single nucleus, which appear to be immigrant blood monocytes (→ in the picture). In addition, individual liver cells are small and shrunken, with striking angular cytoplasm and pyknotic nuclei (→ 2, → 3 acidophilic of single cells).

High magnification, Figure 5–20, **acute viral hepatitis detail** (see also Fig 5–18), shows necrosis of individual cells and the reaction in the liver. At → 1, a necrotic cell with nuclear pyknosis is seen. At → 2 (also ×), there is the ghost of an anuclear cell, a typical eosinophilic body (so-called hyaline or Councilman body, see Fig 5–54). These "hyaline bodies" are not specific for hepatitis, as they are also observed in other conditions. The individual necrotic cells are surrounded by lymphocytes and histiocytes with plump, oval, or slightly indented nuclei. At → 3, there is a swollen Kupffer cell. In the acute stages there are, in addition, bile pigmentation of liver cells and bile casts in the central zones. Mitoses and multinucleated giant cells indicate the onset of liver cell regeneration.

Macroscopic: The liver is enlarged, with rounded edges and spotted, yellow, reddish brown external and cut surfaces.

Chronic hepatitis in 3%–5% of cases develops from an acute hepatitis (chiefly hepatitis B, 15%, and also hepatitis non-A, non-B). It does not develop from hepatitis A. However, there are also cases that begin insidiously without preexisting acute hepatitis. Two forms of chronic hepatitis are recognized:
Chronic active hepatitis (Fig 5–21). This is the most severe form of chronic hepatitis and is manifested by marked inflammatory exudate in the periportal fields, which invades the lamellar boundaries and sends tongue-like projections into the parenchyma (moth-eaten appearance) so that exudate bridges periportal fields, which may lead eventually to cirrhosis. Necrotic liver cells are replaced by an infiltrate of lymphocytes and histiocytes. Within 3–5 years it can develop into cirrhosis of the liver. Thirty percent of cases show a positive

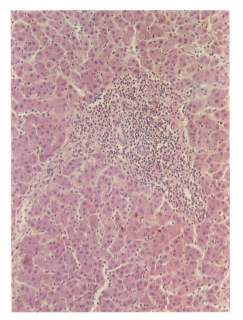

Fig 5–22.—Chronic persistent, recurrent hepatitis (hematoxylin-eosin; 100×).

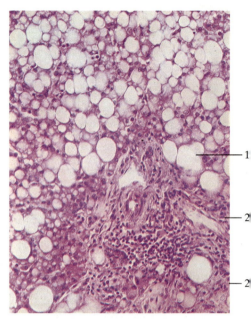

Fig 5–23.—Fatty hepatitis (hematoxylin-eosin; 170×).

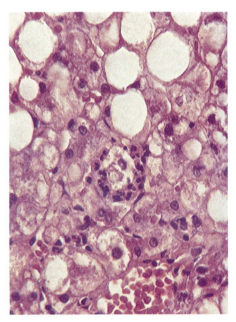

Fig 5–24.—Fatty hepatitis (detail) (hematoxylin-eosin; 400×).

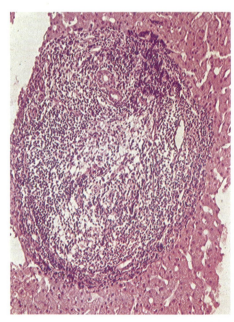

Fig 5–25.—Chronic destructive cholangitis (hematoxylin-eosin; 100×).

reaction with HB antigens. Lupoid hepatitis is a special form of chronic aggressive hepatitis that affects particularly young women (20–29 years). Patients show the LE phenomenon, high antibody titers (IgG, IgA), and antibodies against smooth muscle. HB antigens are absent. Autoaggressive disorder? The inflammatory infiltrate also contains plasma cells.

Macroscopic: Finely granular surface.

Chronic persistent hepatitis (Fig 5–22): The periportal infiltrate consists of lymphocytes, which often form germinal centers, and does not extend into the parenchyma. The parenchyma shows a few necrotic cells and focal or generalized increase in Kupffer cells. Eighty percent of patients have antibodies to HBsAg. The disease may persist many years. Immunoglobulins are not elevated. It usually does not progress to cirrhosis.

Macroscopic: Smooth surface.

Fatty hepatitis (Fig 5–23, 5–24). Liver injury conditioned by alcohol. In the beginning of the disease there is merely fatty change, either focal or diffuse (large or small droplets). Later single cells become necrotic as a result of fat accumulation or balloon-like swelling of liver cells (hydropic and fatty change) or the formation of fat cysts (coalescence of several fatty liver cells, → 1). Characteristically there are **Mallory bodies,** i.e., focal cytoplasmic hyalinization of liver cells (often horn-shaped, Fig 5–26). Mallory bodies are composed of filaments composed of protein related to prekeratin, with diameters of 14–20 nm. The periportal fields are widened (edema, granulocytes, proliferation of bile ducts → 2). Secondarily fibrous proliferation develops in the lobule center (so-called *network fibrosis*) so that solitary cells or a few cells are encased in fibrous tissue. Figure 5–24 shows a necrotic, fatty liver cell which has been resorbed by granulocytes. The Kupffer cells also are increased in number and contain accumulated iron. After 10–15 years of chronic alcohol abuse micronodular cirrhosis may develop (about 10–20% of alcoholics).

Cholangitis: An inflammation of the intrahepatic bile ducts secondary to bile stasis resulting from extrahepatic duct stenosis (gallstones, tumors, scars). Mostly there is an ascending infection with *E. coli* (see Ascending Suppurative Cholangitis earlier this chapter). Primary cholangitis occurs as a **chronic, destructive, nonpurulent cholangitis** (Fig 5–25). Histologically the bile ducts are surrounded by lymphocytes and plasma cells, which are also found in the periportal fields (a similar picture occurs in chronic aggressive hepatitis). Bile ducts are destroyed, the inflammation extends into the parenchyma, and portal biliary cirrhosis may develop.

Clinical: Chiefly women 30–60 years of age. Biliary cirrhosis develops on the average after 7 years. In 98% of cases antibodies against mitochondria can be demonstrated (autoaggression?).

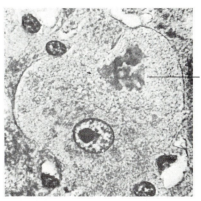

Fig 5–26.—Mallory body (hematoxylin-eosin; 400×).

165

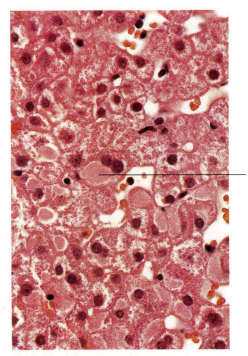

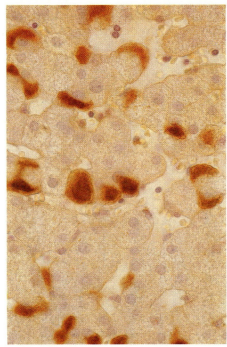

Fig 5–27.—Hepatocytes with ground glass cytoplasm in chronic persistent hepatitis (hematoxylin-eosin; 200×).

Fig 5–28.—Immunohistochemical demonstration of HB surface antigen (HBsAg; 250×).

HBsAg Carriers (Figs 5–27, 5–28). Scattered necrosis of individual hepatocytes, together with increase of reactive Kupffer cells and collections of lymphocytes—occasionally containing germinal centers—suggests progressive disease or activity of the hepatic process. Although such changes can be quite discrete, the presence of ground-glass hepatocytes in the liver and of HBsAg (Australia antigen) indicates persistence of viral infection. Such cases may reflect a balance between immune reaction and virus activity, which in turn may be responsible for the chronicity of persistent hepatitis. HBsAg can be demonstrated immunohistochemically (peroxidase method) in the cytoplasm of hepatocytes (brown reaction product), but not in the nuclei (Fig 5–28).

In carriers of HBsAg, morphological signs of liver damage (necrosis) and the inflammatory reaction (hyperplasia of Kupffer cells, periportal lymphocytic infiltrates) regress while the number of ground-glass hepatocytes increases. If only few and scattered necrotic hepatocytes are to be found, the condition may be termed "minimal hepatitis"; this may be the mildest form of chronic hepatitis.

Other virus-induced liver damage. Parenchymal damage accompanied by mesenchymal reaction also occurs in other viral diseases, for example in infectious mononucleosis (due to Epstein-Barr virus; associated with Kupffer cell hyperplasia), in cytomegalic inclusion disease, and in infection with herpes types A and B viruses.

1. **Chronic active hepatitis.** Disruption of lobular architecture by inflammatory reaction with destruction of the limiting plate. Lymphocytes and plasma cells infiltrate periportal regions. There is piecemeal necrosis of individual hepatocytes as well as groups of hepa-

Normal liver

1. Chronic active hepatitis

2. Chronic persistent hepatitis

3. Chronic destructive cholangitis

4. Nonspecific reactive hepatitis

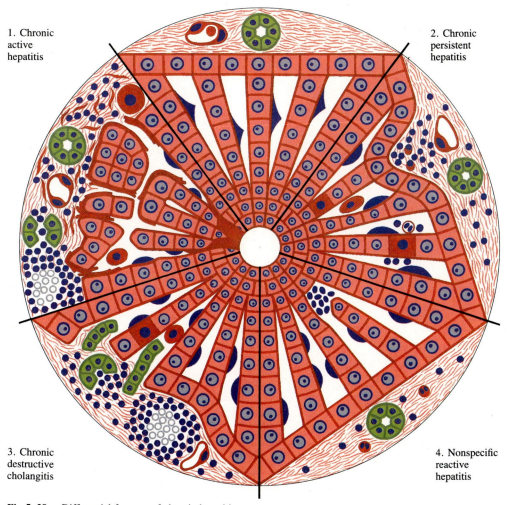

Fig 5–29.—Differential features of chronic hepatitis.

tocytes that is associated with periportal and interstitial fibrosis and a hystiocytic reaction.

2. **Chronic persistent hepatitis.** In this condition the lobular architecture remains intact, but there is infiltration of lymphocytes and plasma cells in the periportal regions. There are ground-glass hepatocytes when the infection is due to hepatitis B virus, and there is proliferation of Kupffer cells.

3. **Chronic destructive cholangitis.** The portal connective tissue around bile ducts is infiltrated by lymphocytes, which may form follicles. There is destruction as well as proliferation of intrahepatic bile ducts.

4. **Nonspecific reactive hepatitis.** The lobular architecture is intact, but there are scattered centroacinar necroses of hepatocytes, in which there are granulocytes and lymphocytes.

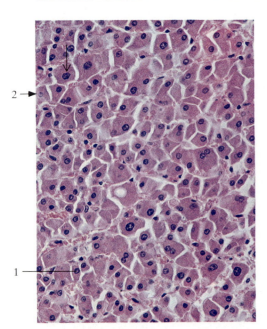

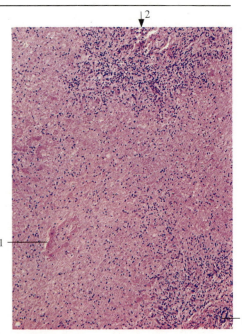

Fig 5–30.—Acute massive liver necrosis showing disorganization of the liver cell cords (hematoxylin-eosin; 270×).

Fig 5–31.—Acute massive liver necrosis (4–6 days old) (hematoxylin-eosin; 110×).

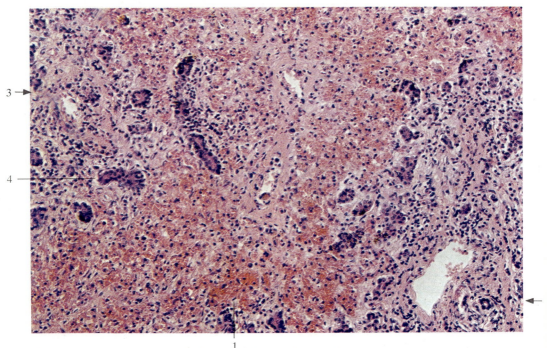

Fig 5–32.—Subacute massive liver cell necrosis (hematoxylin-eosin; 165×).

Massive Liver Necrosis

In **acute massive liver necrosis** (Figs 5–30, 5–31), the whole organ is necrotic. It may be caused by various etiologic agents and may lead to death within a few days. Among causative agents are: 1. *Potent poisons* (e.g., phosphorus, poisonous fungi, arsenic, and others: these cause so-called toxic liver necrosis). In toxic liver injury, a marked degree of fatty degeneration of liver cells is seen at the beginning of the illness. Necrosis develops secondarily and affects the peripheral zones of the lobules preferentially. 2. *Metabolic disturbances* (usually in protein metabolism). 3. *Viral infection.* This causes a *fulminant* or *malignant form of viral hepatitis* and has increased greatly in incidence during the past 20 years (0.5%–5% of cases of acute viral hepatitis). This is so-called acute yellow atrophy of the liver.

The microscopic picture of acute massive liver necrosis varies with the age of the illness and with the time that has elapsed between death and performance of the autopsy. In fresh cases (6–8 hours after death), there is disorganization of the liver cell cords, that is, the individual liver cells have become unattached and appear as separated cellular elements. The cells vary in size, and some are already shrunken (→ 1, Fig 5–30). The cytoplasm is homogeneous and stains more blue than normal (decrease in glycogen content). The nuclei are small and frequently either pyknotic (→) or more faintly stained than normal (karyolysis → 2).

Figure 5–30 shows the liver of a patient who was ill of a clinically obscure "upper abdominal syndrome." At laparotomy, the liver was yellow and slightly reduced in size. An incisional biopsy specimen was taken (see Fig 5–30). Nineteen hours later, the patient died and an autopsy showed the typical picture of massive liver necrosis. Histologically, at autopsy the liver cells were without nuclei and the cytoplasm was faded and finely granular. There was no inflammatory infiltrate.

Acute massive liver necrosis, 4–6 days old (Fig 5–31). If a patient with acute massive liver cell necrosis survives for a few days and then dies, almost complete dissolution of the liver cells occurs. Only homogeneous, eosinophilic material now remains. Intact individual Kupffer cells, however, are still present. The bandlike areas of strongly eosinophilic material (→ 1) still contain anuclear remnants of liver cell cords. The periportal fields (→ 2) are infiltrated with inflammatory cells (lymphocytes) and show occasional proliferated bile ducts (→ 3).

Macroscopic: The liver is small and flaccid and the capsule is wrinkled. The cut surfaces are yellow, yellowish green, or ocher yellow. The liver may weigh as little as 500 gm (normal weight is 1,500 gm). Frequently, crystals of leucine and tyrosine can be seen on the cut surface or on the surface of the capsule (*microscopically:* round granules or crystalline tufts).

Subacute massive liver necrosis (Fig 5–32). When only a part of the liver is affected by the necrosis (e.g., a lobe or a part of a lobe), or if the disease runs a slow course, subacute red atrophy ensues in which cell detritus, the remnants of liver cells, can be seen between the dilated sinusoids (→ 1). Resorption of the necrotic tissue is far advanced and, as as result, the supporting hepatic framework has collapsed and the periportal spaces lie closer to one another (→ 2 and → 3 indicate respectively two portal fields). There are numerous proliferated bile ducts (→ 4) in addition to lymphocytic infiltration. Two central veins can be seen in the middle of the picture between the portal fields. At very low magnification, the increased width of the periportal fields and the proliferation of bile ducts are plainly visible.

Macroscopic: The liver is reduced in size, tough in consistency, and has red and yellow marble-like cut surfaces. The red color is due to hyperemia and pooling of blood. Islands of fatty parenchymous tissue are yellow. This is sometimes called subacute red atrophy of the liver. Duration: 3–8 weeks. Mortality: 40%.

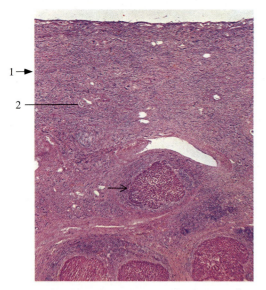

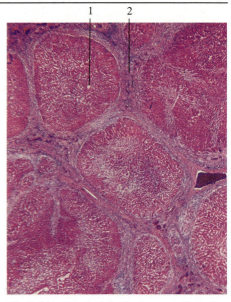

Fig 5–33.—Postnecrotic cirrhosis (hematoxylin-eosin; 15×).

Fig 5–34.—Portal cirrhosis (hematoxylin-eosin; 30×).

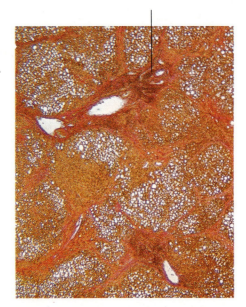

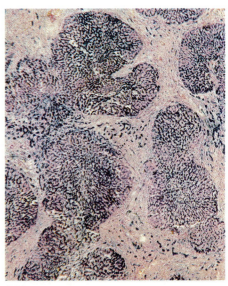

Fig 5–35.—Portal cirrhosis with marked fatty change (van Gieson's stain; 40×).

Fig 5–36.—Pigment cirrhosis (Prussian blue reaction; 30×).

Hepatic Cirrhosis

Postnecrotic cirrhosis (macronodular cirrhosis, Fig 5–33). The results of patchy parenchymatous necrosis are clearly seen in the picture. There is large area of subcapsular tissue destruction (→ 1), the lobular pattern has disappeared, and the periportal zones are collapsed and compressed on one another. This has resulted in large scars that are rich in collagenous tissue and infiltrated with chronic inflammatory cells. The periportal zones also are infiltrated with lymphocytes and, in addition, show bile duct proliferation (→ 2). Islands of remaining parenchyma (→) can still be seen in the scarred tissue. Some of these show central veins or periportal zones, but they no longer have an orderly arrangement, since the necrosis of the lobules has been irregular. The central vein, for example, may lie at the edge of the lobule or the periportal zone may lie in the middle of it *(pseudolobules)*. Other masses of regenerating liver cells have formed nodules with an abnormal architectural arrangement of the liver cell cords.

Macroscopic: The liver is irregularly nodular with depressed large and small scars and coarse nodules (regenerating parenchymal remnants). This type of cirrhosis has large irregular nodules (macronodular cirrhosis): Portal cirrhosis small, uniform, diffuse nodules (diffuse fibrosis). If there is no inflammatory infiltrate, it is called postnecrotic scarring.

Portal or Laennec's cirrhosis (Fig 5–34). Examination with the scanning lens discloses various sized foci of red parenchymatous tissue traversed by bluish red septa of scar tissue. With low-power magnification, the pseudolobules and connective tissue septa connecting the periportal zones can be seen more clearly. Various sized islands of liver tissue with abnormally situated central veins have been formed in this way (→ 1). The connective tissue (→ 2) is infiltrated with cells (lymphocytes, histiocytes, and a few polymorphonuclear leukocytes) and contains proliferated bile ducts. The progress of the cirrhosis is indicated by the degree of involvement of the parenchyma by cellular exudate.

Macroscopic: The liver shows fine, fairly regular nodularity (so-called hobnail liver).

Portal cirrhosis with marked fatty change (Fig 5–35). In this condition, the alteration of architecture develops from the periportal zones just as in portal cirrhosis. With the scanning lens, it is scarcely possible to recognize the tissue as liver. In van Gieson preparations, red connective tissue septa can be seen, while the tissue between has a vacuolated appearance. Low magnification shows lymphocytic infiltration of the periportal fields and bile duct proliferation (→). The liver cells contain round, optically empty droplets (the fat has been dissolved out in the process of preparation). In some places, larger fat cysts have formed (from fusion of fatty cells) (see also Fatty Metamorphosis of the Liver, earlier this chapter). Fatty cirrhosis often develops from fatty hepatitis and occurs frequently in alcoholics. Mallory bodies may be present.

Macroscopic: Large, yellow, finely granular, firm liver. Sixty to seventy percent of all cases of cirrhosis result from malnutrition or toxins (alcohol abuse). Acute viral hepatitis seldom progresses to cirrhosis. The correlation between etiology and the kind of cirrhosis is often uncertain.

Pigment cirrhosis (Fig 5–36). *This occurs mostly as a part of hemochromatosis (bronze diabetes), an illness in which siderin pigment is deposited in the pancreas, spleen, lymph nodes, salivary glands, and many other organs.* Very low magnification of sections treated with Prussian blue shows irregular, bluestained masses of parenchyma traversed by redstained connective tissue septa of various widths. Higher magnification shows granules of blue pigment in the cytoplasm of the liver and Kupffer cells and in the lining cells of proliferated bile ducts.

Macroscopic: The liver is small, firm and brown and shows either fine or coarse granularity.

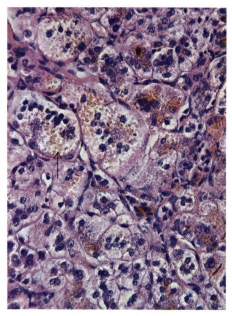

Fig 5–37.—Giant cell hepatitis (hematoxylin-eosin; 300×).

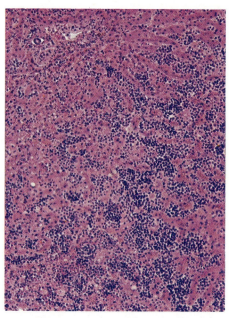

Fig 5–38.—Liver in myeloid leukemia (hematoxylin-eosin; 108×).

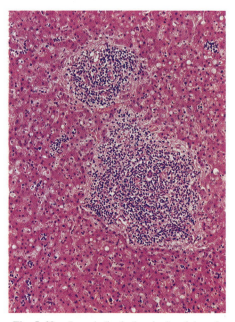

Fig 5–39.—Lymphatic leukemia involving the liver (hematoxylin-eosin; 108×).

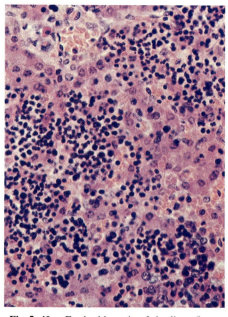

Fig 5–40.—Erythroblastosis of the liver (hematoxylin-eosin; 388×).

Giant cell hepatitis (Fig 5–37). *Giant cell hepatitis of the newborn or infant is the expression of a particular reaction by the infant liver to various noxious stimuli (mainly viral hepatitis, although other causes are possible). The symptoms which are most prominent clinically are those resulting from obstructive jaundice.* Microscopically (Fig 5–37), the normal cords of liver cells are replaced by numerous bizarre multinucleated giant cells (→). They frequently are the width of two or more liver cords. The cytoplasm of these giant cells is vacuolated and often filled with bile pigment (→ in the picture). These giant cells are an expression of faulty regeneration or fusion of cells. Proliferation of connective tissue cells (stellate cells, cells in the periportal fields) is very slight in this phase of the disease. Later, cirrhosis may develop.

Macroscopic: Enlarged liver, with a marked green discoloration.

Chronic myeloid leukemia of liver (Fig 5–35). *In this form of leukemia, there is an unregulated increase in immature early forms of granulocytes in the bone marrow with spillover into the blood. It usually leads to infiltration of the spleen and lymph nodes and to accumulation and increase of myeloblasts, promyelocytes, and myelocytes in the sinusoids of the liver.* The scanning lens reveals preservation of the architecture. Low magnification shows the markedly increased cell content of the sinusoids, most of which are distended and plugged with large, nucleated blood cells (myelocytes with round, vesiculated nuclei and, when more mature, granular cytoplasm; myeloblasts with oval or bean-shaped nuclei). The portal fields are, for the most part, either not involved or only slightly infiltrated with leukemic cells. The liver cells may undergo pressure atrophy and show degenerative changes.

Macroscopic: The liver is enlarged, grayish red, and the lobules are indistinct. In acute leukemia, the periportal zones are especially affected.

Lymphatic leukemia involving liver (Fig 5–39). In contrast to myeloid leukemia, the *periportal zones* in *chronic* lymphatic leukemia are permeated with immature cells (lymphoblasts, lymphocytes), whereas the sinusoids contain only small numbers of nucleated cells. Under low magnification, the markedly increased, blue appearing, spherical periportal zones are at once apparent. Higher magnification shows infiltration of the periportal connective tissue by lymphatic cells, with dense or vesiculated nuclei and scanty cytoplasm.

Macroscopic: The liver is enlarged. The periportal spaces are often visible on the cut surfaces as small, white nodules.

Erythroblastosis of the liver (Fig 5–40). *In this condition, the fetus or newborn infant develops hemolytic anemia as a result of immunization of the mother during pregnancy by fetal red cell antigens inherited from the father. (Most commonly this is Rh incompatibility and less commonly incompatibility of ABO or some other factor.) The anemia results in a marked reactive increase in blood formation in the bone marrow and other hematopoietic tissues of the fetus, including the liver.* Nodules of cellular infiltration are seen in the liver. Under high magnification, these can be identified as foci of intrasinusoidal hematopoiesis. The cells are chiefly erythropoietic (in particular, erythroblasts and normoblasts), with a few from the white cell series and some megakaryocytes. In addition, there is hepatocellular jaundice, since, in most cases, the liver cells are unable to metabolize (conjugate) indirect-reacting bilirubin. Bile casts and siderosis may also be seen.

Macroscopic: A large, red liver. In late stages, there may be generalized edema *(congenital hydrops), anemia* and *severe jaundice* (icterus gravis, often associated with kernicterus).

173

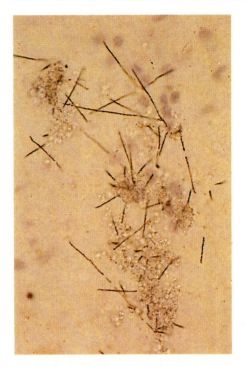

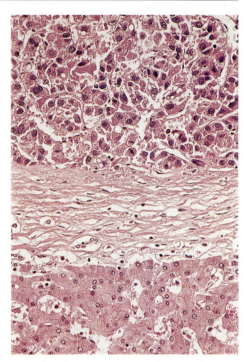

Fig 5–41.—Thorotrast in liver. Autoradiograph of histologic section (200×).

Fig 5–42.—Hepatocellular carcinoma *(top);* normal liver tissue *(bottom)* (hematoxylin-eosin; 150×).

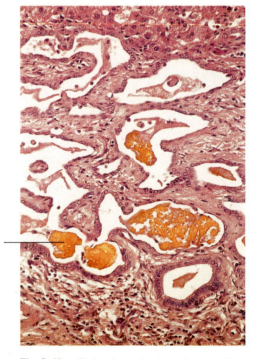

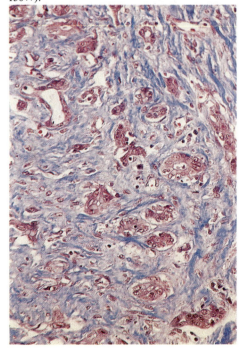

Fig 5–43.—Cholangioma (benign) (hematoxylin-eosin; 150×).

Fig 5–44.—Cholangiocarcinoma (azan stain; 150×).

Thorotrast Storage—Liver Tumors

Effects of thorotrast storage. α-Rays emitted by thorotrast stored by cells over many years produce lesions. Thorotrast, which is a 25% solution of thorium dioxide, is not eliminated after parenteral administration but is stored by reticuloendothelial cells, particularly in the liver. The radiation produces small granulomas in the portal regions, where there are deposits of thorotrasts. Tracks produced by the α-radiation can be made visible by autoradiography (Fig 5–41) and may be as long as 50 μ.

Thorotrast was used as a radiologic contrast medium in the 1930s and 1940s. After a latent period of 10–20 years, lesions were detected in various organs, particularly in the liver, ranging from fibrosis to malignant neoplasms (particularly hemangioendotheliomas).

Hepatocellular carcinoma (malignant hepatoma, hepatocellular type, Figs 5–42, 5–45). This malignant epithelial tumor originates from hepatocytes. It is composed of trabeculae or clusters of cells resembling hepatocytes (Fig 5–42). They frequently have hyperchromatic nuclei, mitotic figures, and indications of cellular atypia. Characteristically, they infiltrate surrounding liver tissue and invade blood vessels. They can produce yellow-brown bile pigment (Fig 5–45).

"Malignant hepatomas" occur most commonly in cirrhotic livers. Among substances carcinogenic in the liver are azo dyes, arsenic, thorotrast, and polyvinylchloride. These carcinogens can cause carcinomas or sarcomas. The latter originate from sinusoidal endothelium and may be termed malignant hemangioendotheliomas.

Cholangioma (benign, Fig 5–43). This is a well-circumscribed, nonencapsulated tumor which arises in portal areas and is composed of cystically dilated bile ducts that contain inspissated bile (→). Most often this tumor is found incidentally at autopsy. When multiple, such tumors have been called microhamartomas (Meyenburg complexes).

Cholangiocarcinoma (Fig 5–44). This type of carcinoma arises from intrahepatic bile ducts. It is composed of neoplastic glands and abundant fibrous stroma. Livers with this tumor may show advanced cholestasis without cirrhosis. Figure 5–44 shows the neoplastic glands, which are lined by cuboidal or cylindrical tumor cells. The azan stain shows the stroma to be rich in collagen.

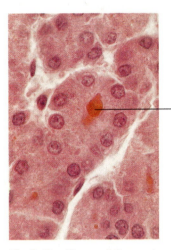

Fig 5–45.—Hepatocellular carcinoma that has produced bile (hematoxylin-eosin; 200×).

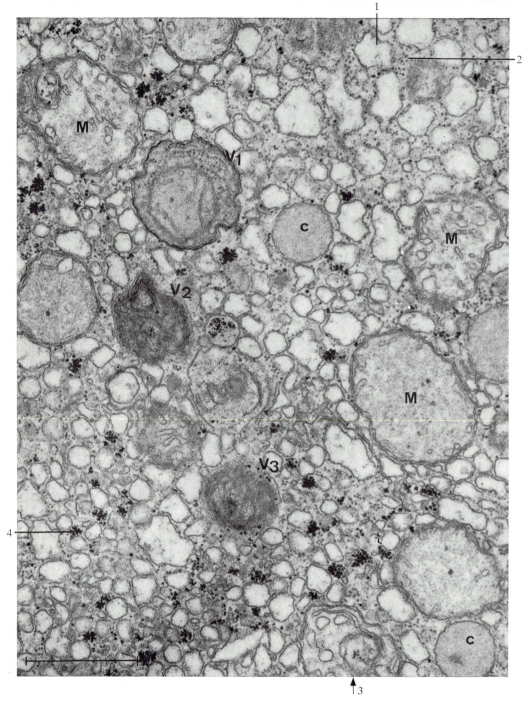

Fig 5–46.—Slight degree of liver cell damage (isolated rat liver perfused with blood containing 10 μg of phalloidin *(Amanita phalloides)* per kilogram of body weight, 30 min.). There is vacuolar dilation of the smooth and rough endoplasmic reticulum (→ 1) and there are ribosomes without membranes (→ 2). There are also autolysosomes (autophagocytotic vacuoles) containing mitochondria (V_1; see also p. 176) and myelin figures (V_2 and V_3) which are presumably a manifestation of the digestion of membranes in these lysosomes. →3: Golgi apparatus; *M*, mitochondria; *C*, peroxisome; → 4: glycogen (32,000 ×). (Miller)

Electron Microscopy of Liver Injury

The electron microscopic changes of the liver cell organelles are rather uniform and, for the most part, nonspecific. Theoretically, all the changes described in the legend to Figure 5–46 may occur. In acute toxic injury (alcohol, carbon tetrachloride, partial hepatectomy, see Fig 5–48) or anoxia, the mitochondria are swollen (cloudy swelling) and the endoplasmic reticulum becomes vacuolated (hydropic degeneration). Glycogen stores disappear, the rough endoplasmic reticulum becomes disorganized and frequently loses its ribosomes (reduction of protein synthesis), and, finally, the cell membranes become fragmented, vacuolated, and are destroyed (see Figs 5–54, 5–55). The lysosomes contain parts of the cellular organelles (Fig 5–47). Similar pictures are seen in acute viral hepatitis, in which hyaline bodies, also called Councilman bodies (see Fig 5–54), appear, i.e., necrotic, shrunken liver cells. Chronic liver toxicity entails primarily focal or diffuse proliferation of the smooth endoplasmic reticulum (intensification of the detoxification process). In chronic *alcoholic intoxication*, focal filamentous masses may be seen (*Mallory bodies*, alcoholic hyalin). Terminally, the endoplasmic reticulum may be entirely disrupted. The smooth endoplasmic reticulum may also appear to form myelin-like whorls (fingerprints). Fat droplets may be seen either in acute or chronic liver damage. In chronic hepatitis, there is also proliferation of collagen fibers in the space of Disse, and a basement membrane may form. In intrahepatic cholestasis (hepatitis, toxic) and extrahepatic cholestasis the bile canaliculi are dilated, the microvilli are swollen at first, then disappear, and the pericanalicular cytoplasm has a denser appearance. Lysosomes, including pericanalicular dense bodies, increase in number and are spread throughout the cytoplasm (activation of acid phosphatase). In addition, bile droplets can be seen in the cytoplasm. Determination of the path of bile reflux into the bloodstream (whether between or through hepatic cells) has not been successful even with the electron microscope. In hepatic cirrhosis, nonspecific changes again are seen (enlargement and clumping of mitochondria, myelin-like degeneration, vacuoles in the endoplasmic reticulum, proliferation of collagen fibers around the liver cells, autophagolysosomes, localized cell destruction, fat deposition, localized glycogen aggregation, pigmentation, bile tubule proliferation, and hemosiderin).

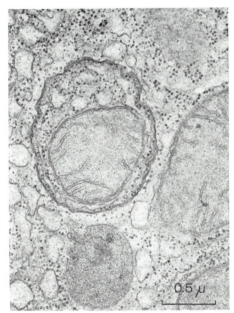

Fig 5–47.—Autophagolysosome, site of focal degradation in a liver cell of a rat. Treatment as in Figure 5–46. Within the surrounding membrane there is a well-preserved mitochondrion and parts of the rough endoplasmic reticulum (ribosomes, membranes) (45,000×). (Courtesy of Miller.)

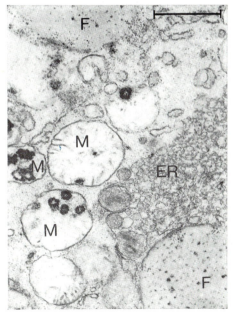

Fig 5–48.—Acute carbon tetrachloride poisoning (after 24 hours, in mouse liver). Note focal proliferation of the smooth endoplasmic reticulum (ER), fat droplets (F), as well as swollen mitochondria with round, black-appearing matrix aggrergates, which are calcium deposits (35,000×). (Hübner)

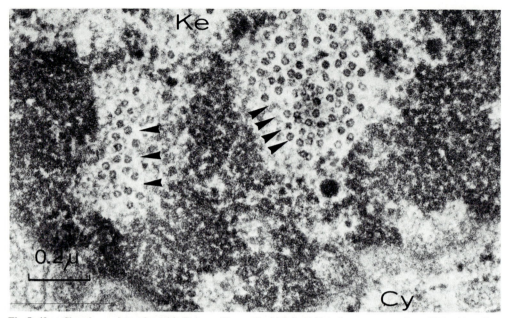

Fig 5–49.—Chronic persistent hepatitis B in an 11-month-old infant. Note hepatocyte nucleus *(KE)* with collections of core antigen particles (HBcAg, *arrows*) of hepatitis B virus.

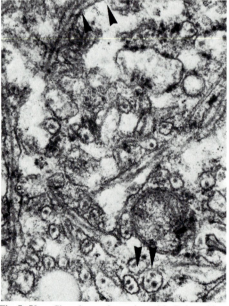

Fig 5–50.—Chronic persistent hepatitis B in a 38-year-old kidney transplant recipient. Note the smooth endoplasmic reticulum *(arrows)* of a hepatocyte with longitudinal and cross sections of HB surface antigen (44,000×). (Kistler)

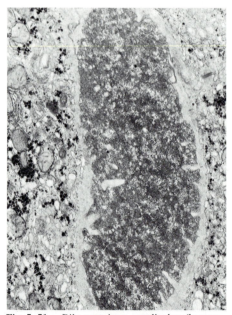

Fig 5–51.—Bile cast in a canaliculus (human, viral hepatitis). There are no microvilli. The lumen is filled with bile pigment (12,000×). (Biava, 1964)

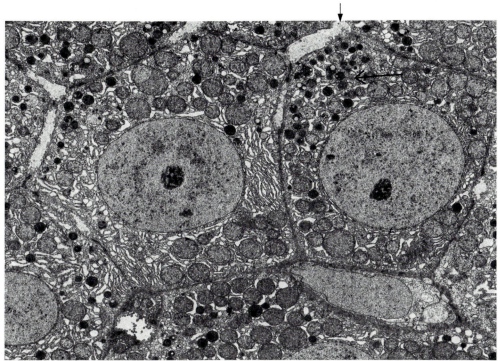

Fig 5–52.—Markedly atrophied liver cells with scanty cytoplasm, tightly packed organelles, and numerous lysosomes (→) in the region of the bile capillaries (*arrow* above). Glycogen is absent (5,000 ×).

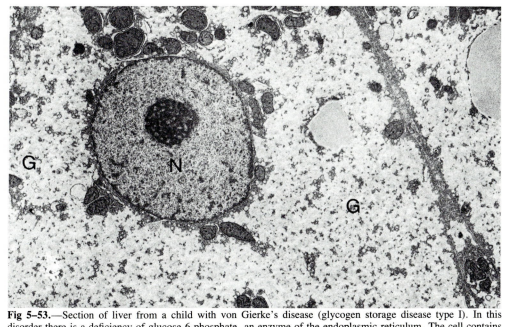

Fig 5–53.—Section of liver from a child with von Gierke's disease (glycogen storage disease type I). In this disorder there is a deficiency of glucose-6-phosphate, an enzyme of the endoplasmic reticulum. The cell contains practically only glycogen and only rudimentary organelles. *N,* nucleus; *G,* glycogen (5,500 ×). (Spycher)

179

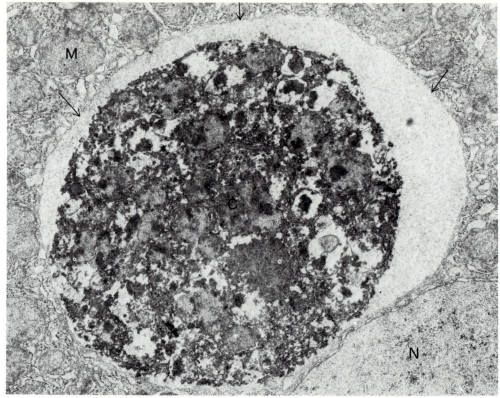

Fig 5–54.—Hyaline (acidophile) body in viral hepatitis. *C,* so-called Councilman body. The necrotic, rounded, and shrunken liver cell contains fragments of organelles and appears to have been engulfed by a hepatocyte. *Arrows* indicate lysosomal membrane. *N,* nucleus; *M,* mitochondria of liver cell (35,000 ×).

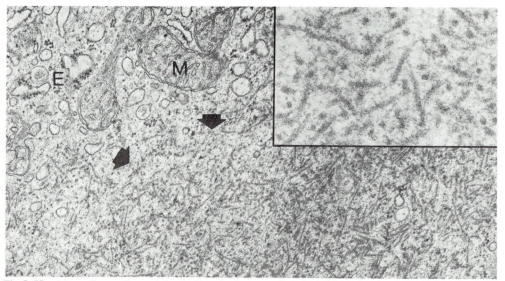

Fig 5–55.—Mouse liver cell containing Mallory bodies, so-called alcoholic hyalin (administration of griseofulvin). Notice the nodular arrangement of the microfilaments (→ and *inset*). This is probably a pathologic protein. *M,* mitochondria; *E,* endoplasmic reticulum (22,000 ×; *inset,* 39,000 ×). (Denk)

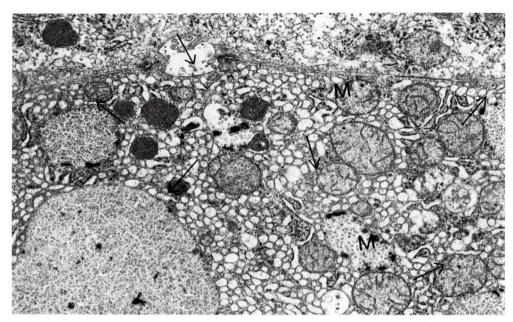

Fig 5–56.—Section of a liver cell from a child with Pompe's disease (glycogen storage disease type II). In this disorder there is a deficiency of the lysosomal enzyme α-1,4-glycosidase. There are gigantic storage vacuoles packed with glycogen *(arrow)*. *M,* mitochondria (1,000×). (Spycher)

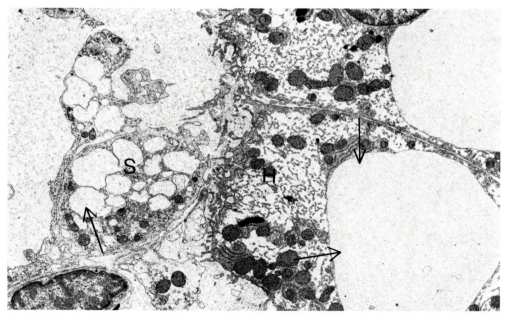

Fig 5–57.—Section of parts of liver cells from a child with GM-1 gangliosidosis, absence of lysosomal enzyme β-galactosidase. Large storage vacuoles filled with GM-1 ganglioside (→) are present in the cytoplasm of the hepatocytes *(H)* and Kupffer cells *(S)* (5,300×). (Spycher)

181

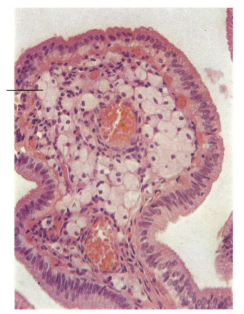

Fig 5–58.—Cholesterolosis of the gallbladder (hematoxylin-eosin; 350×).

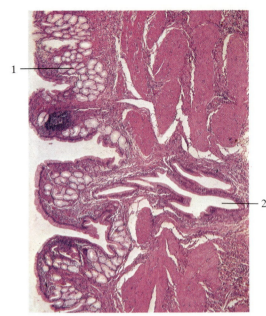

Fig 5–59.—Chronic hypertrophic cholecystitis (hematoxylin-eosin; 80×).

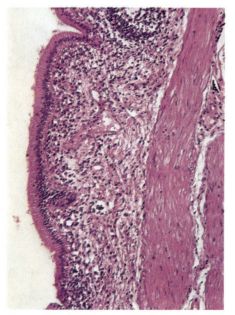

Fig 5–60.—Chronic atrophic cholecystitis (hematoxylin-eosin; 100×).

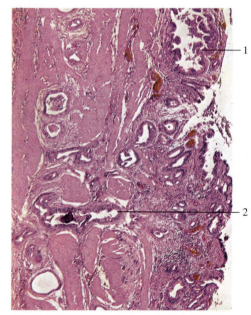

Fig 5–61.—Adenocarcinoma of the gallbladder (hematoxylin-eosin; 60×).

Gallbladder Disease

Introduction: The gallbladder is a hollow, thin walled organ lined with mucous membrane and a net-like layer of smooth muscle. The mucosa consists of delicate stromal folds covered on the surface with a single layer of cylindrical epithelium. Occasional aberrant bile ducts *(Luschk's crypts)* occur in the outer portions of the gallbladder wall.

Cholesterolosis of the gallbladder (Fig 5–58). *This is a metabolic disorder (localized lipidosis) and manifests histologically by the appearance of pseudoxanthoma cells in the mucosal folds.* Figure 5–58 shows the marked enlargement of the distended tips of a mucosal fold that is covered by columnar epithelium. The underlying subepithelial stroma is thick and contains large cells with central nuclei and finely granular or vacuolated cytoplasm. Macrophages (→) filled with cholesterin and cholesterin esters (dissolved during the preparatory process of paraffin embedding).

Cholesterosis (''strawberry'' gallbladder) is found in 5%–40% of resected gallbladders. It is particularly common in women 40–70 years old. Cholesterosis has few if any clinical manifestations.

Cholecystitis (Figs 5–59, 5–60) *in most cases is a chronic, recurrent, and nonspecific inflammation of the gallbladder.* Acute inflammations characteristically show mural necrosis, hemorrhage, diffuse inflammation of the gallbladder wall (severe inflammations may be phlegmonous or gangrenous), and empyema. In chronic inflammation the mucosa may become thick (**chronic hypertrophic cholecystitis,** Fig 5–59) and the mucosal folds broad because of lymphocytic infiltration, fibrosis, and scar tissue. The surface epithelium shows transformation to mucous glands reminiscent of *Brunner's glands (intestinal metaplasia → 1).* Increased luminal pressure in the gallbladder causes diverticulum-like mucosal outpouchings *(Rokitansky-Aschoff sinuses → 2).* They appear as empty spaces lined with columnar epithelium and extend through the muscularis. In long-standing chronic cholecystitis scarring and flattening of the mucosal folds are prominent (**chronic atrophic cholecystitis,** Fig 5–60). Finally, the gallbladder wall may become completely fibrotic and rigid *(porcelain gallbladder).*

Chronic cholecystitis occurs frequently in elderly obese women and in 90% of cases is accompanied by cholelithiasis. In the early stages, chronic cholecystitis is usually abacterial and results from interference with the blood supply (e.g., impacted cystic stone). Bacterial infection develops later by way of the bile ducts, bloodstream, or lymphatics.

Carcinoma of the gallbladder (Fig 5–61) *is a malignant epithelial tumor arising from the mucosa and occurs almost exclusively in a scarred gallbladder. Histologically it may be an undifferentiated carcinoma, a well-differentiated adenocarcinoma, or an adenoacanthoma (carcinoma with a mixture of squamous and glandular epithelium).* Figure 5–61 shows the darker staining strands of carcinoma cells replacing mucosa (→ 1) and infiltrating deeply into the wall (→ 2).

Gallbladder carcinomas form about 1.5% of all malignant tumors. They are diagnosed in nearly 4% of resected gallbladders. Macroscopically they are either diffusely infiltrating or nodulopapillary.

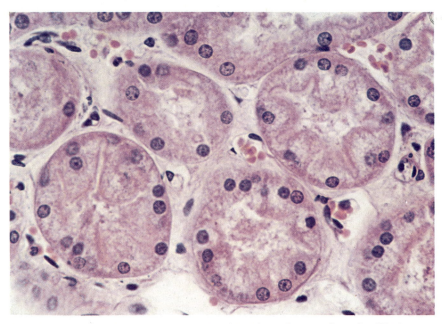

Fig 6–1.—Cloudy swelling of proximal tubules of the kidney (hematoxylin-eosin; 600×).

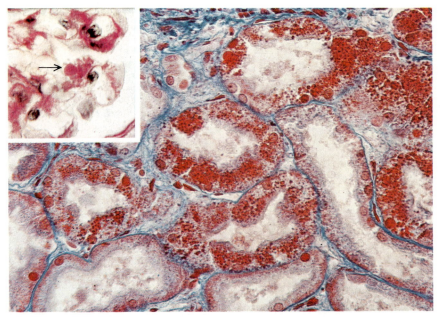

Fig 6–2.—Hyalin droplets in proximal tubules (reabsorbed protein in phagolysosomes) (azan stain; 456×). *Inset:* Hyalin droplets in the investing epithelium of a glomerulus (rat); experimental glomerulonephritis (PAS; about 500×).

6. Kidney

Histologic examination of kidney sections should proceed according to the following guidelines. Evaluation of the *thickness of cortex and medulla* in the specimen. *Alterations of vessels:* especially at the corticomedullary junction and in the afferent arterioles. *Glomeruli:* cellularity, the condition of the basement membrane, capsular lining epithelium, focal or diffuse necrosis of the glomerulus. *Tubules:* size of lumen, size of cells, cytoplasmic deposits, segments affected. *Interstitium:* cellular and fibrous content.

Cloudy swelling (Fig 6–1). *This is a disturbance of the ionic milieu of the cell that entails uptake of water and sodium with concomitant loss of potassium from the cells, which then begin to swell.* The swelling affects mitochondria particularly. The resulting increase in the size of particulate matter leads to increased dispersion of light and, thereby, to a Tyndall effect, i.e., to cloudiness. Figure 6–1 shows proximal tubular epithelium, the cytoplasm of which is filled with fine, pale droplets (swollen mitochondria), giving rise to a finely honeycombed appearance. Fine, granular, coagulated protein material is also seen in the narrowed lumina of the tubules. The same changes occur also in postmortem specimens and are differentiated only with difficulty from antemortem cloudy swelling. If the tissue sections are treated with dilute acetic acid, the contents of the mitochondria precipitate on the mitochondrial membrane, and the cytoplasm again becomes clear.

Macroscopic: Enlarged, soft organ with dull cut surfaces. The parenchyma bulges above the cut surface. Cloudy swelling occurs, especially with toxic injury (e.g., diphtheria).

In *hydropic degeneration,* the process is similar—free water accumulates in the cells and forms vacuolar spaces in mitochondria, endoplasmic reticulum, and ground substance. Microscopically, the cytoplasm is filled with large and small optically empty vacuoles. In some instances, perinuclear halos also appear. Hydropic degeneration is seen particularly in cases of acute anoxia, toxic inhibition of enzymes (e.g., cyanide poisoning), substrate depletion, or inhibition of oxidative phosphorylation (e.g., barbiturate poisoning). All these conditions cause deficiency of ATP with resulting failure of the sodium pump to work.

Hyalin droplet accumulation (Fig 6–2 and Fig 5, section on General Pathology, and accompanying text). *Protein droplets appear in the cytoplasm of proximal tubular epithelial cells due to tubular reabsorption, e.g., in glomerulonephritis.* Histologically, medium magnification reveals swelling of the proximal tubular cells due to infiltration of deep red-staining and somewhat refractile protein droplets. The lumen contains hyalin casts or granular precipitates of protein. At this stage, single epithelial cells, filled with protein-containing droplets, are also found in the lumen.

In rare cases, hyalin droplet accumulation also involves the epithelial cells of glomerular loops, which are, of course, related morphologically to the tubular epithelium. The inset in Figure 6–2 shows experimental glomerulonephritis in a rat in which there is marked thickening of the basement membrane and proliferation of epithelial and endothelial cells. The arrow points to an epithelial cell with round hyalin droplets in the cytoplasm.

Macroscopic: Enlarged, pale grayish white kidneys (large, white kidney), e.g., in amyloidosis or myeloma (myeloma nephrosis).

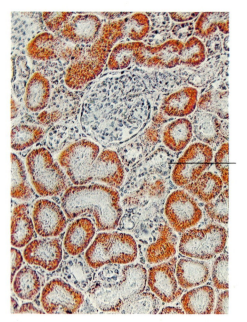

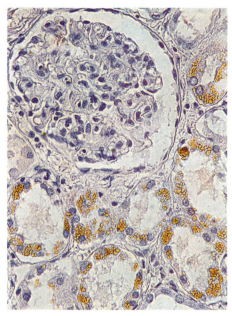

Fig 6–3.—Fatty degeneration of the proximal tubules of the cortex (Sudan-hematoxylin; 160×).

Fig 6–4.—Cholemic (bile) nephrosis (hematoxylin; 459×).

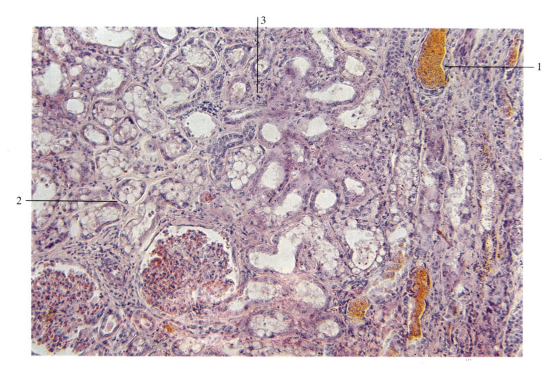

Fig. 6–5.—Hypoxic nephrosis with hypopotassemia (hematoxylin-eosin; 111×).

Noninflammatory Kidney Disease (Nephrosis)

Formerly the term "nephrosis" was used to describe degenerative changes in the renal tubules in inflammatory kidney disease. This limited definition is no longer tenable. At the present time the following are recognized. (1) Clinically: nephrotic syndrome: kidney disease with proteinuria, hypoalbuminemia, hyperlipemia, and generalized edema. Causes: chiefly glomerulonephritis, amyloidosis, diabetic glomerulosclerosis, mercury or other poisons. (2) Pathologically: noninflammatory kidney disease which may or may not be accompanied by the nephrotic syndrome, and in which there are lesions in either the glomeruli (glomerulonephrosis, e.g., Kimmelstiel-Wilson disease, amyloid disease) or the tubules (tubular nephrosis, e.g., cholemic nephrosis).

Fatty degeneration of proximal of the cortex (Fig 6–3). *Deposition of neutral fats and lipids in the tubular epithelial cells can result either from resorption by the tubular cells (e.g., lipoid nephrosis associated with diabetes), from hypoxia, or from toxic injury.* The figure shows fatty changes resulting from the hypoxia of anemia. Scanning the section at low magnification reveals accumulation of the Sudan stain in the cortex. The medullary border is sharply delineated, and with intermediate magnification (Fig 6–3) the loops of Henle are seen to be mostly spared. Fine lipid droplets are deposited in the epithelial cells of the proximal convoluted tubules of the cortex. The lipid droplets either lie in the basal portion of the cell or completely fill it. The cells are swollen. The tubular lumen is narrowed. The portions of the distal tubules next to the glomeruli (→) are not involved.

Lipid nephrosis (see Fig 6–13), when it occurs as an independent disease, is also characterized by marked fatty changes of the tubular system with deposition of neutral fats and lipids (doubly refractile). In addition, fatty deposits are found in the interstitium.

Macroscopic: The kidney is slightly enlarged and the cortex is yellow.

Bile, or cholemic, nephrosis (Fig 6–4) *signifies degenerative changes and deposition of bile pigments in the proximal tubular epithelial cells during the course of jaundice (reabsorption, see Fig 6–12).* Hematoxylin stain brings out very well the yellow to green color of the bile pigment. Medium magnification reveals granular deposits of bile pigment in the cytoplasm of the proximal tubular epithelium. In addition, there are degenerative changes such as cloudy swelling and slight fatty changes. Occasional shed cells can also be found in the lumina of the tubules. Bile-stained hyaline casts are present in the collecting ducts. The glomeruli are not affected.

Macroscopic: Slightly enlarged kidney, green to yellowish brown cortex and medulla.

Hypoxic nephrosis with hypokalemia (Fig 6–5). *(Synonyms: hemoglobinuric nephrosis, myoglobinuric nephrosis, crush kidney, shock kidney in trauma, lower nephron nephrosis.) This is an acute process that may be caused by various injurious agents (trauma, poisons) and is characterized by the onset of severe shock, hemolysis or myolysis, and degeneration and necrosis of renal tubules. The term vascular-tubular syndrome describes the two essential components: vascular collapse (disturbance of perfusion) and toxic tubular degeneration.* Microscopically, the most striking finding is the presence of proteinaceous casts containing hemoglobin or myoglobin (brown casts in the collecting ducts, → 1) in the distal tubules, Henle's loops, and collecting ducts. Proximal convoluted tubules may show focal necrosis. In addition, degenerative changes of the tubular epithelium may be seen (cloudy swelling, fatty degeneration). If there is an accompanying hypokalemia (polyuric phase of the shock kidney) cystic dilation of the base of the tubular epithelial cells (proximal) develops, which microscopically gives the impression of vacuolar degeneration (→ 2). Later, tubular rhexis develops (rupture of kidney tubules). The epithelium of the proximal tubules in Figure 6–5 is for the most part flattened (a sign of insufficiency). The interstitial tissues are swollen by edema (→ 3). The glomeruli are hyperemic and have wide basement membranes.

Macroscopic: Enlarged kidneys, dirty grayish brown color.

187

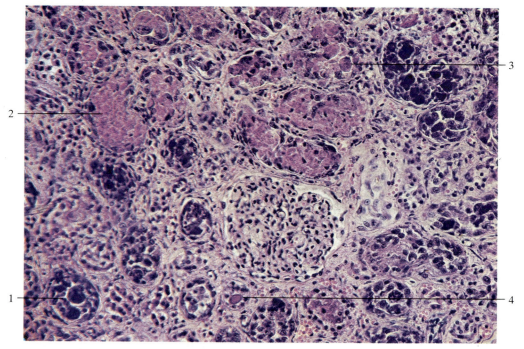

Fig 6–6.—Mercuric bichloride nephrosis (hematoxylin-eosin; 200×).

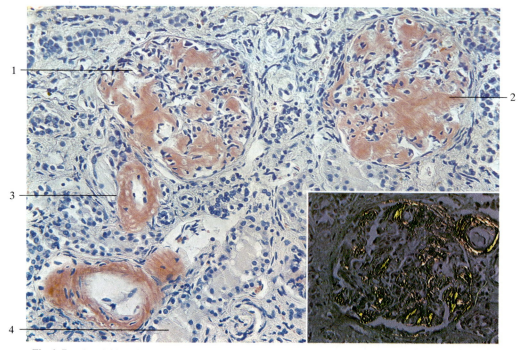

Fig 6–7.—Amyloid nephrosis (Congo red–hematoxylin; 200×). *Inset:* Amyloid under polarized light.

Mercuric bichloride nephrosis (Fig 6–6). *Corrosive mercuric bichloride produces a marked, necrotizing nephrosis, with secondary calcification of necrotic tubular cells.* It involves particularly the proximal convoluted tubules. There is considerable controversy concerning the pathogenesis and site of action of the mercury, but, if death occurs during the acute phase, necrosis of the proximal convoluted tubules is seen. Within a few days, deposits of calcium can be found in the necrotic areas (matrix aggregates). Regeneration of tubules follows survival of the acute phase, as evidenced by the marked proliferation of flat epithelial cells, which may be the predominant feature of the microscopic picture.

Microscopic examination of the cortex in the acute and subacute stages reveals necrotic red-staining tubules and dark blue-staining deposits of calcium. Medium magnification (Fig 6–6) shows irregular blue calcium deposits of varying size as well as calcified epithelial cells that have been partly shed into the lumen (→ 1), with the result that cross sections of the tubule may appear completely filled. In other areas, tubules are filled with granular, eosinophilic masses (→ 2). Here, the epithelium is necrotic and, together with the shed epithelial cells (→ 3) and protein casts, forms a homogeneous concrement. Other segments of the tubules also contain casts (distal tubule, → 4). The interstitium is edematous. The glomeruli are bloodless, normally cellular, and have delicate basement membranes.

Macroscopic: Enlarged, soft kidney with dull red or grayish white external and cut surfaces.

Amyloid nephrosis (Fig 6–7). *This is a glomerulonephrosis due to amyloidosis (spleen, liver, adrenal, and intestine, etc., are also involved) and is manifested by deposition of abnormal protein, amyloid, in the glomeruli and afferent arterioles.*

Examination of a hematoxylin-eosin–stained section with a scanning lens reveals large, homogeneous, eosinophilic, hyalinized cortical glomeruli. Medium magnification shows arterioles with homogeneous, hyalinized walls. The hyaline protein material stains readily with Congo red: the red stain is specific for amyloid. The amyloid accumulation appears first as a fine red streak lying between the basement membrane and the endothelium of the glomeruli (→ 1). With increasing deposition, the glomerular loop thickens and the lumen is narrowed. As a result, the loops take on a homogeneous, anuclear appearance. Adjacent affected loops may merge to produce a uniformly red area (→ 2). The end stage is an obliterated glomerulus. The same process occurs in the media of the arcuate arteries and afferent arterioles (→ 3). The muscle cells deteriorate, and the media appears as a smooth red ring. Secondarily, amyloid is deposited in the pericapillary interstitial tissues and the tubular basement membranes. Many of the proximal convoluted tubules are dilated and contain casts which are Congo red negative (→ 4). Amyloid stained with Congo red is doubly refractive in polarized light (Fig 6–7, inset). Hyaline droplet accumulation occurs frequently (compare Figs 6–13 and 6–14). The amyloid kidney often becomes contracted due to the glomerular involvement and the subsequent atrophy of the tubular system and the proliferation of interstitial connective tissue.

Macroscopic: The kidney is large, firm, white, and waxy. The cut surface is dry and translucent; the medulla is usually reddish and the line of demarcation from the swollen cortex is preserved. The contracted amyloid kidney is small and gnarled.

189

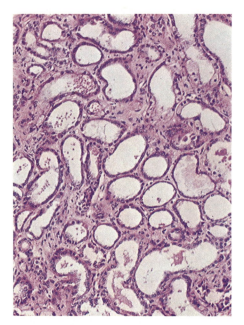

Fig 6–8.—Shock kidney with dilated tubules (hematoxylin-eosin).

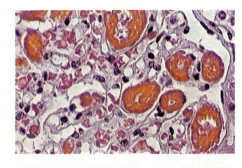

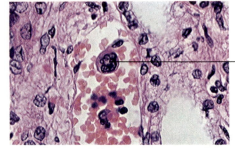

Fig 6–9.—Top, fibrin and platelet thrombi in glomerular capillaries (Goldner stain). Bottom, megakaryocyte inside interstitial capillary (hematoxylin-eosin).

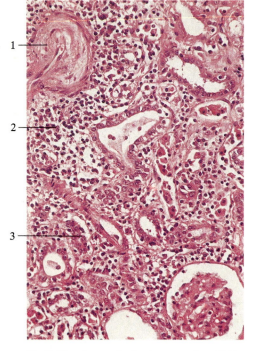

Fig 6–10.—Acute rejection in a transplanted kidney (hematoxylin-eosin; 150×).

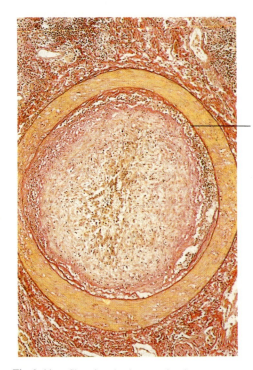

Fig 6–11.—Chronic rejection reaction in a transplanted kidney (elastica–van Gieson's stain; 150×).

Shock Kidney—Rejection Reaction in Transplanted Kidney

Shock kidney (Figs 6–8, 6–9). In various forms of shock (after severe trauma, burns, myocardial infarction, hemorrhage, in eclampsia, and in endotoxin shock) there are structural changes in the kidneys. These are consequences of diminished vascular perfusion, but accumulation of immature blood cells in renal capillaries may also be noted. Ectasia (widening) of renal tubules occurs frequently and is usually inconspicuous (Fig 6–8). Microscopically, there is dilation of tubules that are lined by flattened epithelial cells and whose lumina are empty. Furthermore, one sees interstitial edema with scattered infiltration of lymphocytes.

Intravascular coagulation (Fig 6–9, top) occurs mainly in endotoxin shock. The Goldner stain shows orange-red fibrin and platelet thrombi in capillary lumina, especially those of glomeruli. This particular lesion is inconspicuous in hemorrhagic shock or in shock associated with myocardial infarction. Another histologic change is the presence of immature blood cells in the lumina of capillaries at the corticomedullary junctions (Fig 6–9, bottom). The arrow in Figure 6–9 indicates a megakaryocyte.

Hyaline fibrin and **platelet thrombi** are signs of disseminated intravascular coagulation. This leads to plugging of blood vessels and to "consumption coagulopathy." Atypical fibrin polymers may be formed in the lumina of medium-sized veins (hyaline spheres, "shock bodies").

Rejection reaction in transplanted kidney (Figs 6–10, 6–11). Rejection reactions result from immunologic differences between the transplanted organ and the recipient. Distinctions are made on the basis of the rapidity of the immune reactions: *hyperacute reaction, 24–48 hours after transplantation; acute reaction,* days after transplantation; *chronic reaction;* rejection reaction evolving during a period of several weeks.

Acute rejection reaction (Fig 6–10). Exudative inflammation and necrosis predominate. There is interstitial edema with lymphocytic infiltration (→ 2), also edema in the intima of arterioles (→ 1), as well as scattered necrosis of tubular epithelial cells (detached cells with pyknotic nuclei and eosinophilic cytoplasm, → 3).

Chronic rejection reaction (Fig 6–11). Proliferative lesions in the medium-sized renal arteries are conspicuous, principally proliferation of intimal connective tissue with abundant collagen. There is progressive closure of the vascular lumen. In contrast to the early acute lesions, the chronic lesions are irreversible. The elastica–van Gieson's stain shows the intimal proliferation especially well (Fig 6–11). Note the yellow medial smooth muscle and the dark brown internal elastica (→) that delimits the original border of the lumen.

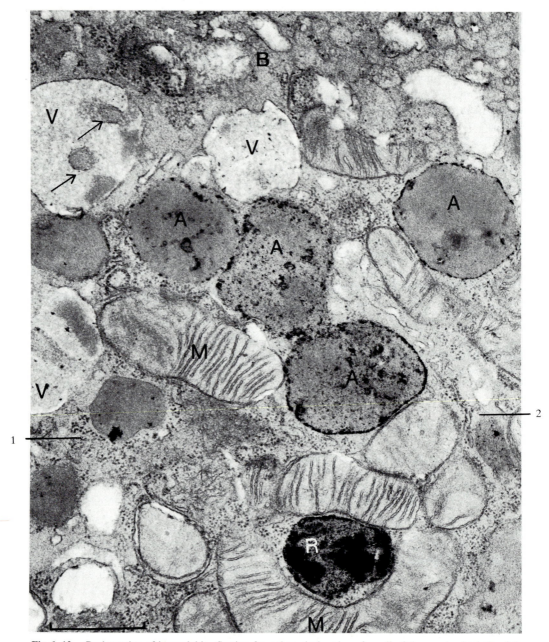

Fig 6–12.—Reabsorption of hemoglobin. Section from the apical region of a cell of the proximal tubule of the kidney (mouse, 1 hour after intraperitoneal injection of ox hemoglobin). *B,* lower margin of brush border. All stages of the uptake and concentration of the hemoglobin can be followed in this picture from the top to the bottom. The vacuoles *(V)* contain, in addition to granular protein, hemoglobin droplets (→). In the absorption droplets *(A)* the hemoglobin is concentrated into bodies limited by a single membrane. The black particles are precipitates of lead phosphate (= histochemical reaction for acid phosphatase). These organelles can thus be identified as lysosomes. *R,* residual body with strong acid phosphatase activity and marked concentration of hemoglobin; *M,* mitochondria; → 1, ribosomes and polysomes; → 2, rough endoplasmic reticulum (24,000×). (Miller et al.)

Fine Structure of Tubular Reabsorption

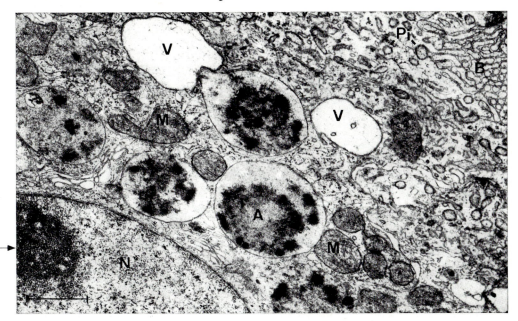

Fig 6–13.—Protein reabsorption droplets in the proximal tubules in protein nephrosis in man. Part of a tubular epithelial cell with a section of the brush border *(B)*. There are pinocytotic vesicles *(Pi)* near the brush border. These deliver absorbed protein to vacuoles *(V)*. The protein reabsorption droplets *(A)* develop from these. *M*, mitochondria; *N*, nucleus; →, nucleolus (16,000×). (Thoenes)

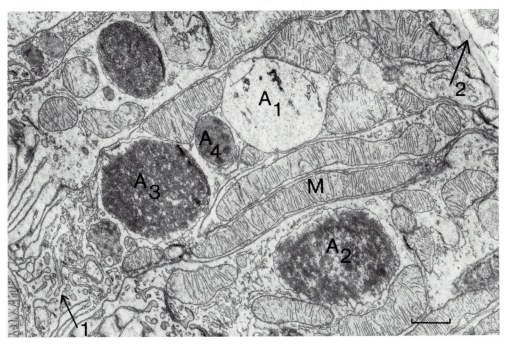

Fig 6–14.—Protein reabsorption droplets (protein storage phagoosomes) in the proximal renal tubular epithelium in lead poisoning of rat following several intraperitoneal injections of lead acetate (cumulative dose, 50 mg). Note large bodies bounded by a single membrane and with a fine granularity (A_1) as well as contents of increased electron density $(A_2–A_4)$. *M*, mitochondria. There are numerous pinocytotic vacuoles at the base of the brush border (→ 1). → 2, peritubular basement membrane (10,500×). (Dr. Totovic)

Vascular Disorders of the Kidney

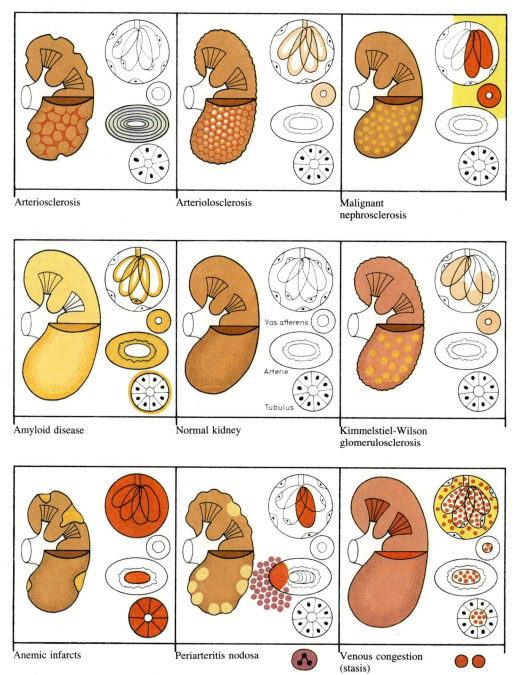

Fig 6–15.—Schematic representation of the gross and microscopic changes encountered in vascular disorders of the kidney.

Vascular Renal Disorders

Vascular diseases in the kidney (Fig 6–15) involve either large arteries or the arterioles. The glomeruli almost always become involved secondarily, and ultimately the tubules.

Arteriosclerosis (see Fig 6–16) may uncommonly involve the main *renal arteries* at the junction with the aorta or just beyond (fibromuscular dysplasia), and the resulting obstruction leads to ischemia of the kidney and renal hypertension *(Goldblatt mechanism)*. Involvement of arteries of the interlobular and arcuate type is manifested by concentric fibrosis and elastosis which narrows the lumen. The severity of the glomerular lesion (hyaline degeneration) depends on the extent of the arterial sclerosis.

Macroscopic: The surface is red and shows retracted small scars.

Arteriolosclerosis or arteriolar nephrosclerosis (see Fig 6–18) usually shows hyalinization of *afferent arterioles* with narrowing of the lumina. Decreased vascular perfusion leads to hyalinized thickening of the capillary loops, terminating in complete obliteration of the glomerulus. The hyalin is probably formed by cells of the mesangium (mesangial matrix, see Glomerulonephritis, later this chapter). Marked involvement leads to contraction of the kidney: *red granular atrophy (primary contracted kidney)*. Arteriosclerosis and arteriolosclerosis frequently occur together (arterio-arteriolonephrosclerosis).

Macroscopic: Fine granularity of the surface with small reddish scars, resulting eventually in marked shrinkage of the entire organ, notably the cortex (primary contracted kidney, red granular atrophy). When combined with arteriosclerosis, there also are large, red scars.

Malignant nephrosclerosis (see discussion later this chapter) is characterized by fibrinoid necrosis of the walls of small arteries, afferent arterioles, and glomerular loops. It may be superimposed on preexisting arteriolar nephrosclerosis or arise de novo in unaffected vessels.

Amyloidosis cannot rightly be considered a vascular renal disorder, but it is considered here so as to allow comparison with the gross and histologic pictures of other renal disorders.

Kimmelstiel-Wilson glomerulosclerosis (see discussion later this chapter) represents a special sort of arteriolar nephrosclerosis. It goes hand in hand with hyalinization of the afferent and efferent arterioles, as well as with diffuse hyaline thickening of the capillary loops, and gives rise to characteristic hyaline nodules in the glomerular loops. The gross appearance usually resembles arteriolar nephrosclerosis. Often there is also fatty degeneration of tubules giving a variegated appearance (red and yellow spots).

An **anemic infarct** most commonly results from embolic or thrombotic occlusion of an artery. There is a wedge-shaped, sharply demarcated, pale yellow area of necrosis that becomes depressed, contracted and white with increasing scar formation.

The acute stage of **periarteritis nodosa** (Figs 2–8, 2–10, p. 80) in the kidney shows a yellowish gray mottled pattern. Eventually, fine, speckled, contracted scars develop (older areas of necrosis). There is fibrinoid necrosis of the arteries, with granulomatous inflammation and scarring.

The **congested kidney** is enlarged, dusky red, particularly in the medulla, and the surface veins are spider-like. The glomeruli are congested and there are protein deposits in Bowman's space. In addition, there is interstitial edema.

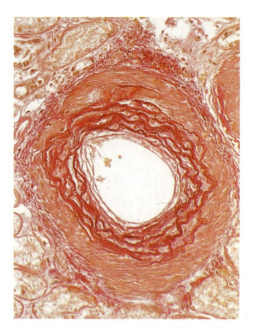

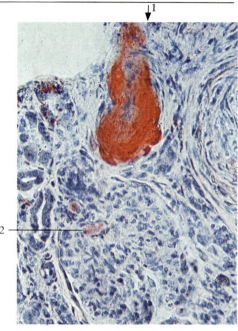

Fig 6–16.—Arteriosclerosis of the kidney (elastica–van Gieson's stains; 100×).

Fig 6–17.—Arteriolar nephrosclerosis (Sudan-hematoxylin; 380×).

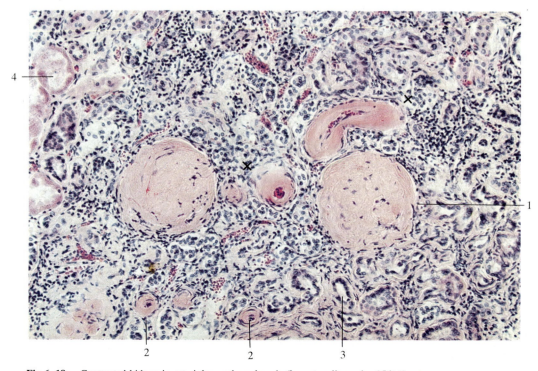

Fig 6–18.—Contracted kidney in arteriolar nephrosclerosis (hematoxylin-eosin; 156×).

Arteriosclerosis of the kidney (Fig 6–16). Histologically, this is actually the same process that we observed in arteriosclerosis in the heart vessels (see Coronary Arteriosclerosis, chap. 2), although the lesion is not crescentshaped, but rather has a concentric configuration. At first glance, one notices the very thick walls of the larger arteries, especially in the medulla. Medium magnification reveals hyperplastic proliferation of the elastica in the intima. This is due not only to multiplication and splitting of elastic fibers (black in the section) but also to an increase of acellular fibrous tissue (sclerosis), all of which lead to marked narrowing of the lumen. Glomeruli are partially hyalinized and the corresponding tubules have atrophied, with interstitial fibrosis and lymphocytic infiltration. Local hyalinization of several glomeruli with concomitant atrophy of tubules leads to interstitial fibrosis and formation of contracted surface scars (arteriosclerotic scar). It is difficult for the beginner to differentiate arteriosclerotic scars and the associated lymphocytic infiltration from chronic pyelonephritis—but the striking arterial changes and comparatively scant lymphocytic infiltration should lead to a correct interpretation.

Arteriolosclerosis (Fig 6–17, see also chap. 2). In arteriolosclerosis (arteriolarsclerosis) hyalin appears between the intima and media with lumenal narrowing and medial atrophy. The changes are the same in the kidney as in the brain, cardiac muscle, or spleen. Hematoxylin and eosin stains reveal red, homogeneous, and anuclear arteriolar walls (see Fig 6–18). The hyalinized vessels become very conspicuous when stained for fat. Inspection of the section with the scanning lens reveals several reddish dots in the cortex that can be identified, with higher magnification, as afferent arterioles (→ 1), the wall of which is infiltrated by neutral fats. The media is markedly atrophic—isolated nuclei are still visible in the outermost parts of the media (see also Fig 6–18, → 2). The lumen of the arteriole, barely discernible by means of a few preserved endothelial cell nuclei, is markedly narrowed. Note the deposits of fat (Fig 6–17) in the glomerular connective tissue (→ 2: mesangium). Tubules in the proximity of affected glomeruli have atrophied.

Contracted kidney in arteriolar nephrosclerosis (Fig 6–18). If hyalinization of the afferent arterioles progresses so that a majority of the vessels are affected and if, in addition, there is concomitant sclerosis of medium-sized arteries, obliteration of large numbers of glomeruli and tubules will follow. Examination with a scanning lens discloses thinning of the cortex as well as numerous reddish discoid lesions that higher magnification shows to be glomeruli with eosinophilic concentric laminations containing a few isolated nuclei (→ 1). The afferent arterioles surrounding these glomeruli have characteristic lesions in the wall (×)—the intima is greatly thickened, the lining endothelial cells are barely discernible, and the lumen is narrowed. The muscle fibers of the media are markedly atrophic or have disappeared. With hematoxylin-eosin stains, the appearance of the tissue resembles that found in amyloidosis. The Congo red stain, however, is negative, and van Gieson's stain brings out the red hyalinized glomeruli and arterioles (fresh hyalin is yellow, see Fig 10,A, section on General Pathology). Figure 6–18 shows a longitudinally sectioned lesion in an afferent arteriole (× upper right); → 2 and × in the center point to arteriolar lesions cut in cross section. As a result of hyalinization of the glomeruli, there is atrophy of the dependent tubular system (→ 3), shown by shrunken tubules with narrow lumina and atrophy of lining epithelium. Several tubules have been obliterated. There is compensatory proliferation of interstitial fibrous tissue and lymphocytic infiltration (scars). Areas of the cortex that contain intact glomeruli undergo compensatory hypertrophy. Grossly, such areas can be seen as projecting nodules.

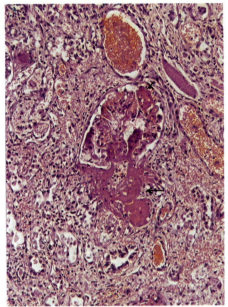

Fig 6–19.—Malignant nephrosclerosis (hematoxylin-eosin; 120×).

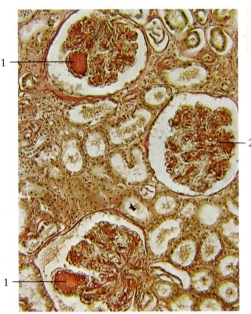

Fig 6–20.—Kimmelstiel-Wilson glomerulosclerosis (van Gieson's stain; 120×).

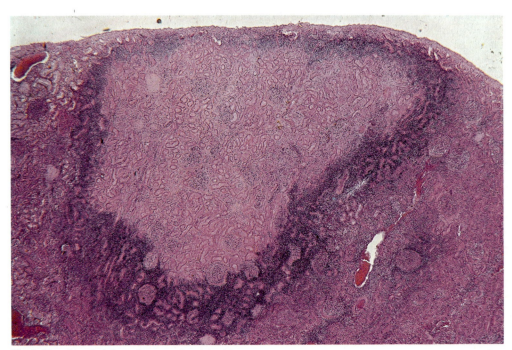

Fig 6–21.—Anemic infarct (hematoxylin-eosin; 30×).

Malignant nephrosclerosis (Fig 6–19) *consists of a rapidly progressive fibrinoid necrosis of the walls of small renal arteries, afferent arterioles, and glomerular loops.*

Histologically, the walls of arterioles appear to be hyalinized, so that the walls appear homogeneous and the lumens are narrowed (→). The ''hyaline'' material stains strikingly bright red with hematoxylin-eosin. With van Gieson's stain, it is yellow (see Figs 10,A and B, section on General Pathology, and discussion earlier this chapter). There is nearly always an accompanying polymorphonuclear infiltration although it may be very slight. Frequently there are erythrocytes in the fibrinoid material, indicative of rapid intrusion of blood into the vessel wall. The fibrinoid necrosis almost always involves adjacent glomerular loops (×), so that either single loops of the glomerulus or groups of them are affected. Should malignant nephrosclerosis be superimposd on arterio- or arteriolonephrosclerosis, there will be a combination of sclerosis of medium-sized vessels and hyalinization of arterioles, in addition to the foci of fibrinoid necrosis. But malignant nephrosclerosis can develop without preexisting hypertension. It has been proposed that in such cases there is primary endothelial damage (endotheliotropic nephroangiopathy) that is connected with the hemolytic-uremic syndrome (HUS).

Macroscopic: Variegated, speckled kidney with indistinct gray-white foci on a reddish background. *Clinically,* when malignant hypertension develops in young people it follows a rapidly fatal course, leading to uremic or apoplectic death. Older patients (50–60) may manifest malignant hypertension as a sequel to a previously benign course, in which case the history shows a combination of arteriolosclerosis and malignant nephrosclerosis.

Kimmelstiel-Wilson glomerulosclerosis (Fig 6–20) *occurs as a complication in approximately 20% of cases of diabetes mellitus. Typically, there is hyalinization of the glomerular loops. Clinically, the patients have proteinuria, hypertension, and sometimes slight renal failure.*

Histologically, there is a very characteristic lesion. Numerous glomeruli show hyalinization of single or several capillary loops, resulting in the formation of rounded ball-like structures (in van Gieson's stain, red or yellowish red, → 1). The remaining glomerular loops are either free of any changes or else show the early stages of hyalinization. Some glomeruli also exhibit a diffuse thickening of the capillary wall (→ 2). The basement membranes are often frayed. In addition, the hyalinization frequently involves the afferent and *efferent arterioles.* Electron microscopically there is thickening of basement membranes, especially in the mesangium.

Macroscopic: Finely granular, slightly contracted kidney.

Anemic infarct (Fig 6–21). *This is caused by embolic obstruction of a branch of the renal artery, resulting in a wedge-shaped area of coagulation necrosis.*

Examination of the section with a scanning lens reveals a pale red, wedge-shaped area, surrounded by a bluish, highly cellular zone outside of which there is a thin red rim. Observation of the central portion of the wedge-shaped area reveals the typical signs of *necrosis:* the nuclei are achromatic and the cytoplasm is homogeneous or finely granular. The nuclei in the interstitium and the glomeruli appear as shadows of their former selves. On the whole, early infarcts will still show the faint outlines of tubules and glomeruli. Higher magnification reveals *polymorphonuclear leukocytes* in the *peripheral cellular zone* as well as all the phases of nuclear disruption: pyknosis, rhexis, lysis, and finely scattered nuclear debris. Surrounding the cellular zone there is usually a *zone of reactive hyperemia:* however, this is not conspicuous in our section. Note the thin, subcapsular strip of preserved parenchyma which receives its blood supply from the capsular vessels.

Macroscopic: Yellow, dry firm area. Older foci are contracted (resorption by granulation tissue), the final result being a deeply contracted, white scar. The emboli most frequently come either from a verrucous endocarditis, a mural thrombus in the heart (e.g., myocardial infarct), or from the aorta. Other causes: thrombotic arteriosclerosis, periarteritis nodosa.

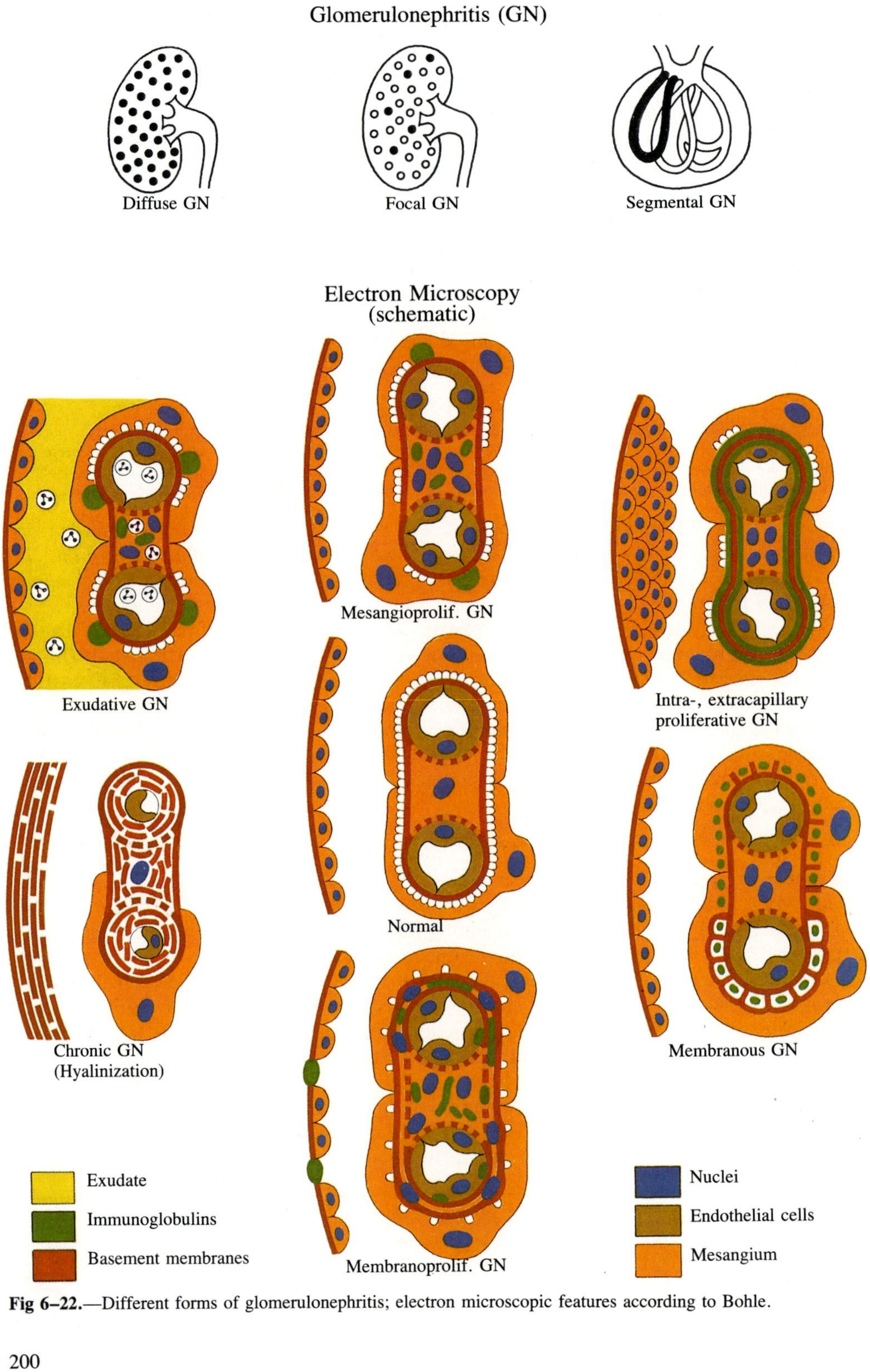

Glomerulonephritis (GN)

Diffuse GN   Focal GN   Segmental GN

Electron Microscopy
(schematic)

Exudative GN

Mesangioprolif. GN

Intra-, extracapillary
proliferative GN

Chronic GN
(Hyalinization)

Normal

Membranous GN

Membranoprolif. GN

▮ Exudate	▮ Nuclei
▮ Immunoglobulins	▮ Endothelial cells
▮ Basement membranes	▮ Mesangium

Fig 6–22.—Different forms of glomerulonephritis; electron microscopic features according to Bohle.

TABLE 6–1.—CLASSIFICATION OF GLOMERULONEPHRITIS (GN)

TYPE	MORPHOLOGY	PATHOGENESIS, IMMUNOLOGY	CLINICAL FEATURES
Exudative GN (Acute exudative and proliferative GN)	Granulocytes; exudation and slight mesangial and endothelial proliferation	**Postinfectious** (streptococcal infection, scarlet fever, sore throat), also serum sickness; **Immune complex nephritis:** subepithelial immune body deposits ("humps")	Early: high antistreptolysin O titer, hypocomplementemia, albuminuria, hematuria; BP ↑; often good prognosis; healing via mesangioproliferative GN
Mesangioproliferative GN (Intracapillary GN) acute → chronic	Proliferation of mesangium and endothelium	**Postinfectious** (*Streptococcus, staphylococcus,* viruses) IgA-, IgG-nephritis; immune complex nephritis; subepithelial immune deposits on glomerular loops ("humps") and/or mesangium	Hematuria, proteinuria; most common type of GN; steroid therapy +; **good prognosis,** frequently a nephrotic course; 90% recover
Proliferative intra-extracapillary GN (Extracapillary GN) rapid progression	Proliferation of parietal capsular epithelial cells, semilunar crescents; little proliferation of both endothelium and mesangium, variant: necrotizing type	**Antibasement membrane nephritis,** e.g., in Goodpasture's syndrome; immunoglobulins line basement membrane diffusely	**Poor prognosis** Rapidly progressive, "subacute"; proteinuria, hematuria; prognosis better in children; BP ↑
Membranous GN (Peri- or epimembranous GN)	Basement membrane much thickened, so-called spikes; later: reduplication of basement membrane; little cellular proliferation	**Immune complex nephritis** (autoantibodies?), subepithelial immune deposits, spikes; virus? (Aleutian mink); after gold therapy	**Nephrotic syndrome** Steroid therapy (+); 30% heal, 50%–70% persist; may be induced by drugs
Membranoproliferative GN (Mesangiocapillary GN)	Basement membrane thick (double contour), proliferation of mesangium; mesangial cells between reduplicated basement membrane	**Hypocomplementemia,** subendothelial or intramembranous immune deposits	70% have nephrotic syndrome; steroid therapy +; immunosuppression +; prone to heal
Minimal GN ("Minimal change GN" lipoid nephrosis)	Glomeruli not remarkable on light microscopy or only minimal increase of mesangium	*a.* Healing stage of mesangioproliferative GN; IF-positive cases *b.* Minimal change GN, IF-negative cases	True lipoid nephrosis; steroid therapy (+); 60% heal
Focal and/or segmental GN	Single glomeruli affected and/or single groups of loops; proliferative or sclerotic (fibrous tissue)	Idiopathic or postinfectious or Schönlein-Henoch purpura, lupus erythematosus; Goodpasture syndrome, sarcoidosis	Proliferative form: chiefly favorable prognosis; sclerotic form: chiefly with nephrotic syndrome and poor prognosis

201

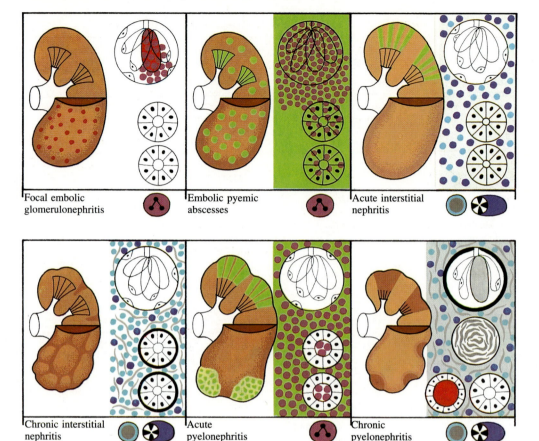

Focal embolic glomerulonephritis

Embolic pyemic abscesses

Acute interstitial nephritis

Chronic interstitial nephritis

Acute pyelonephritis

Chronic pyelonephritis

Fig 6–23.—Diagrammatic survey of the gross and histologic characteristics of inflammatory renal diseases (except glomerulonephritis).

Focal embolic glomerulonephritis (see Fig 6–37) shows patchy fibrinoid necrosis of single or groups of glomerular loops.

Macroscopic: Slightly enlarged kidney with discrete petechiae.

Embolic pyemic kidney abscesses (see Fig 6–38) appear as small abscesses in the region of a single glomerulus.

Macroscopic: Diffusely scattered yellow foci surrounded by a zone of hyperemia.

If the bacteria have gained access to the medullary parenchyma, there are numerous yellow, linear streaks which microscopically correspond to elongated abscesses with bacterial colonies.

Acute interstitial nephritis may be either *suppurative or nonsuppurative.* The interstitial tissues are distended by exudate (e.g., in burns, see shock kidney) or show streaklike infiltration of lymphocytes and histiocytes.

Macroscopic: Enlarged, yellowish gray kidney.

Chronic interstitial nephritis is characterized by the infiltration of lymphocytes and histiocytes. There is accompanying proliferation of connective tissue.

Macroscopic: Grayish red, gnarled, contracted kidneys.

Acute or chronic **pyelonephritis** (see discussion later this chapter) results in damage to one or more kidney segments.

The inflammation is either descending, following bacteremia, or ascending, when there is obstruction to urinary flow (kidney stones, tumors, etc.). In the acute stage there are groups of abscesses and streaky cellular infiltrates; in the chronic stage there are flat, reddish or gray-white scars that retract the cortex.

Glomerulonephritis (GN)

Glomerulonephritis is an inflammation of glomeruli that affects either all the glomeruli of both kidneys uniformly (diffuse GN) or single glomeruli focal GN (see Fig 6–22). Most frequently all the glomerular loops are involved and less frequently only some of the loops (segmental involvement), as for example in focal embolic glomerulonephritis.

The inflamed glomeruli show the usual signs of inflammation: exudation due to leakage of blood plasma and migration of granulocytes (exudative GN). Cells of the mesangium and endothelium proliferate either alone (mesangial or intracapillary proliferative GN) or in association with proliferation of the glomerular and capsular epithelial cells (intra/extra-capillary proliferative GN). In so-called membranous GN the basement membrane is conspicuously thickened. Cellular proliferation is very limited. In membranoproliferative GN there are both thickening of the basement membrane and cellular proliferation.

Because immune complexes can be detected either in or on the basement membrane at some stage in nearly all forms of GN, it is thought that an antigen-antibody reaction is the chief underlying cause of the injury. Activation of complement (c_1-c_9) takes place at the same time. These facts seem to explain many of the morphological features, such as exudation, accumulation of granulocytes, and even necrosis.

In chronic glomerulonephritis, regardless of the form of GN from which it develops, there is thickening of the mesangial matrix which advances beneath the endothelium on the basement membrane until the lumina of the capillary loops are completely obstructed (damaged glomeruli become hyalinized), resulting in diminution and finally loss of glomerular filtration.

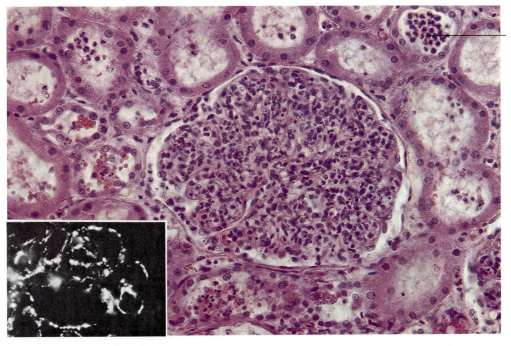

Fig 6–24.—Acute exudative glomerulonephritis (hematoxylin-eosin; 300×). *Inset:* Deposits of immunoglobulin and complement in the mesangium and along the basement membrane (immunofluorescence).

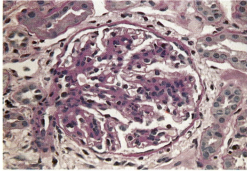

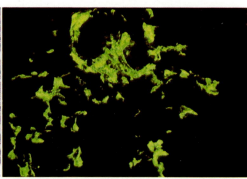

Fig 6–25.—Mesangioproliferative glomerulonephritis (PAS-hematoxylin; 220×).

Fig 6–26.—Deposits of immunoglobulins (IgA, IgG) in the mesangial matrix in mesangioproliferative glomerulonephritis (immunofluorescence 280×).

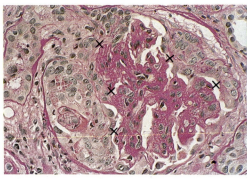

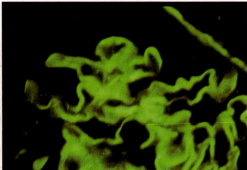

Fig 6–27.—Intracapillary and extracapillary proliferative glomerulonephritis (× marks border of extracapillary proliferation) (PAS-hematoxylin; 260×).

Fig 6–28.—Deposits of immunoglobulin (IgG) along the basement membrane in anti-glomerular basement membrane nephritis (immunofluorescence; 280×).

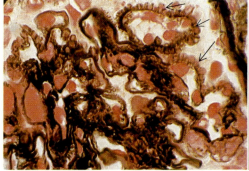

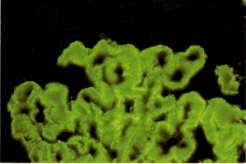

Fig 6–29.—Membranous glomerulonephritis (→, spikes) (Jones chromotrope R stain; 400×).

Fig 6–30.—Granular deposits of immunoglobulin (IgG) on the external surface of the glomerular basement membrane in membranous glomerulonephritis (280×).

Acute exudative glomerulonephritis. Figure 6–24 shows the **acute stage of exudative glomerulonephritis.** Only the magnification provided by a scanning lens is needed to see the enlarged, highly cellular glomeruli. The glomerular tuft fills Bowman's space completely; capillary loops are dilated and filled with neutrophils. Erythrocytes, protein, and polymorphonuclear leukocytes are present both in the capsular space and the tubules (→). Interstitial tissues are edematous and swollen. Tubular epithelial cells are enlarged and often show cloudy swelling.

Macroscopic: The kidneys are swollen and the cut surfaces bulge beyond the edges of the tense capsule. Flea-bite hemorrhages are present on the surface.

Mesangioproliferative glomerulonephritis (Figs 6–25, 6–26). This condition has also been termed mesangiocapillary glomerulonephritis and lobular glomerulonephritis. Figure 6–25 shows the essentials, as indicated by the PAS stain. The mesangium is markedly thickened and clearly visible, whereas the glomerular basement membrane appears delicate. Mesangial cells are increased in number, endothelial cells less so but may be enlarged. The capsular epithelium is unchanged. As indicated in Table 6–1, this form of GN can be acute, with associated hematuria and proteinuria, and can then take a chronic course. Figure 6–26 shows immunofluorescent staining of deposits of immunoglobulin and complement in the mesangium.

Intraextracapillary proliferative glomerulonephritis (idiopathic crescentic glomerulonephritis, or rapidly progressive glomerulonephritis, Fig 6–27). The capsular spaces of glomeruli contain crescents resulting from proliferation and enlargement of parietal epithelium of Bowman's capsule (× × ×). Loops of glomeruli are compressed by these proliferated cells. Endothelial and mesangial cells have also proliferated. In time, the crescents acquire collagen fibrils and the glomerular loops become acellular. The interstitium near the glomerulus may show a serous exudate and moderate lymphocytic infiltrates. The epithelial cells in proximal convoluted tubules show hyalin droplets. A similar type of glomerular nephritis can be produced in rabbits (Masugi nephritis, anti-glomerular basement membrane nephritis), with deposits of anti-basement membrane IgG along the glomerular basement membrane (Fig 6–28).

Macroscopic: Enlarged red to yellow kidneys with red petechial hemorrhages.

Membranous glomerulonephritis (epi- or perimembranous GN, Fig 6–29). In the early stage of this condition granular immune complexes are deposited on the epithelial side of the glomerular basement membrane (see Fig 6–30). Later the basement membrane develops spikes between these deposits. Neighboring spikes may fuse, thereby producing ''duplication'' of stretches of basement membrane. There is little cell proliferation. The most prominent clinical feature is a nephrotic syndrome.

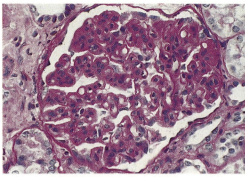

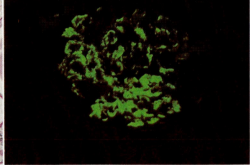

Fig 6–31.—Membranoproliferative glomerulonephritis (PAS-hematoxylin; 240 ×).

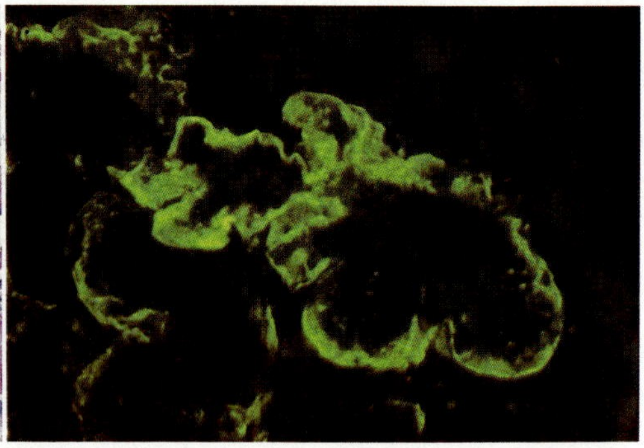

Fig 6–32.—Lumpy deposits of IgM along the basement membrane in membranoproliferative glomerulonephritis (immunofluorescence; 320 ×).

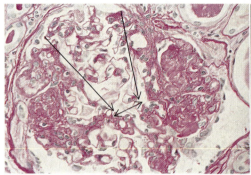

Fig 6–33.—Segmental glomerulosclerosis (left and right side of the glomerulus). Note the minimal involvement between the arrows (PAS-hematoxylin; 260 ×).

Fig 6–34.—Focal and segmental deposits of IgM in the mesangium and along the basement membrane (immunofluorescence; 220 ×).

Membranoproliferative glomerulonephritis (Fig 6–31). There is proliferation of mesangial cells along with subendothelial and intramembranous deposition of immune complexes. The immune complexes split up segments of basement membrane. They are also deposited along the basement membrane toward the peripheries of capillary loops. Immunofluorescence (Fig 6–32) reveals deposits of immunoglobulins and complement along and within the membrane. This condition is frequently associated with a nephrotic syndrome and persistent hypocomplementemia.

Segmental glomerulosclerosis (focal segmental glomerulonephritis, focal sclerosing glomerular lesions, Fig 6–33). Individual loops of glomeruli and/or scattered individual glomeruli are affected in this condition. The picture shows hyalinosis of glomerular loops and augmentation of mesangial matrix. Figure 6–34 shows segmental deposits of immune complexes. There is only minimal cell proliferation in the nearly uninvolved segments of glomeruli.

Minimal change glomerular disease (lipoid nephrosis, NIL disease, idiopathic nephrotic syndrome). In this condition there is virtual absence of cell proliferation, and minimal increase in mesangial cells may be the only glomerular abnormality. At times the basement membranes may be slightly thickened. The condition is associated with classic lipoid nephrosis, and immune deposits are absent. Minimal change disease must be distinguished from residua of mesangioproliferative glomerulonephritis, in which there may be immune deposits.

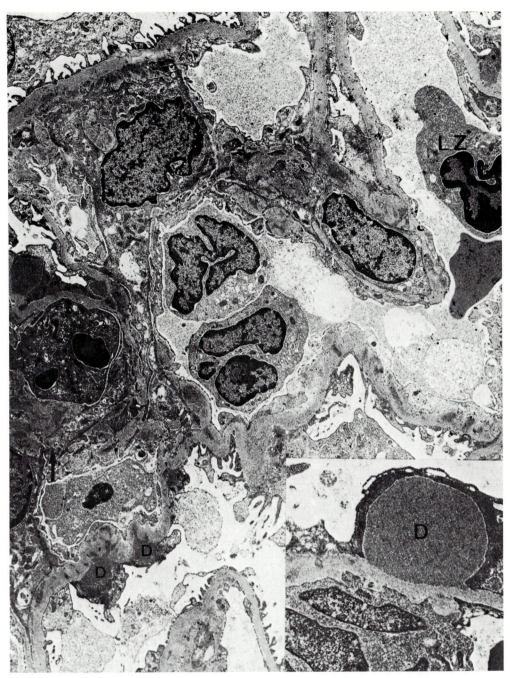

Fig 6–35.—Acute exudative proliferative glomerulonephritis (diffuse proliferative glomerulonephritis). Note immune complex deposits in mesangium and on the epithelial side of the basement membrane (*D*, ''humps''). The capillary lumen and the mesangium contain granu-locytes (6,500×). *Inset:* Membranous glomerulonephritis in a patient with nephrotic syndrome. *D*, immunoglobulin deposit between fused spikes of basement membrane (toward epithelial side) (14,000×).

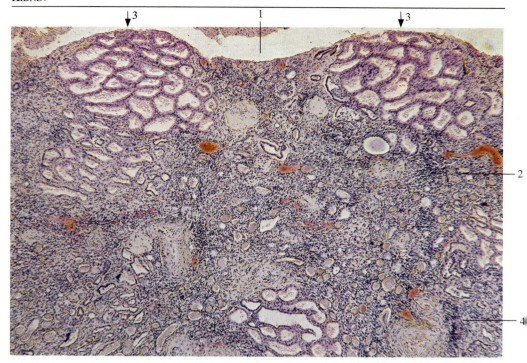

Fig 6–36.—Chronic glomerulonephritis (hematoxylin-eosin; 40×).

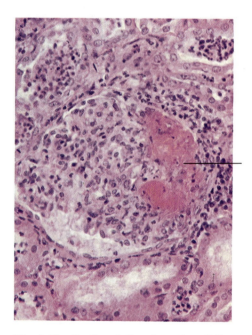

Fig 6–37.—Focal embolic glomerulonephritis (hematoxylin-eosin; 280×).

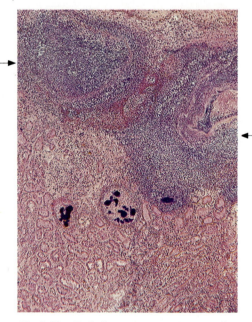

Fig 6–38.—Embolic renal abscess (hematoxylin-eosin; 72×).

Chronic glomerulonephritis (Fig 6–36). Survey of the preparation with a scanning lens reveals noticeable thinning of the cortex. Some areas show scarring of the surface and accumulations of inflammatory cells, while other areas show small cystic spaces and cellular paucity. Under medium magnification, most of the glomeruli are seen to have been replaced by hyalinized nodules. Frequently, the crescent-shaped lesions of intra/extracapillary glomerulonephritis are still preserved. The attached tubules are markedly atrophic (→ 1), lined with flattened epithelium, and filled with hyaline casts (→ 2). The interstitial tissue is increased in amount and infiltrated by lymphocytes. In addition to areas of scarring (resulting in retraction of the surface, → 1), there are also areas of compensatory hypertrophy (→ 3), with fully preserved glomeruli and dilated tubules lined with cuboidal epithelium. Aside from the completely hyalinized glomeruli, there are also some in which the inflammatory changes are recent. The vessels often show arteriosclerosis and arteriolosclerosis (→ 4). In the end stages, the various types of glomerulonephritis cannot be differentiated. Kidneys contracted by arterionephrosclerosis or arteriolonephrosclerosis may also be difficult to differentiate.

Macroscopic: Small, firm kidneys with yellow or gray granular surfaces. Sometimes the surface may be smooth, especially in cases of chronic mesangioproliferative glomerulonephritis.

In focal embolic glomerulonephritis (Fig 6–37), *there is inflammation of isolated loops of single glomeruli. It is seen particularly in cases of subacute bacterial endocarditis.* In the acute stages, there is fibrinoid necrosis of isolated capillary loops or groups of loops. They appear as homogeneous, anuclear, eosinophilic masses (→). Erythrocytes can often be seen in the fibrinoid material. This material involves the wall of the glomerular loops and also actually lies in the loops (fibrin thrombi). The unaffected loops are intact, showing, at most, slightly increased cellularity and thickening of the basement membrane. Bowman's space and the tubules contain granular casts, possibly erythrocytes and polymorphs. Healing of the lesions leads to focal scar formation and fusion of the loops with the parietal epithelium.

Macroscopic: The kidneys are slightly enlarged and present a flea-bitten appearance.

Embolic renal abscesses (Fig 6–38). *Hematogenous spread in septicemia or pyemia leads to the formation of abscesses in the cortex and focal, streaklike suppuration in the medulla.* The scanning lens reveals scattered, highly cellular lesions in the cortex. Intermediate magnification reveals focal collections of polymorphs in the cortex along with necrosis (→: abscesses). In other parts, there are clusters of bacteria in glomerular and other capillary loops, and the surrounding parenchyma is infiltrated by leukocytes and partly necrotic. The interstitial connective tissue also contains leukocytes. The proximal tubules contain granular casts.

The *foci of suppuration in the medulla* result from passage of bacteria through the glomeruli and their accumulation in the medulla, where they form streaklike abscesses containing central bacterial colonies (blue), frequently surrounded by an area of necrosis and a peripheral zone of leukocytes.

Macroscopic: Yellow or gray abscesses (1–2 mm) are scattered throughout the cortex, on the surface of the kidney, and as streaks along the medullary rays.

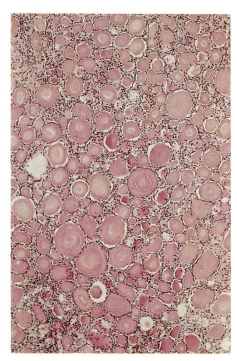

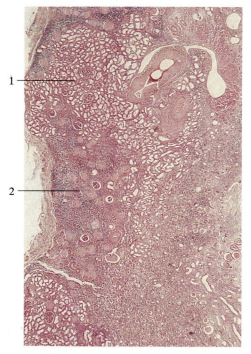

Fig 6–39.—Chronic pyelonephritis (hematoxylin-eosin; 40×).

Fig 6–40.—"Thyroid kidney" in chronic pyelonephritis (hematoxylin-eosin; 100×).

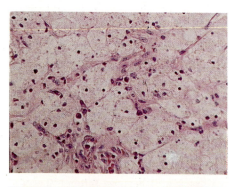

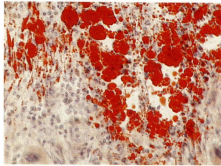

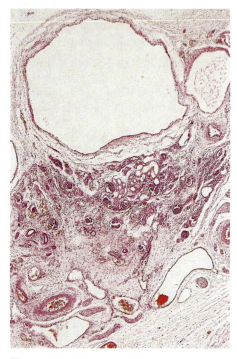

Fig 6–41.—Xanthomatous pyelonephritis (top, hematoxylin-eosin; bottom, Sudan; 150×).

Fig 6–42.—Polycystic kidney (hematoxylin-eosin; 40×).

Pyelonephritis—Xanthomatous Pyelonephritis—Polycystic Kidney

Chronic pyelonephritis (Figs 6–39, 6–40). This condition may be called "destructive chronic interstitial nephritis" because interstitial inflammation leads to destruction of kidney parenchyma with scarring. Inspection with a scanning lens (Fig 6–39) reveals focal, mainly subcapsular scars composed of fibrous tissue, lymphocytes, and hyalinized glomeruli (→ 2). In these foci the cortical surface of the kidney is retracted; surrounding tubules are dilated—an expression of compensatory hyperfunction. Rather characteristic of chronic pyelonephritis is the presence of thyroid-like areas (Fig 6–40). These are groups of tubules whose lumina contain densely eosinophilic, concentrically layered protein casts, and thus the tubules resemble thyroid follicles that are filled with colloid. The histologic changes in chronic pyelonephritis also include alterations in blood vessels: arteriosclerosis, intimal fibrosis, arteriolosclerosis, and, less frequently, arteriolonecrosis and arteriolitis proliferans.

Xanthomatous pyelonephritis (Fig 6–41). This is a special form of pyelonephritis in which chronic, purulent inflammation is linked with the presence of xanthomatous cells. The condition affects renal parenchyma, pelvis, and the hilar adipose tissue. Microscopy reveals granulation tissue with newly formed capillaries, and many lymphocytes and plasma cells. Pseudoxanthoma cells are characteristic. After staining with hematoxylin-eosin (Fig 6–41, top), one sees large cells with pale-staining cytoplasm and small nuclei. The Sudan stain (Fig 6–41, bottom) reveals the cytoplasm to be filled with red-staining fat. These cells are macrophages, but sometimes their differentiation from the cells of hypernephroma (clear cell carcinoma of the kidney) may be difficult.

Xanthomatous pyelonephritis is somewhat more frequent in men than in women, particularly in the third decade. Excretory urograms may simulate a tumor. Macroscopically one sees a golden-yellow, broad zone, 1–5 mm in thickness, that surrounds the granulation tissue.

Other forms of pyelonephritis:
1. **Pyelonephritis in children.** Frequent inflammatory condition (about 5% of all childhood illnesses), often associated with varied and misleading symptoms, and rarely diagnosed correctly in its early stage. Asymptomatic cases predominate.
2. **Pyelonephritis in women.** About 5% of pregnant women develop an asymptomatic but significant bacteriuria. The pyelonephritis usually begins in the second month but becomes clinically manifest only in the fifth to eighth month. An unrecognized pyelonephritis during pregnancy may cause fetal death in 17% of cases and perinatal mortality of infants in 28%.
3. **Pyelonephritis in men** develops mainly in more advanced years and is generally related to obstruction to urinary flow (hyperplasia of the prostate, tumors of the prostate or bladder, ureteral and urethral strictures).
4. **Specific pyelonephritis.** This term includes pyelonephritis due to specific organisms, particularly the tubercle bacillus. In tuberculous pyelonephritis the renal parenchyma is destroyed and there is extensive caseous necrosis.

Polycystic kidney (Fig 6–42). This is most commonly a bilateral, congenital disorder, with formation of multiple cysts. One form of the disease, in which the cysts are relatively small, occurs in infants and causes early death. Another form, more commonly detected in juveniles or adults, is characterized by large cysts. Microscopically the numerous cysts are lined by flat epithelium. Between cysts a small amount of preserved renal parenchyma may be seen. The interstitial connective tissue is relatively loose. Some of the larger cysts may contain trapped eosinophilic urine. In some instances there is bleeding.

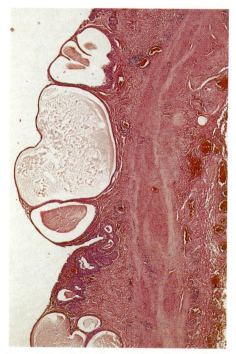

Fig 6–43.—Ureteritis cystica (hematoxylin-eosin; 40×).

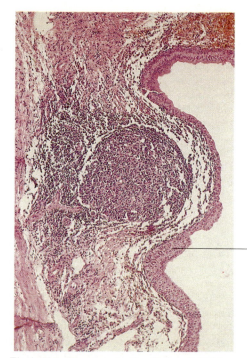

Fig 6–44.—Chronic ureteritis with lymphoid follicle (ureteritis follicularis) (hematoxylin-eosin; 60×).

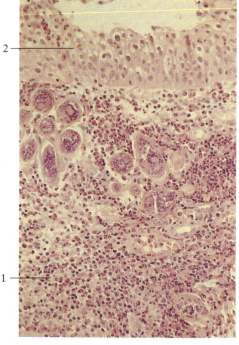

Fig 6–45.—Schistosomiasis of urinary bladder (bilharziasis; 150×).

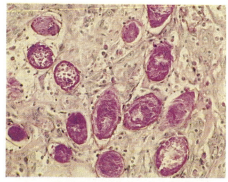

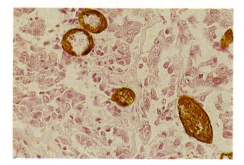

Fig 6–46.—Ova of *Schistosoma haematobium* in wall of urinary bladder (bilharziasis) (**top,** PAS; **bottom;** von Kossa's stain; 150×).

Inflammation of Urinary Tract—Urinary Bladder

Ureteritis cystica (Fig 6–43). This is a special form of chronic ureteritis in which there are numerous cysts in the ureteral mucosa. The condition represents the terminal stage of chronic inflammation. In the early stage there are small solid nests of transitional epithelium (hyperplastic epithelial nests of von Brunn). These develop central spaces that become cystically enlarged. In the fully developed condition there are larger cysts which protrude above the mucosal surface and are lined by layers of epithelium. These cysts contain eosinophilic amorphous material.

Follicular ureteritis (Fig 6–44). Chronic inflammation of the ureteral mucosa may produce focal lymphocytic infiltrates. These elevate the overlying transitional cell epithelium (→). Sometimes the lymphocytic foci contain germinal centers. A similar sort of chronic inflammation also occurs in the renal pelvis and the urinary bladder. Grossly it is seen in the form of tiny white nodules or stipples and is to be distinguished from tuberculosis.

Bilharziasis, schistosomiasis (Figs 6–45, 6–46). Schistosomiasis is a group of parasitic diseases caused by three different parasites (trematodes) distributed in different parts of the world. *Schistosoma haematobium* causes bilharziasis of the urinary bladder; *S. japonicum* and *S. mansoni* affect gut, mesenteric veins, and liver. Bilharziasis occurs in the Nile Valley (Egypt). The stroma of the urinary bladder shows marked inflammation in which eosinophilic leukocytes are most prominent (Fig 6–45,→ 1). The overlying bladder epithelium is somewhat hyperplastic (→2). Ova of the parasite lie in the inflamed stroma and can be demonstrated selectively with the PAS stain (Fig 6–46, top). When dead, the ova become encased in calcium salts and are stained dark brown to black by the von Kossa method (Fig 6–46).

Vital eggs are excreted in the urine. In water (rivers, lakes, etc.) they develop into larvae **(miracidia),** which enter water snails. After several weeks **cercaria** develop, which swarm into the water. These can penetrate the human epidermis and reach the pelvic venous plexus via lymphatics and blood vessels. The disease manifests itself clinically several months after the invasion by cercaria. Initially there is an acute, later a chronic, cystitis; finally, scarring may cause contraction of the bladder. The chronic inflammation may lead to carcinoma of the urinary bladder.

Specific inflammations of the urinary bladder include **tuberculosis** that may be associated with tuberculosis elsewhere in the urogenital tract. In this condition, there are tiny white, irregularly distributed nodules or undermined ulcers in the bladder mucosa. Elderly women develop a form of chronic cystitis that may be caused by *E. coli* and may be secondary to insufficiency of the urethral orifice.

Cystitis emphymsematosa is a condition caused by gas-forming bacilli. It causes acute inflammation in the vicinity of the gas bubbles in the wall of the bladder (to be distinguished from postmortem changes). **Endoxan bladder** is a collective term for severe hemorrhagic cystitis that develops in consequence of therapy with cytostatic or cytotoxic drugs.

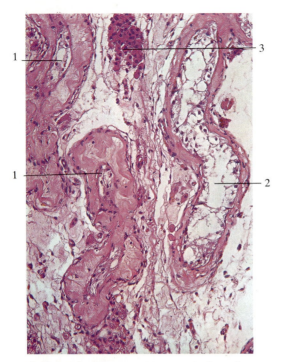

Fig 7–1.—Testicular atrophy (hematoxylin-eosin; 100×).

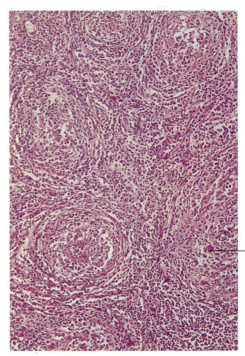

Fig 7–2.—Granulomatous orchitis (hematoxylin-eosin; 80×).

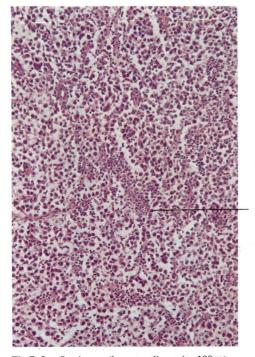

Fig 7–3.—Seminoma (hematoxylin-eosin; 100×).

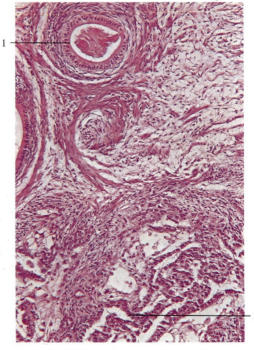

Fig 7–4.—Malignant teratoma of testes, intermediate type (MTI) (hematoxylin-eosin; 90×).

7. Genitalia—Pregnancy

Male Genitalia: Testis

Testicular atrophy (Fig 7–1) *results from either local or generalized injury which causes wasting of testicular tubules and either partial or complete arrest of spermatogenesis.* Figure 7–1 shows two completely hyalinized and wasted tubules (→ 1). A third testicular tubule (→ 2) has a thick basement membrane that is only partially lined by *Sertoli cells* and no longer contains spermatozoa. The loose and relatively increased connective tissue resulting from the testicular atrophy contains islands of hyperplastic, eosinophilic *Leydig cells* (→ 3).

The testis is one of the most sensitive of organs. It reacts with marked, rarely reversible atrophy to mechanical (trauma), chemical (chemotherapy), and thermal (heat: intra-abdominal or inguinal testes) stimuli, inflammations (gonorrhea), hormones (e.g., hyperestrogenism of liver cirrhosis or hormone therapy for prostatic carcinoma), and irradiation. In the aged testicular involution develops *(involution—physiologic process, atrophy—pathologic process!).* Testicular atrophy may also be genetically conditioned, as for example in Klinefelter syndrome (men with an eunuchoid stature, gynecomastia, sterility, XXY chromosomes).

Granulomatous orchitis (Fig 7–2) *is a chronic inflammation of the testis, presumably of multiple causes, that is manifested pathologically by granulomatous inflammation with giant cells and clinically simulates a tumor.* Histologically the normal structure of the testis is completely destroyed and replaced by granulomatous inflammation with lymphocytes, plasma cells, histiocytes, and solitary, multinucleated giant cells (→) that occasionally resemble *Langhans' giant cells.*

Granulomatous orchitis occurs preferentially in the 50 to 60-year-old age group. Causes include escape of spermatozoa from the tubules (sperm granulomas account for 40% of cases), specific and nonspecific bacterial and mycotic inflammations, trauma, and autoimmune disorders, as well as primary vascular lesions.

Preliminary remarks about testicular tumors: The most frequent tumors arise from germinal epithelium; among these are seminomas and teratomas. Among the nongerminal tumors are androgen-producing *Leydig cell tumors* (sexual precocity when they arise in children), *Sertoli cell tumors,* tubular adenomas (adenoma tubulare testis, corresponding to *Sertoli cell hyperplasia* in cryptorchidism), as well as lymphomas and mesenchymal tumors. Tumors of the testis may appear at all ages. About 6% of tumors arise in an undescended testis.

Seminoma (Fig 7–3) *typically consists of clear cells arranged in islands or cords surrounding collections of lymphocytes* (→).

Testicular tumors showing only a seminomatous component (cut serial sections to exclude a teratocarcinoma) have a relatively good prognosis. They mestastasize preferentially by way of the lymph stream.

Teratoma of the testis (Fig 7–4) *is composed of tissue of various degrees of maturity and organoid structure derived from the three germ layers.* Differentiated teratoma (TD) contains adult-type tissues, such as differentiated glands, respiratory epithelium, smooth and stripped muscle fibers, cartilage, and bone. Malignant teratoma, anaplastic (MTU—embryonic or undifferentiated carcinoma) shows no evidence of differentiation. An intermediate form, malignant teratoma, intermediate type (MTI), is shown in Figure 7–4 in which there are differentiated glands (→ 1) and cords of solid, anaplastic tumor (→ 2).

Malignant trophoblastic teratoma (MTT), corresponding to chorionepithelioma, has a different clinical and prognostic significance. It consists of multinucleated giant cells and macroscopically is hemorrhagic. Clinically it is characterized by gonadotropin production and a high grade of malignancy (early hematogenous metastasis). Seminoma, teratoma, and chorionepithelioma may present in combination (see p. 224).

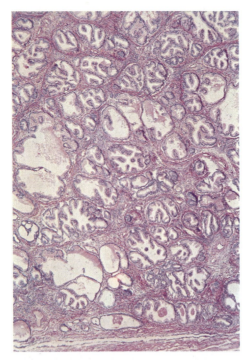

Fig 7–5.—Adenomatous hyperplasia of prostate (so-called prostatic hypertrophy) (hematoxylin-eosin; 20×).

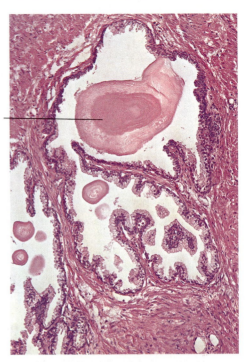

Fig 7–6.—Prostatic concrement (corpora amylacea) (hematoxylin-eosin; 120×).

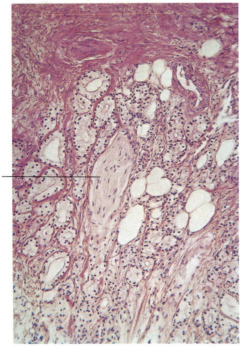

Fig 7–7.—Well-differentiated carcinoma of prostate (hematoxylin-eosin; 100×).

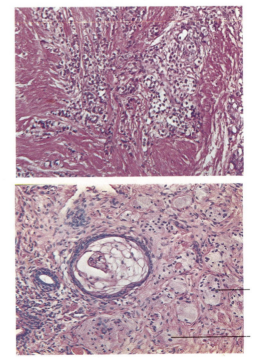

Fig 7–8.—**Top,** undifferentiated carcinoma of prostate. **Bottom,** involution of a prostatic carcinoma with squamous metaplasia after estrogen therapy (hematoxylin-eosin; 100×).

Prostate

Adenomatous hyperplasia of the prostate (so-called prostatic hypertrophy, Figs 7–5, 7–6) *is a hormonally conditioned* hyperplasia and hypertrophy of the periurethral glands of the prostate (so-called internal prostatic glands) accompanied by either diffuse or nodular increase in the smooth muscle fibers.* The external prostatic glands (site of origin of prostatic carcinoma!) are pushed to the periphery and form the so-called surgical capsule. Histologically, under **low magnification** (Fig 7–5) the apparently hyperplastic and dilated glands are easily seen. **Higher magnification** (Fig 7–6) shows irregularly shaped lumina resulting from pseudopapillary infolding of the lining epithelium, which is composed of cylindrical cells with clear cytoplasm and basally situated nuclei. The single cell layer is preserved. The stroma contains elongated eosinophilic muscle fibers. Often a prostatic nodule will show a purely leiomyomatous pattern (hard consistency may clinically simulate carcinoma). The lumina of the glands contain amorphous, eosinophilic secretory masses, inflammatory cells, and occasional concentrically layered, calcified protein bodies *(corpora amylacea or prostatic concrements, →).*

Adenomatous hyperplasia is a disease of elderly men. Macroscopically both lateral lobes are enlarged and commonly a pseudo-middle lobe develops. Not infrequently the condition is accompanied by *sclerosis of the sphincter. Histologically* this shows bandlike hypertrophy of the musculature of the sphincter by connective tissue rich in collagen fibers. Only rarely does malignancy develop in adenomatous hyperplasia.

Introductory remarks about carcinoma of the prostate. Carcinoma of the prostate likewise is a disease of older men. For all practical purposes it appears after about 50 years of age and increases progressively with age. *Histologically,* for prognostic and therapeutic purposes, the following kinds are distinguished: *well-differentiated carcinomas* (clear or occasionally eosinophilic cell adenocarcinoma), *moderately well-differentiated,* and *undifferentiated carcinomas.*

Less usual types are cribriform carcinoma, squamous cell carcinoma (very rare), transitional cell carcinoma (corresponding to carcinoma of the urinary bladder), and mucinous carcinoma (suspect a rectal carcinoma!). Mesenchymal and metastatic carcinomas in the prostate are rare.

Well-differentiated carcinoma of the prostate (Fig 7–7) shows a diffuse spreading and infiltrating growth pattern with cords of closely packed glands with narrow lumina and composed of clear cells. Perineural invasion by the tumor is typical but not pathognomonic (the arrow points to a nerve). Well-differentiated adenocarcinoma has the best prognosis. Frequently it is discovered accidentally in older men (after 70 years of age) during prostatectomy for adenomatous hyperplasia. If they are silent clinically they are described as *latent carcinoma* (in *occult carcinoma* the site of a primary tumor which has produced metastases is not known; examples include carcinomas of stomach, breast, prostate and lung.)

Undifferentiated carcinoma of the prostate (Fig 7–8, top) *consists of solid masses or cords of tumor cells with cytologic signs of wild growth (pleomorphic cells and nuclei, hyperchromatic nuclei, mitoses).*

Undifferentiated prostatic carcinoma appears frequently before the 60th year and runs a progressive and malignant course. It infiltrates the prostatic capsule (stage T_2) and invades neighboring organs (T_3 invasion of the urinary bladder and T_4 invasion of periprostatic organs). Later there is lymphatic (N_1) and hematogenous (M_1) spread with distant metastasis (especially osteoplastic metastases to bones).

Squamous metaplasia (Fig 7–8, bottom) *develops in the prostate, particularly in the region of an infarct, or after estrogen therapy for carcinoma.* In the middle of the picture there is an island of epithelium showing squamous epithelial differentiation. Surrounding it are groups of degenerating carcinoma cells resulting from hormone therapy (shrivelled glands with pyknotic nuclei). Originally this was a well-differentiated clear cell prostatic carcinoma (→).

---

*Probably not (or not only) estrogens, but androgens (5α-dihydroxytestosterone).

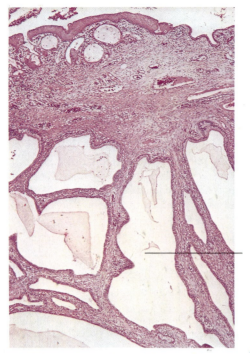

Fig 7–9.—Ectropion (hematoxylin-eosin; 20 ×).

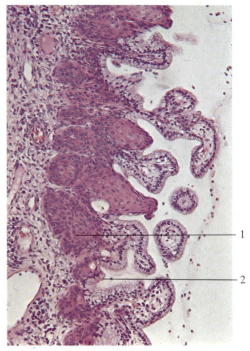

Fig 7–10.—Squamous metaplasia of the cervical mucosa (hematoxylin-eosin; 110 ×).

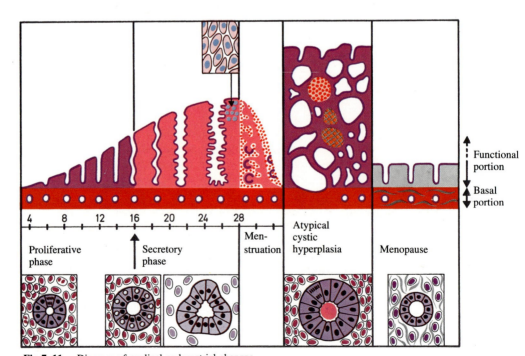

Fig 7–11.—Diagram of cyclical endometrial changes.

Female Genitalia: Ectropion—Squamous Metaplasia—Menstrual Cycle

Ectropion of the external os (Fig 7–9). *This is eversion of the cervical mucosa in the direction of the surface of the cervical os.* The cylindrical epithelium of the endocervical mucosa, which is very sensitive to mechanical and chemical stimuli, is gradually replaced by squamous epithelium. Such transformation may take place by extension from the periphery *(ascending overgrowth)* as well as developing locally. A fully developed **squamous covering of a pseudoerosion** *(ectropion with contiguous overgrowth* (Fig 7–10) shows multilayered noncornified squamous epithelium on the surface with extension into the cervical glands (→). As a result secretion of mucus by the cervical glands is obstructed and retention cysts develop *(Nabothian follicles).*

In an **erosion** there is a true defect of the mucosa which, however, seldom causes reddening of the surface of the os. More commonly the mucosal defect is only simulated. The hyperemic blood vessels and cervical glands are clearly visible through the thin everted cervical mucosa. This is called a *glandular pseudoerosion* and is the consequence of papillary transformation caused by chronic irritation *(glandulopapillary pseudoerosion).*

As a result of chronic local irritation (e.g., chronic inflammation) the normal cylindrical epithelium of the cervical mucosa may change to **metaplastic squamous epithelium** (Fig 7–10). This metaplasia results from an increase of the basal reserve cells that normally are present in the mucosa and progressively lift up and finally push off the cylindrical epithelium. Figure 7–10 shows the bulky, villous structure of the cervical mucosa which in parts is replaced (→ 1) or invaded by (→ 2) metaplastic squamous epithelium.

Normal cyclical changes in the endometrium (Fig 7–11). The endometrium is made up of a *functional portion* (with a superficial compact layer and an underlying spongiosa), both the structure and function of which are under the control of the ovarian hormone, and a narrow basal layer lying on the myometrium which remains after menstruation and so acts as a base for regeneration. In the **normal menstrual cycle** between the 4th and 14th day following activation of the follicular hormone *(estradiol)* the **proliferative phase** appears. The endometrial glands increase and thicken and cellular stroma becomes prominent. At 15 days rupture of the follicle occurs. Between the 15th and 28th day of the cycle the influence of the corpus luteum (progesterone) is established—the **secretory phase.** On the 28th day the period of **menstruation** starts and generally lasts for 3 days. During a normal cycle the tissue and cellular changes in the different phases are quite characteristic.

Proliferative phase (4–14 days). The tubular glands elongate and the stromal cells are compact. In cross sections the glands are seen to have small rounded, optically empty lumina lined by dark, cubical to cylindrical cells. Mitoses are common in both glands and stromal cells.

Secretory phase (15–28 days). Small vacuoles containing glycogen situated basally or retronuclearly in glandular epithelium are the first sign of secretion. During the secretory phase, the endometrial glands become tortuous, thin, and irregular. The cytoplasm of the epithelium is clear and the nuclei migrate to the bases of the cells. The stromal cells are loosened and large (pale stroma). At the end of the secretory phase the compact layer (under the mucosa) shows large pseudodecidual cells (pseudodecidual transformation, see Fig 7–22).

Menstruation (1–3 days). After the secretory phase, bleeding occurs and all but the basal layers of the endometrium are shed. The glandular epithelium and stromal fragments can be easily identified in the blood. There are no evidences of coagulation (fibrin thrombi).

Senile involution. A physiologic process (not to be confused with atrophy) which sets in with the menopause. The entire uterine mucosa becomes thin. The stromal cells and fibers are compactly arranged and the glands small, round, and numerically increased. Frequently the lumina of the glands are dilated, filled with eosinophilic material, and lined with beveled cuboidal epithelium.

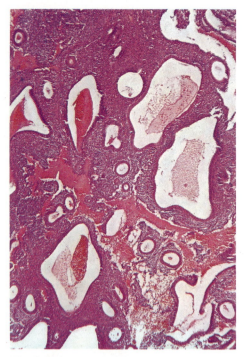

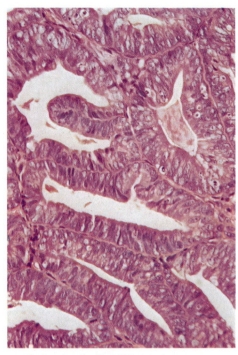

Fig 7–12.—Cystic hyperplasia (grandular-cystic) of the endometrium (hematoxylin-eosin; 32 ×).

Fig 7–13.—Adenomatous hyperplasia of the endometrium (hematoxylin-eosin; 200 ×).

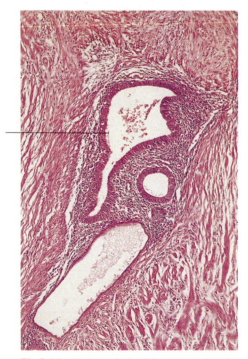

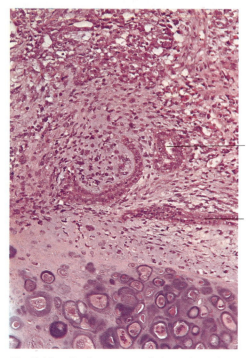

Fig 7–14.—Endometriosis of the myometrium (hematoxylin-eosin).

Fig 7–15.—Carcinosarcoma of the endometrium (hematoxylin-eosin; 90 ×).

Diseases of the Endometrium

Cystic hyperplasia of the endometrium ("Swiss cheese endometrium" Fig 7–12) *is a stromal and glandular hyperplasia induced by hyperestrogenism*. The diagnosis is usually made by curettage, which yields large pieces of tissue embedded in blood. On inspection by the naked eye, the microscopic section is remarkable for the abundance of the material and the large size of the individual fragments. Higher magnification shows endometrium in the proliferative stage and a compact stroma. Cystic dilation of the endometrial glands that are lined by a single layer of cylindrical epithelial cells is a prominent feature. Intermingled with the intact endometrium are small fragments of aglandular stroma as well as loosened and detached glands and epithelium which may have resulted from the surgical scraping. Of diagnostic significance, if present, are small, eosinophilic, homogeneous or finely granular fibrin thrombi which indicate a disorder of endometrial blood flow.

Cystic hyperplasia is caused by hormonal imbalance as a result of which estrogen secretion is both increased and prolonged. The most common cause of this estrogen excess is *persistence of the follicle,* which is especially prominent in the premenopausal period (after 40 years of age). In young women changes similar to cystic hyperplasia may be seen in the first period after a preceding pregnancy (so-called *adjustment hyperplasia*). In older women in the menopause a hormone-producing ovarian tumor (granulosa cell tumor or thecoma) may be present.

Following prolonged estrogen stimulation, cystic hyperplasia can change to **adenomatous** or **atypical hyperplasia** (Fig 7–13). Histologically the endometrial glands are small and not dilated lying "back to back." Individual glands consist of a disorderly layer of tall epithelium showing many mitoses. Adenomatous hyperplasia is a "precancerous" condition and—especially in very marked cases—cannot be distinguished from a well-differentiated adenocarcinoma. Particularly in young women the differential diagnosis is important both for prognostic and therapeutic reasons, because in this age group adenomatous hyperplasia has the potential of regression. Carcinomas of the fundus of the uterus are either glandular or anaplastic carcinomas. *Adenocanthoma* has a glandular pattern plus areas of squamous metaplasia.

Uterine endometriosis interna (adenomyosis uteri, Fig 7–14) *indicates either deep endometrial penetration or ectopic endometrium in the uterine wall*. Histologically there are small collections of endometrial glands (→) in the myometrium surrounded by stroma. The quiescent appearance of the cells in the glands and surrounding stroma rule out a diagnosis of carcinoma.

Endometriosis occurs most frequently in the myometrium where it may cause focal *(adenomyosis)* or more often *diffuse muscular hyperplasia* (thickness of wall in excess of 20 mm). Endometriosis, however, may occur in other organs (external endometriosis), e.g., ovary (chocolate cysts), small intestine, navel and dermal scars. It is a benign lesion which very seldom becomes malignant (adenoacanthoma in endometrial cysts of the ovary).

Carcinosarcoma (Fig 7–15) *is a malignant neoplasm with both carcinomatous and sarcomatous components*. Histologically there are ill-defined cords of glandular carcinomatous tissue (→) lying in a polymorphocellular stroma. In the lower third of the figure the stroma shows cartilaginous differentiation.

Carcinosarcomas are very rare tumors. Adenomyosarcoma, or Wilms' tumor of the kidney, is one of the best-known malignant mixed tumors, and carcinosarcomas also are known to occur in the endometrium, lung, esophagus, breast, and thyroid. By age and sex, these tumors are distributed as the corresponding carcinomas. Distant metastases—of frequent occurrence—can be purely sarcomatous, carcinomatous, or a mixture. Pathogenetically one should differentiate among *collision tumors* (accidental collision of a sarcoma and a carcinoma), *compositional tumors* (simultaneous origin from the stroma and the parenchyma of an organ), and *combination tumors* (origin from the same neoplastic parent tissue but with different differentiation, e.g., Wilms' tumor).

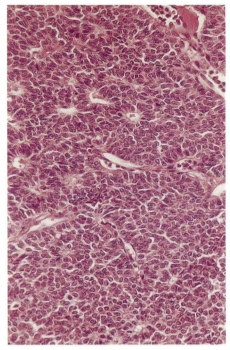

Fig 7–17.—Granulosa cell tumor of the ovary (hematoxylin-eosin; 200×).

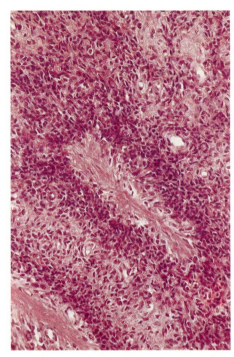

Fig 7–18.—Theca cell tumor of the ovary (hematoxylin-eosin; 200×).

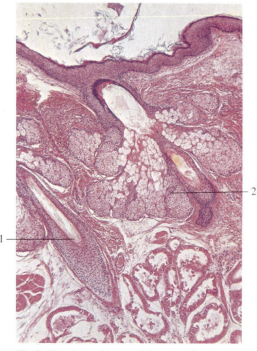

Fig 7–19.—Dermoid cyst of the ovary (hematoxylin-eosin; 45×).

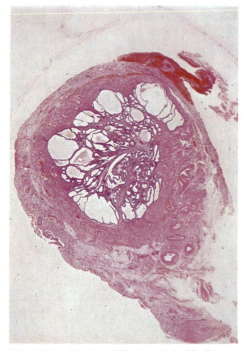

Fig 7–20.—Chronic, follicular salpingitis (hematoxylin-eosin; 15×).

Ovarian Cysts—Tumors—Salpingitis

Ovarian cysts (Fig 7–16) are of very common occurrence but are uncommonly a cause of clinical illness. The cysts can be derived from follicles, corpora lutea, embryonal rests (epoophoron), or the peritoneum (serous cysts). Usually, however, the origin of an ovarian cyst cannot be determined at the time of its discovery and so it is called a *simple ovarian cyst.* Figure 7–16 shows three cysts of the ovary: both of the upper ones are **follicular cysts,** the lower one is a **corpus luteum cyst** (the distinction between a cystic corpus luteum and a corpus luteum cyst is arbitrary). As a rule ovarian cysts are a chance finding. Complications are unusual, e.g., rupture, hemorrhage, or torsion with infarction of the cyst. If the organ is studded with cysts it is called a polycystic ovary. *Stein-Leventhal syndrome:* large, white polycystic ovaries with a thickened capsule, absence of a corpus luteum, sterility, and hirsutism.

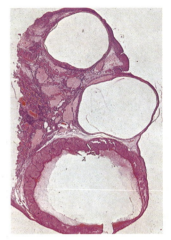

Fig 7–16.—Follicle and corpus luteum cysts in an ovary (hematoxylin-eosin; 15×).

Introductory remarks on ovarian tumors: Systematic consideration of ovarian tumors takes into account the numerous variants in their pathologic and clinical aspects. There are tumors that arise from *paramesonephric coelomic epithelium* (e.g., cystoma, *Brenner tumor),* tumors that arise from *undifferentiated gonadal mesenchyme* (benign and malignant mesenchymal tumors), tumors that arise from *sexually differentiated gonadal mesenchyme* (granulosa and theca cell tumors, androblastoma, hilus cell tumor, gynandroblastoma), tumors that arise from *embryonic cells* (dermoid cyst, teratoma), and tumors that arise from the *mesonephric system* (mesonephroma). In addition, metastatic tumors may occur in the ovary, especially from stomach *(Krukenberg tumor)* and breast carcinomas.

Granulosa cell tumor of the ovary (Fig 7–17) *belongs to a group of facultative malignant tumors that are derived from differentiated ovarian mesenchyme and usually manifest endocrine activity (estrogen secretion).* Histologically the tumors are richly cellular and have solid trabeculae, microfollicles, or a sarcoma-like structure. Characteristically the tumor cells form rosettes surrounding hollow spaces *(Call-Exner bodies).*

Granulosa cell tumors occur at any age. About 30% of them show evidence of malignancy (metastases are uncommon); in the remaining 70% recurrence may occur. Histologially a diagnosis of granulosa cell tumor cannot always be made with certainty.

Theca cell tumors (Fig 7–18) are also germinal tumors (differentiated ovarian mesenchyma) showing endocrine activity. Histologically, elongated cells are arranged in whirls surrounded by abundant collagen fibers. Marked fatty change is typical and gives these fibroma-like tumors a yellow color. About 3% become malignant.

Dermoid cyst of the ovary (Fig 7–19) *is a dysontogenetic neoplasm arising from embryonic cells and containing epidermis, skin appendages, and not infrequently bone and teeth.* Histologically there is a large cystic space lined with a layer of epidermal-like squamous epithelium, beneath which there are hair follicles (→ 1) and sebaceous glands (→ 2). In the lower third of the figure there are dilated sweat glands.

Chronic follicular salpingitis (Fig 7–20) *is the end product of previous chronic interstitial salpingitis and is the result of growth of remnants of the mucosa into the wall with formation of a labyrinth of epithelial sinuses.* Histologically, with low-power magnification, the tube is seen to contain numerous glandular spaces of various sizes.

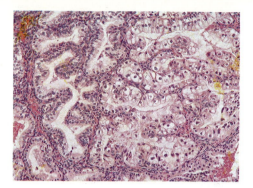

Fig 7–21.—Secretory endometrium in extrauterine pregnancy (Arias-Stella phenomenon) (hematoxylin-eosin; 80×).

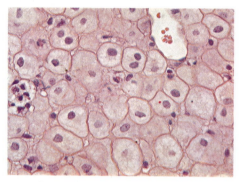

Fig 7–22.—Decidual cells (hematoxylin-eosin; 250×).

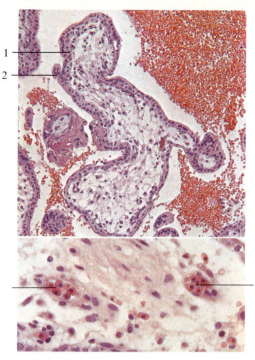

Fig 7–23.—**Top,** placental villi (hematoxylin-eosin; 100×). **Bottom,** nucleated erythrocytes (hematoxylin-eosin; 250×).

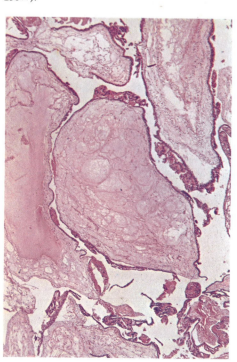

Fig 7–24.—Hydatidiform mole (hematoxylin-eosin; 20×).

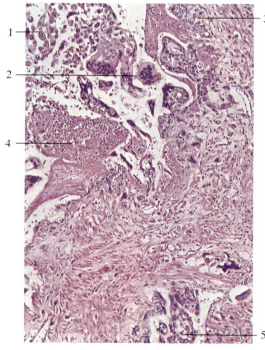

Fig 7–25.—Choriocarcinoma (hematoxylin-eosin; 100×).

Pregnancy: Abortion—Hydatidiform Mole—Choriocarcinoma

Abortion or miscarriage (Figs 7–21 through 7–23) is the intrauterine death and expulsion of an embryo before the 28th week of pregnancy. Histologically the aborted material shows secretory or postsecretory endometrium returning to the resting phase (Fig 7–21), decidual reaction of the stroma (Fig 7–22), and placental villi (Fig 7–23). Frequently there is also marked infiltration of polymorphonuclear leukocytes, which as a rule are not a response to bacteria but rather to disintegration and separation of the endometrium.

In pregnancy the endometrium is the secretory phase—due to the presence of a corpus luteum of pregnancy—and returns to normal after death of the embryo. At this time star-shaped glands are seen having projecting cells with clear cytoplasm and dark, pyknotic nuclei. Such changes, particularly when marked, are referred to as the **Arias-Stella phenomenon** (Fig 7–21) and are solely the result of delayed expulsion of an embryo which has been the cause of the pregnancy. When the curettage shows evidence of incomplete expulsion but no placental villi, then the possibility of an extrauterine pregnancy must be considered. NOTE: extrauterine pregnancy can neither be excluded nor established with certainty by histologic examination of endometrium.

Decidual cells (Fig 7–22) are large stromal cells having distinct borders, abundant cytoplasm, and a round, centrally placed nucleus. They make up the maternal portion of the placenta. Since placental cells are influenced also by exogenous hormones, they are not pathognomonic evidence of pregnancy.

Placental villi (Fig 7–23) are histologic evidence of abortion which can be lacking in extrauterine pregnancy and after completed miscarriages. The villi are composed of a delicate, cell-poor stroma that contains capillaries. In the mature placenta these capillaries contain nucleated erythrocytes (Fig 7–23, lower arrows). The surface of the placental villi consists of an inner layer of cuboidal cells (cytotrophoblasts-Langhans' cells,→ 1) and an outer layer of large, multinucleated giant cells without definable borders (syncytial trophoblasts,→ 2).

Hydatidiform mole (Fig 7–24) is presumed to result from absent or defective formation of fetal vessels leading to ballooning of the stroma of the villi and marked proliferation of trophoblasts. Histologically there are markedly enlarged villi showing lakelike transformation of the stroma which is poor in cells and fibers and shows nodules of proliferated chorion epithelium on the surface (Figs 7–24, 7–26).

Choriocarcinoma (Fig 7–25) is a malignant tumor of placental chorionic villi. The tumor has cytohistolytic trophoblastic activity giving rise to destructive growth and it metastasizes early. In Figure 7–25 the myometrium is invaded by large masses of cells (→ 1). Polymorphous, multinucleated giant cells (→ 2) as well as small clusters of cuboidal cells (→ 3: derived from the Langhans' cells) are also seen. Finally, there are areas of necrosis and fibrin deposition (→ 4). Of diagnostic significance is invasion of veins (→ 5: tumor in vein).

Most choriocarcinomas arise on the basis of a hydatidiform mole (about 60% of cases). Both the primary tumor and its metastases are unusually hemorrhagic. The tumor produces gonadotropin (its detection is important for both diagnosis and prognosis). Choriocarcinomas also occur in the testis in men.

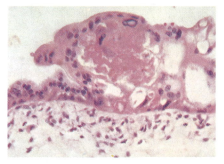

Fig 7–26.—Hydatidiform mole (hematoxylin-eosin; 200 ×).

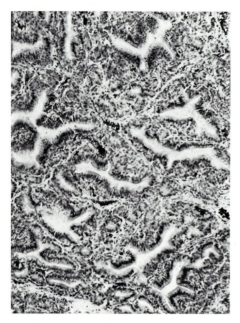

Fig 8–1.—Simple goiter (hematoxylin-eosin; 99×).

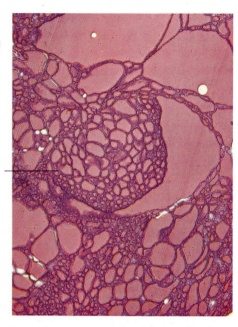

Fig 8–2.—Nodular colloid goiter (hematoxylin-eosin; 38×).

1

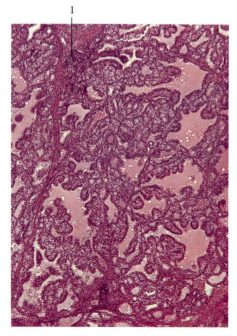

Fig 8–3.—Primary thyrotoxicosis; Graves' disease (hematoxylin-eosin; 38×).

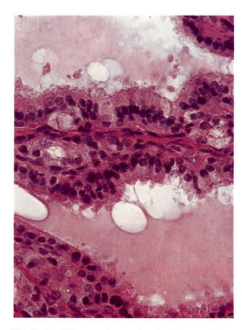

Fig 8–4.—Primary thyrotoxicosis; Graves' disease (hematoxylin-eosin; 396×).

8. Endocrine Glands

Consideration of disturbances of the endocrine glands will be limited to illustrations of a few typical cases, since a thorough description would exceed the scope of this book. Hyperfunction is ordinarily associated with enlargement of the gland and hyperplasia, the proliferation and enlargement of the cells and nuclei ultimately bringing about an adenomatous appearance. Hypofunction, on the other hand, is associated with atrophy of the organ, hypoplasia of cellular elements, and interstitial fibrosis.

Goiter: *Any enlargement of the thyroid in excess of the normal weight for adults of 20–25 gm. The enlargement may result from disturbances of thyroid function (decrease or increase), inflammations, or tumors.*

Diffuse colloid goiter in the adult (euthyroid nodular goiter) develops from simple goiter, i.e., simple diffuse hyperplasia of the thyroid (Fig 8–1) which is common during childhood to puberty (especially in females). Microscopically the thyroid lobules are enlarged and consist of either colloid-free follicles and branching glands lined by tall cylindrical epithelium or of solid cell masses.

Nodular colloid goiter (Fig 8–2). *Nodular thyroid hyperplasia and thyroid adenomas appear to be endemic in certain regions (e.g., the Great Lakes region, Switzerland) but may also be sporadic and are usually regarded as compensatory hyperplasia due to iodine insufficiency* (amino acid deficiency?, inhibition of thyroxin synthesis?) Colloid goiter shows a variety of morphological features. The illustration (Fig 8–2) shows a section of a macrofollicular nodular colloid goiter. A survey of the microscopic section with the scanning lens shows that the nodules are composed of many different-sized follicles and are surrounded by a dense fibrous capsule. The follicles are filled with colloid and lined with flat cuboidal epithelium. Higher magnification reveals cushion-like excrescences of epithelium, which may be so pronounced that new follicles arise within the excrescence (→). Degenerative changes (e.g., central necrosis, cysts, hemorrhages, scars, calcifications) arise as a result of vascular insufficiency and compression of the proliferating colloid nodules against the connective tissue capsule in which lies the nutrient vasculature (oxygen deficiency).

Macroscopic: Enlarged, nodular thyroid. The cut surface shows glistening nodules and focal yellow lesions (degenerative changes). Chiefly occurs in men. *Pathogenesis:* Iodine deficiency leads to diffuse hyperplasia (excess TSH)-with increase in iodine certain areas develop enriched colloid → colloid nodules. The reason for focal distribution is not clear. *Toxic adenomatous goiter* is a hormone-producing adenoma. Histologically there is no correlation between ^{131}I activity and the morphological signs of activity (tall, clear epithelium and decreased colloid).

Primary thyrotoxicosis or Graves' disease (Figs 8–3, 8–4). *In this condition, hyperfunction of the gland produces increased amounts of thyroid homones* (thyrotoxicosis). At low magnification the histologic section (Fig 8–3) reveals large and small, highly branched follicles of various shapes with little or no colloid. The irregular configuration of the follicles is due to the cushion-like overgrowth of the epithelium (pseudopapillary proliferation) which, in places, shows fibrous stalks (papillary proliferation). The colloid, particularly near the surface of the epithelial cells, contains numerous vacuoles. Isolated foci of lymphocytes, in which there are some plasma cells, are quite characteristic (→ in Fig 8–3). **High magnification** (Fig 8–4) shows tall columnar epithelium with pale cytoplasm and basally placed nuclei. In some places, the epithelium is stratified. The so-called resorption vacuoles stand out clearly in this picture. These are artifacts of fixation, indicating that the colloid has a thin consistency.

The cause of hyperthyroidism is not known. An increase in production of thyrotropin-releasing factor (TRF) in the midbrain or of thyroid-stimulating hormone (TSH) has not been proved. A long-acting thyroid stimulator, an IgG (immunoglobulin), called LATS, is produced and becomes bound to cell membranes of the thyroid glands and, like TSH, increases activity. Circulating antibodies against thyroglobulin and the presence of lymphocytes and plasma cells in thyrotoxicosis (Graves' disease) suggest an autoimmune disorder.

Macroscopic: The thyroid is enlarged, and the cut surfaces resemble pancreas.

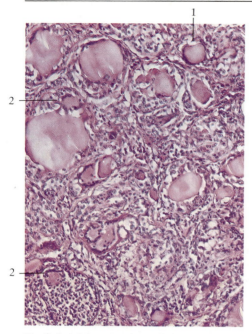

Fig 8–5.—Subacute, nonsuppurative thyroiditis (de Quervain) (hematoxylin-eosin; 160×).

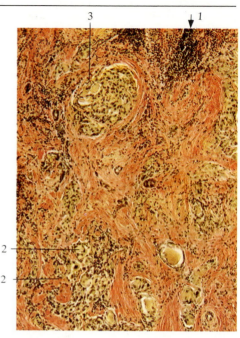

Fig 8–6.—Riedel's struma (van Gieson's stain; 102×).

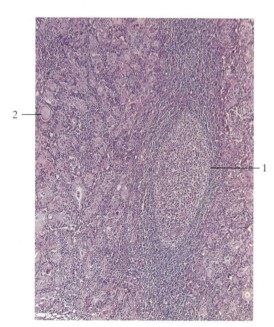

Fig 8–7.—Hashimoto's struma (struma lymphomatosa) (hematoxylin-eosin; 60×).

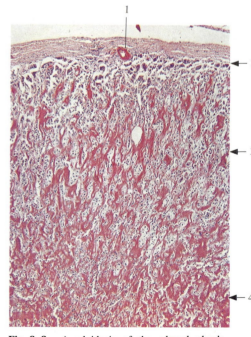

Fig 8–8.—Amyloidosis of the adrenal glands (Congo red stain; 120×).

Thyroiditis

The nonspecific inflammations of the thyroid, although rare, do present an impressive and characteristic histologic picture. In addition to *acute* or *subacute suppurative* and *nonsuppurative inflammations* (*thyroiditis* of de Quervain) there are two types of *chronic thyroiditis*—chronic hypertrophic thyroiditis, or *Riedel's struma* (Riedel), and *struma lymphomatosa* (Hashimoto's disease or lymphadenoid goiter).

Subacute nonsuppurative thyroiditis (de Quervain) (Fig 8–5). Histologically, there are follicles of different sizes lined by cuboidal to columnar epithelium, which, in part, has a cushion-like appearance. Scattered about are smaller follicles without colloid. The relatively viscous colloid and colloid masses (→ 1) have been resorbed by giant cells partly derived from epithelium and partly from mesenchyma (→ 2, a foreign body reaction). Small numbers of lymphocytes, plasma cells, and occasional polymorphonuclear leukocytes can be seen between the follicles. No hypothyroidism. Often a past history of viral infection (mumps).

Chronic hypertrophic thyroiditis or Riedel's struma (Fig 8–6). This form of chronic thyroiditis is accompanied by thyroid enlargement. The organ is firm and the cut surface reveals dense, white sclerotic scar tissue. The predominant features, microscopically, are hyalinized streaks of scar tissue and focal lymphocytic infiltration (→ 1). The follicles, except for some small remnants, are destroyed. A few isolated groups of intact follicles (→ 2) may undergo regenerative proliferation, thus giving rise to small adenomas (→ 3). An important diagnostic feature is the extension of the chronic sclerosing inflammation into the soft tissues of the neck, in particular the muscles. Sometimes only a single thyroid lobule is affected.

Struma lymphomatosa (Hashimoto) (Fig 8–7). This is a chronic, progressive inflammation characterized by lymphocytic infiltration and atrophy of thyroid follicles and destruction of follicular epithelium. Figure 8–7 shows diffuse interstitial lymphocytic infiltration (often there are plasma cells), with formation of a typical lymphoid follicle having a reaction center (→ 1). The thyroid follicles are small; some contain inspissated colloid (→ 2) and others are empty.

Clinical: Hypothyroidism, sometimes myxedema.

Macroscopic: Slightly swollen, firm, brownish cut surface flecked with white.

Pathogenesis: 65% of the cases of chronic thyroiditis show autoantibodies against thyroid tissues when tested immunologically (autoimmunity). Also antibodies against gastric parietal cells and intrinsic factor (40% of all patients have pernicious anemia) may be seen. It can be shown in animal experiments that injection of thyroid extract causes a thyroiditis that histologically resembles very closely struma lymphomatosa. Thyroid carcinoma occurs in 3% of cases. A similar mechanism (autoaggression) has been suggested for many other diseases: allergic encephalitis, lupus erythematosus, immune hemolytic anemia, agranulocytosis, thrombocytopenia, chronic glomerulonephritis, cirrhosis of liver, myasthenia gravis, ulcerative colitis.

Amyloidosis of the adrenal gland (Fig 8–8). *Amyloid deposition in the adrenal cortex occurs regularly in cases of general amyloidosis (kidney, spleen, liver). Clinical adrenal cortical insufficiency can develop in severe cases.* The section shows a small artery (→ 1) in the capsule, in the wall of which a homogeneous, red-stained deposit can be seen. In the cortex, the amyloid is deposited around capillaries. The zona glomerulosa is unaffected (→ 2). Broad bands of amyloid in the zona fasciculata (→ 3) and reticularis (→ 4) have caused pressure atrophy of the cortical cells.

Macroscopic: The adrenals are enlarged and appear glassy.

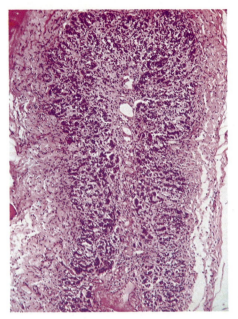

Fig 8–9.—Atrophy of the adrenal cortex (hematoxylin-eosin; 66×).

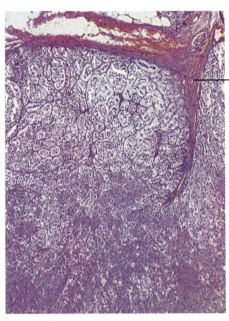

Fig 8–10.—Hyperplasia of the adrenal cortex in Cushing's disease (hematoxylin-eosin; 64×).

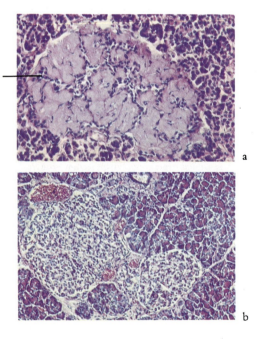

a

b

Fig 8–11.—**Top,** hyalinization of an islet of Langerhans (diabetes mellitus) (hematoxylin-eosin; 170×). **Bottom,** islet hyperplasia (newborn of a diabetic mother) (hematoxylin-eosin; 127×).

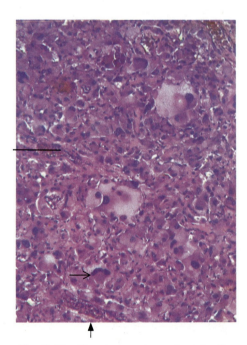

Fig 8–12.—Pheochromocytoma (hematoxylin-eosin; 130×).

Atrophy of adrenal cortex (Fig 8–9). Adrenal insufficiency may result from manifest disease of the adrenal cortex (tuberculosis, cytotoxic contraction, hemorrhage, and unknown causes), so-called *primary adrenal insufficiency*. Clinically, the picture is that of *Addison's disease*. On the other hand, adrenal insufficiency may be *secondary to insufficient hypophyseal stimulation* (ACTH deficiency) as in postpartum pituitary necrosis or scarring, or after infections or trauma.

Figure 8–9 is from a patient with *Sheehan's syndrome* and *secondary cortical atrophy*. The cortex is much reduced and the various zones are completely disorganized. The cortex consists solely of clumps and groups of cells, the arrangement of which is faintly reminiscent of the zona glomerulosa. There is also proliferation of interstitial fibrous tissue.

Macroscopically, the adrenal cortex is paper-thin. *Clinically,* there is panhypopituitarism, so-called Simmond's disease.

Adrenal cortical hyperplasia in Cushing's disease (Fig 8–10): In Cushing's syndrome, there is overproduction of adrenocortical hormones (glucocorticoids), with metabolic transformation from protein manufacture to production of glucose and fat. In 30% of cases, the adrenal cortex shows hyperplasia which is dependent on increased ACTH production by a basophilic or chromophobic pituitary adenoma. Usually, however, no pituitary tumor can be found (primary hyperplasia of unknown cause). True adrenal cortical adenomas (or carcinoma in children) may also cause the syndrome.

Figure 8–10 shows great widening of the adrenal cortex (compare this with Fig 8–9, which is at the same magnification) which is so great that only a portion of the cortex can be shown. The zona fasciculata extends to the connective tissue capsule; in its upper part there are lipid-laden cells (the fat has been dissolved in preparation of the section), arranged in clusters,→: radiating septum of connective tissue (beginning adenoma formation, nodular hyperplasia).

Macroscopic: Enlarged adrenals showing a wide, yellow cortex and nodular hyperplasia or adenomas. *Clinical:* Obesity of the trunk, full-moon visage, thick neck, striae, hypertension, osteoporosis, diabetes.

Islet hyalinization in diabetes mellitus (Fig 8–11, top). Hyalinization of the capillaries of the islets of Langerhans may be found, particularly in diabetes in elderly persons (not in young persons!). Whether this is the cause or the consequence of the diabetes is disputed. The hyaline material (amyloid) is deposited in the wall of the capillaries, obstructs the lumen, and secondarily causes atrophy of the islet cells (→).

Islet hyperplasia (newborn of a diabetic mother) (Fig 8–11, bottom). This is considered an adaptation hyperplasia of the islets of Langerhans of the fetus to the hyperglycemia of the diabetic mother. The richly cellular giant islets can be easily seen under low magnification. Higher magnification shows, in addition, greatly enlarged nuclei and often multinucleated giant cells (β-cell hyperplasia).

Pheochromocytoma (Figs 8–12, 8–13). This is usually a benign tumor (malignant examples are rare) of the adrenal medulla (most unilateral, 40–50 years). Most have endocrine activity (periodic outpouring of adrenalin and noradrenalin. *Clinical:* Increase in blood pressure, hyperglycemia).

The histologic picture shows epithelial tumor tissue arranged in strands or cellular clusters, often situated perivascularly (→: vessel). The cells are large, round or polygonal, and pleomorphic and frequently have eccentrically situated nuclei. Giant cells are seen frequently. Wide hemorrhage is common. The brown color produced by the chromate reaction (dichromate salts) demonstrates adrenalin (fine granules) and noradrenalin-producing cells (large granules) (Fig 8–13). Noradrenalin can be identified with potassium iodide. Commonly there is hemorrhage and resulting deposition of hemosiderin (Fig 8–13).

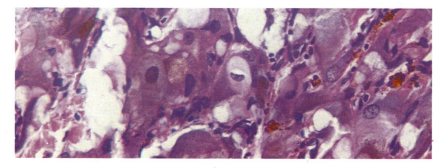

Fig 8–13.—Pheochromocytoma after chromation (hematoxylin-eosin; 375 ×).

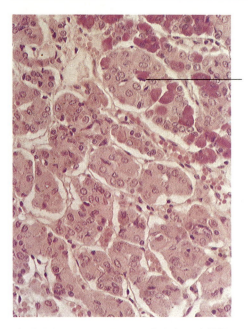

Fig 8–14.—Focal hyperplasia of pituitary ACTH cells (hematoxylin-eosin; 400×).

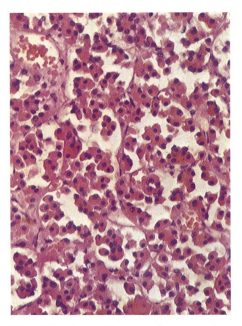

Fig 8–15.—Eosinophilic adenoma of the anterior lobe of the pituitary (hematoxylin-eosin; 130×).

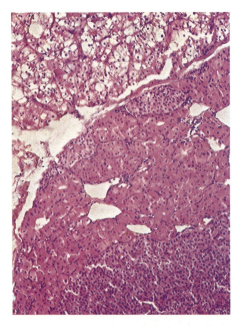

Fig 8–16.—Parathyroid adenoma (hematoxylin-eosin; 130×).

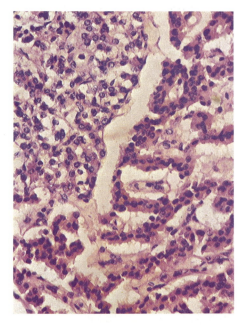

Fig 8–17.—G-cell adenoma of pancreas in Zollinger-Ellison syndrome (hematoxylin-eosin; 400×).

Focal hyperplasia of pituitary ACTH cells in primary adrenal cortical insufficiency (Fig 8–14). The illustration is of the margin of a hyperplastic focus of ACTH-stimulating cells. Stained by hematoxylin-eosin, the cells appear large and polygonal and have granular gray-appearing cytoplasm. Since the ACTH granules do not stain clearly they have been called chromophobe cells, amphophiles, or neutrophils. The ACTH cells for the most part show a follicular arrangement and enclose a drop of colloid. In the upper right-hand corner of the figure there are some bright red acidophilic TSH cells (growth hormone).

The classic division of cells of the anterior lobe of the hypophysis (adenohypophysis) into acidophiles, basophiles, and chromophobes, which was based on hematoxylin-eosin stains, no longer is appropriate for our modern functional and morphological ideas. With the help of fluorescence antibody techniques and new histologic staining methods it is possible to make a truly functional classification of the different types of cells of the anterior lobe of the hypophysis. Thus the classic "basophils," which are identical to the periodic acid–positive mucoid cells, can be subdivided into TSH cells (thyroid-stimulating hormone, alcian blue–positive "S" cells), FSH (follicle-stimulating) and LH cells (luteinizing hormone, alcian blue–negative, purple staining cells), ACTH cells (alcian blue–negative, faintly purple staining "R" cells), and MSH cells (melanocyte-stimulating hormone).

Eosinophilic adenoma of the anterior lobe of the pituitary (Fig 8–15). About 30% of anterior pituitary adenomas are composed either entirely or predominantly of eosinophilic (acidophilic) cells. Histologically, in sections stained with hematoxylin-eosin, they are compactly arranged, medium-sized, uniform, polygonal cells with bright red cytoplasm (Fig 8–15). The spaces between the cell groups are artifacts due to shrinkage during preparation.

Eosinophilic adenomas may show increased hormone activity and thus cause *acromegaly* or *gigantism*.

Parathyroid adenoma (Fig 8–16). Histologically, adenomas of the parathyroid glands, in contrast to hyperplasia, are nodules consisting of the three cell types that compose the glands: (1) small chief cells (bottom of picture), (2) oxyphil cells with abundant eosinophilic cytoplasm (middle of picture), and (3) water-clear chief cells (top of picture). The chief cells contain glycogen which has been washed out by the aqueous fixatives and stains. Water-clear chief cells constitute the functionally active parathormone-producing cells, while oxyphil cells are thought to be involutional forms of chief cells.

Autonomous, benign parathyroid adenomas are the cause of 90% of all cases of *primary hyperparathyroidism*. The remaining 10% are due to primary hyperplasia and hypertrophy of the parathyroids or to a functionally active parathyroid carcinoma.

G-cell tumors of pancreatic islets in the Zollinger-Ellison syndrome (Fig 8–17). Histologically, these are solid tumor nodules composed of nests and cords of uniform epithelium with eosinophilic cytoplasm. Usually pseudoacini are prominent, in contrast to true glands, and contain scanty, shrunken stroma. In the top left-hand part of the picture there is exocrine pancreas.

G-cell tumors are tumors of gastrin-secreting cells that occur chiefly in the pancreatic islets. *Gastrin* is a polypeptide hormone that can be cytochemically localized in certain polypeptide-secreting endocrine cells (APUD series*). Other APUD cells are ACTH cells, MSH cells, α cells (glucagon), β cells (insulin) of the islets of Langerhans, C cells of the thyroid (calcitonin) as well as argyrophiles and the enterochromaffin cells of the small intestine. G-cell tumors with *Zollinger-Ellison syndrome* (clinical triad: pancreatic tumor, hypersecretion, and hyperacidity of gastric juice; therapeutically intractable; and commonly recurrent ulcers typically located in stomach or duodenum or atypically in jejunum).

---

*APUD = amine precursor uptake and decarboxylation.

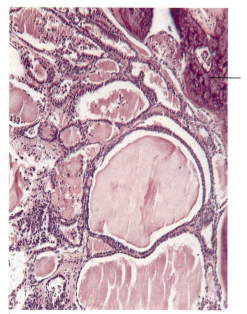

Fig 8–18.—Follicular carcinoma of thyroid; metastasis (hematoxylin-eosin; 80×).

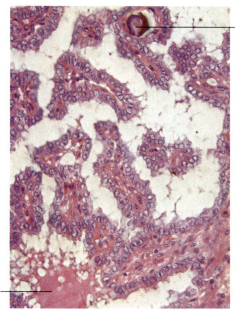

Fig 8–19.—Papillary carcinoma of thyroid (hematoxylin-eosin; 200×).

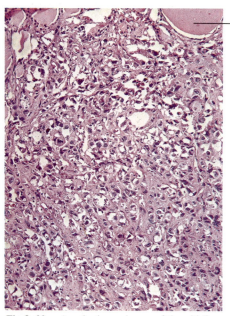

Fig 8–20.—Anaplastic carcinoma of thyroid (hematoxylin-eosin; 100×).

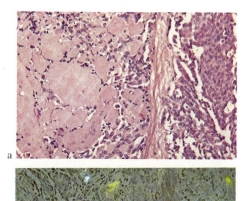

Fig 8–21.—**Top,** medullary carcinoma of thyroid with amyloid stroma (hematoxylin-eosin; 100×). **Bottom,** doubly refractive amyloid in polarized light (Congo red stain; 80×).

Malignant Thyroid Tumors

Malignant tumors of the thyroid may arise either from follicular epithelial cells or parafollicular epithelium (calcitonin-producing C cells). Tumors derived from follicular epithelium include well-differentiated, organoid carcinomas as well as undifferentiated or anaplastic carcinomas. Oncocytoma is a cytologic variant of these. Malignant thyroid tumors account for 0.1% of deaths from all malignant tumors and are about eleventh in the tumor fatality list. They appear mostly between 40 and 60 years of age: organoid neoplasms earlier, undifferentiated carcinomas later. Women are affected 2–3.5 times more frequently than men.

Follicular carcinoma (Fig 8–18) *belongs to the organoid malignant neoplasms of the thyroid and frequently is first detected by the presence of a metastasis from a seemingly normal thyroid gland or encapsulated thyroid nodule or adenoma.* (For this reason it was formerly called "metastasizing adenoma.") Figure 8–18 shows a vertebral metastasis of a follicular carcinoma of the thyroid having follicles of different sizes which are filled with homogeneous eosinophilic colloid (the metastases may store ^{131}I). The arrow points to the bluish-staining bony trabeculae of the vertebra (decalcified).

Papillary thyroid carcinoma (Fig 8–19) consists of ramifying stromal septa covered by a single layer of epithelium. The nuclei of these cells are poor in chromatin and occasionally enclose a large, round, faintly acidophilic vacuole (invagination of cytoplasm). The stroma (Fig 8–19) contains bluish, concentrically layered calcium deposits (psammoma bodies, → 2). Small colloid masses lie between the strands of tumor (→ 2).

Papillary carcinoma of the thyroid chiefly occurs in children and young persons. At first it grows very slowly and metastasizes to cervical lymph nodes, which not uncommonly may be the first and only clinical sign of the tumor for many months. NOTE: Solitary thyroid nodules are more frequently malignant in the young than in adults. For prognostic and therapeutic purposes, papillary tumors should always be diagnosed as malignant tumors.

Anaplastic thyroid carcinoma (Fig 8–20) *is an undifferentiated tumor showing no organoid structure.* Histologically the tumor shows all the signs of malignancy: cellular and nuclear pleomorphism and many mitoses, some of which are atypical. Occasionally anaplastic thyroid carcinoma cannot be differentiated from a spindle cell carcinoma (sarcoma-like growth of a carcinoma). Figure 8–20 shows a very pleomorphic carcinoma which has invaded and destroyed the thyroid follicles (→).

Anaplastic thyroid carcinomas are particularly malignant. They occur preferentially in older people (after 60) and invade the capsule, blood vessels (→ hematogenous metastases → lung) and trachea early. Histologically the following types are recognized: spindle cell, round cell, pleomorphic (polymorphous), and clear cell (corresponding to hypernephroid renal carcinoma).

Oncocytomas are composed of large cells with finely granular eosinophilic cytoplasm (rich in mitochondria) and round chromatic nuclei. Oncocytomas are either adenomas or carcinomas and show no clinical manifestations different from follicular or anaplastic carcinomas. Oncocytes (= swollen cells) appear also in other organs (e.g., in parathyroid and salivary glands, trachea, liver, etc.) Thyroid oncocytomas formerly were called *Hürthle cell tumors.*

Medullary thyroid carcinoma with amyloid stroma (Fig 8–21) *is a slow-growing, late-metastasizing carcinoma which arises from C cells.* The tumor forms medullary islands surrounded by homogeneous, eosinophilic stroma (Fig 8–21, top). Preparations stained with Congo red and examined with polarized light show the greenish yellow double refraction characteristic of amyloid.

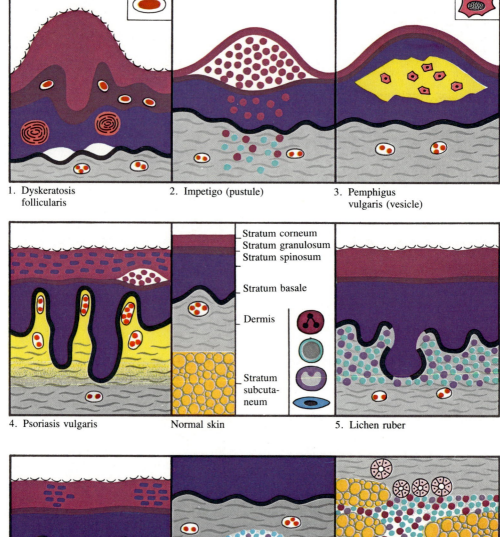

1. Dyskeratosis
   follicularis

2. Impetigo (pustule)

3. Pemphigus
   vulgaris (vesicle)

4. Psoriasis vulgaris

Normal skin

Stratum corneum
Stratum granulosum
Stratum spinosum

Stratum basale

Dermis

Stratum
subcuta-
neum

5. Lichen ruber

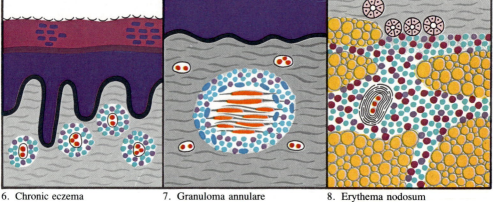

6. Chronic eczema
   (neurodermatitis)

7. Granuloma annulare

8. Erythema nodosum

Fig 9–1.—Diagram of examples of different skin lesions.

9. Skin—Soft Tissues—Breast

The histopathology of the skin constitutes a difficult and complicated area of knowledge. As a rule the tissue changes can only be interpreted correctly with knowledge of the clinical (age, sex, duration) and gross findings (localization, onset, appearance, color, etc.). Only a few skin diseases, chosen for their clinical or theoretical significance, can be discussed in this chapter because of limitations of space.

1. **Disturbances of cornification.** There are numerous congenital and acquired skin and general diseases. In *ichthyosis congenita,* which differs from ichthyosis vulgaris only in the severity of the changes, hyperkeratosis and atrophy of the granular cell layer are conspicuous. Hyperkeratosis also occurs in local chronic irritation *(calluses)* or in viral warts, cutaneous horns, chronic arsenic poisoning (palmar and plantar hyperkeratosis), and from other causes.

In **dyskeratosis follicularis of Darier** (Fig 9–1/1) are found both hyperkeratosis and dyskeratosis leading to suprabasal splitting (acantholysis) with formation of vesicles and lacunae. Typically there are "corps ronds" (large eosinophilic cells with distinct borders and basophilic nuclei in the stratum granulosum and stratum spinosum) as well as "grains" (small cells with elongated nuclei) localized in the horny layer.

2. **Epidermal lesions. Impetigo** (Fig 9–1/2) is a bacterial skin infection (staphylococci and streptococci) manifested by vesicle formation in the horny layer. The vesicles contain polymorphonuclear leukocytes. Vesicle formation (bullous eruption) is also a prominent feature of **pemphigus vulgaris** (Fig 9–1/3). There are intraepidermal acantholytic cells with degenerate prickle cells (so-called Tzanck cells). The dermal papillae in the floor of the vesicles are hyperplastic and covered with a layer of persistent basal cells.

3. **Disturbances of epidermis and corium: psoriasis vulgaris** (Fig 9–1/4). A familial, progressive disease which presents as sharply delimited erythematous, maculopapillary eruptions overlaid with pale silver scales. The microscopic picture shows parakeratosis (nucleated scales), acanthosis (prolongation of the epidermal columns), and papillomatosis (extension of dermal papillae nearly to the horny layer). Dilated vessels, perivascular edema, and infiltration of lymphocytes, histiocytes, and granulocytes are seen in the stratum papillare and stratum reticulare. Microabscesses, which are not always found, contain compacted neutrophilic leukocytes just below the stratum corneum.

Lichen ruber planus (Fig 9–1/5) is a dermatitis accompanied by marked itching and irregularly marginated, livid red papules. The principal histologic features are thickened, hyperkeratotic epidermis and a bandlike infiltrate composed predominantly of lymphocytes. It occurs in the basal cell layer, which shows vacuolar degeneration and has a moth-eaten appearance.

Chronic eczema (Fig 9–1/6) is a common form of dermatitis and is classified according to either etiology, course, or morphology. Histologically there are chiefly hyperkeratosis, lichenification, and occasional islands of parakeratosis. Rete pegs are elongated, the dermis showing a prominent perivascular infiltrate.

4. **Disturbance of dermis and subcutis.** In this category are inflammatory, degenerative diseases as well as infiltrations (e.g., amyloidosis of skin). **Granuloma annulare** (Fig 9–1/7) shows nodular degeneration of collagen in the dermis together with inflammation and fibrosis. The nodules result from coagulation necrosis, homogenization and fragmentation of collagen fibers and are infiltrated with lymphocytes, histiocytes, and fibroblasts. The lesion must be differentiated from lipoid necrobiosis and rheumatic nodules. **Erythema nodosum** (Fig 9–1/8) consists of slightly raised nodules underneath the skin, situated in the upper subcutaneous tissues. When fresh, the lesions contain small infiltrates composed of neutrophiles and lymphocytes. There is similar inflammation in the walls of small veins, together with proliferation of endothelium. Older lesions may contain focal collections of histiocytes and multinucleated foreign body giant cells.

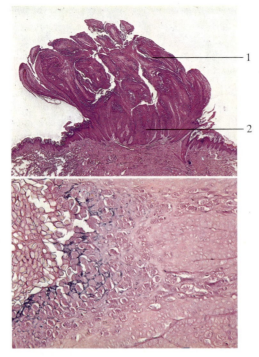

Fig 9–2.—**Top,** common wart (hematoxylin-eosin; 8×). **Bottom,** molluscum contagiosum (hematoxylin-eosin; 80×).

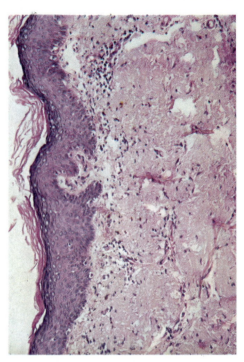

Fig 9–3.—Senile elastosis (hematoxylin-eosin; 100×).

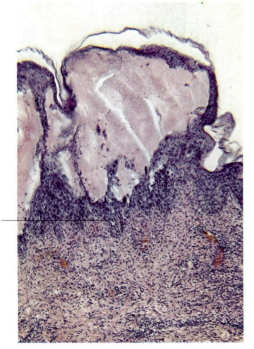

Fig 9–4.—Vesicular eruption in chickenpox (varicella) (hematoxylin-eosin; 60×).

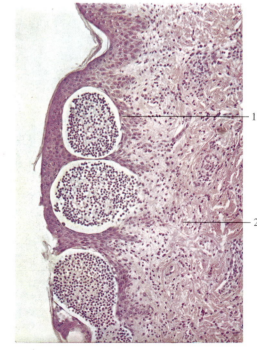

Fig 9–5.—Dermatitis herpetiformis (hematoxylin-eosin; 80×).

Verruca vulgaris (common wart, Fig 9–2) *occurs chiefly in children and young persons. It is a benign, virus-caused neoplasm of the skin, manifested by hyperkeratosis, acanthosis, papillomatosis, and cellular inclusions.* Histologically there is a mixture of hyperkeratotic and parakeratotic (persistence of nuclei in the horny layer) cornification (→ 1). The underlying epidermis shows acanthosis and papillomatosis (→ 2), and prominent keratohyaline granules. In the upper layers of the stratum spinosum and corneum many cells are ballooned by edema. Verruca vulgaris shows two types of inclusions: basophilic, intranuclear, DNA-containing (positive Feulgen reaction) inclusions and eosinophilic, Feulgen negative, cytoplasmic inclusions that derive from keratohyaline granules.

There are several types of viral warts which differ in their localization and morphology. *Verruca plantaris,* the plantar wart, develops beneath the surface of the skin. *Horny mucous warts* (e.g., on the lip) show only slight cornification. *Verruca plana juvenilis* shows prominent acanthosis and hyperkeratosis, lacks papillomatosis, and may convert to verruca vulgaris. **Molluscum contagiosum** or venereal wart (Fig 9–2, bottom) may be described as an infectious acanthoma lying beneath the skin surface. Typically there are molluscum bodies: cornified epithelial cells containing nuclear remains and viral elementary bodies. They are eosinophilic and at first show septa but later are homogeneous.

Senile elastosis (Fig 9–3) *consists of homogeneous degeneration of collagen fibers in the upper corium.* The tissue has a uniform appearance and stains intensely with elastica stains. The overlying epidermis is variably widened with slight hyperkeratosis.

Senile elastosis is a degenerative lesion and should be distinguished from **senile keratosis** in which there are marked epidermal changes: parts are atrophic and other parts hypertrophic. There is pronounced superficial hyperkeratosis and the underlying epidermis shows cellular atypia and mitoses (so-called dysplasia). These changes, occurring particularly in the elderly and in persons exposed excessively to the sun or weather (farmers, seamen, etc.), may be precancerous lesions.

Vesicular eruption in chickenpox (Fig 9–4). *This is a virus disease characterized by a generalized vesicular and pustular exanthem.* Histologically, there is intraepidermal vesicle formation just as in smallpox, herpes zoster, and herpes simplex. Figure 9–4 shows such a vesicle containing homogeneous protein material. The uppermost epidermal layer forms the outer margin, and a thin basal layer (→) delimits the vesicle from the dermis. The dermis is slightly infiltrated with lymphocytes. The intraepidermal vesicle is formed from the deterioration of epidermal cells. Intranuclear inclusion bodies are present. Similar vesicles, but without inclusion bodies, are seen in the skin in burns and freezing.

Dermatitis herpetiformis (Fig 9–5). *This is a dermatitis of allergic origin which causes an irritating pruritus. The disease involves particularly the trunk, buttocks, and scalp.* In contrast to pemphigus vulgaris (= intraepidermal vesicles), the microscopic picture of dermatitis herpetiformis reveals mainly subepidermal vesicles or bleb formations. In the vesiculobullous eruptions, many eosinophilic leukocytes are found (→ 1). The dermal connective tissue forming the floor of the vesicles shows an inflammatory reaction (→ 2). Edema, dilated blood vessels, eosinophilic leukocytes, and lymphocytes are present.

Macroscopic: The clinical picture is pleomorphic. Erythema, urticaria, vesicles, and bullae occur. Often the eruption is herpetiform. A symmetric distribution is often apparent.

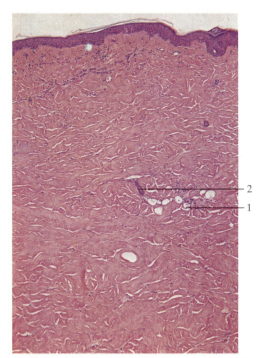

Fig 9–6.—Scleroderma (hematoxylin-eosin; 40×).

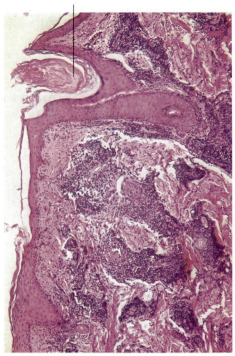

Fig 9–7.—Chronic discoid lupus erythematosus (hematoxylin-eosin; 30×).

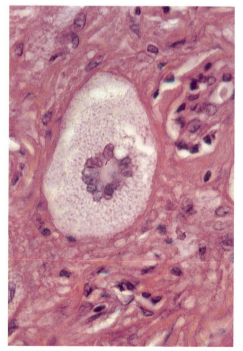

Fig 9–8.—Touton giant cell in xanthoma (hematoxylin-eosin; 320×).

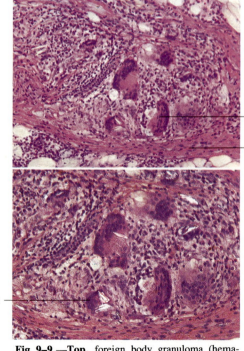

Fig 9–9.—Top, foreign body granuloma (hematoxylin-eosin; 80×). Bottom, doubly refractile foreign bodies in polarized light (hematoxylin-eosin; 100×).

Scleroderma (Fig 9–6) *may be either isolated or generalized and belongs to the group of collagen or, more properly, connective tissue diseases. Clinically it is manifested by thickening of the dermis due to increase in collagen fibers.* Histologically there is distinct thinning of the epidermis. The underlying corium contains bundles of numerous thick and sclerotic collagen fibers. Fibroblasts are numerically diminished and skin appendages are absent (atrophy). Trapped fat cells (→ 1) and sweat glands (→ 2) suggest that the corium is increased in thickness at the expense of the fat panniculus.

Clinically a distinction is made between *circumscribed, localized benign scleroderma* and the *progressive, diffuse, generalized form* with involvement of internal organs (heart, muscle, intestine, esophagus, kidneys). Transitions between the two forms do not occur. They are indistinguishable histologically. *Macroscopically* there is an irregularly shaped nodule of thick and retracted skin. It occurs particularly on the hands and face *(acrosclerosis)*.

Disseminated **lupus erythematosus** (Fig 9–7) also belongs to the group of connective tissue diseases. It can be manifest as an acute, generalized disorder or as a chronic ailment limited to the skin. In *chronic discoid lupus erythematosus* the following changes in the skin are seen: (1) Hyperkeratosis of *epidermis,* hypergranularity (increase in keratohyaline granules), atrophy of prickle cells, and focal liquefaction of basal cells. (2) Atrophy of *skin appendages* as well as follicular plugging by keratin (→). (3) Lymphocytic infiltration in the *corium* extending into the epidermis and hair follicles. Telangiectasis, edema, and destruction of elastic fibers are also present.

In acute lupus erythematosus there is fibrinoid degeneration of the collagen fibers of internal organs (heart, kidney, spleen) and involvement of the skin is seldom prominent.

Touton giant cells (Fig 9–8) are multinucleated foam cells (resulting from fine fat droplets in the cytoplasm). Characteristic of these cells are the centrally placed, wreath-shaped nuclei and the surrounding eosinophilic cytoplasm. Foam cells are seen in numerous metabolic disturbances and inflammatory, posttraumatic, and neoplastic diseases, e.g., in primary hypercholesterolemic xanthomatosis, xanthoma and fibroxanthoma, histiocytoma, giant cell tumors of bone, in fatty deposits (xanthelasma of the eyelids), in cholesterosis and inflammation of the gallbladder, and in the pelvis of the kidney and other organs.

Foreign body granuloma (Fig 9–9) *has a peripheral zone of scarring (→ 1) and a central zone rich in inflammatory cells* (lymphocytes, histiocytes, blood vessels) as well as *typical foreign body giant cells.* They contain *foreign bodies (→ 2)* of various sizes. Doubly refractive foreign bodies (talc crystals) can be clearly demonstrated in polarized light (Fig 9–9, bottom). Other foreign bodies include *endogenous material* (cholesterin crystals, extruded epithelial mucus, horny lamellae from a ruptured atheroma) as well as *exogenous* material (wood, talcum, metal, oily materials, paraffin). Fat-soluble foreign bodies often appear as crystal-like spaces.

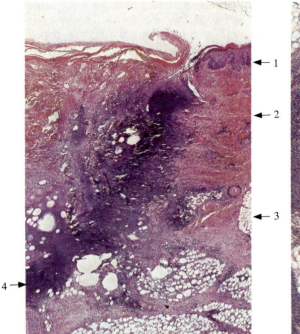

Fig 9–10.—Decubitus (hematoxylin-eosin; 15×).

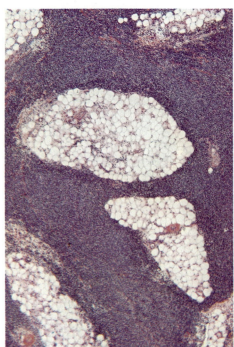

Fig 9–11.—Acute phlegmonous inflammation of subcutaneous fat tissue (cellulitis) (hematoxylin-eosin; 42×).

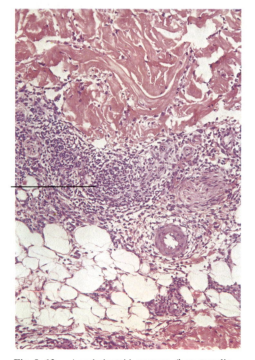

Fig 9–12.—Anaphylactoid purpura (hematoxylin-eosin; 80×).

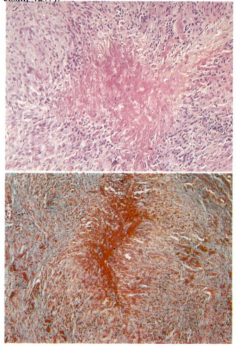

Fig 9–13.—Rheumatoid nodule (**top,** hematoxylin-eosin; **bottom,** azan stain; 80×).

Decubitus (Fig 9–10). *This is an example of cutaneous necrosis due to local tissue death resulting from prolonged pressure. This type of necrosis occurs most frequently over the ischium in bedridden patients or patients with spinal cord injuries and is due to compression of blood vessels and eventual ulceration.* The histologic picture reveals preserved epidermis (→ 1), dermis (→ 2) and subcutaneous tissues (→ 3). A blue-staining zone of leukocytes and cellular debris cuts transversely through the section (→ 4). This blends into another necrotic, anuclear zone. Later, granulation tissue will delimit and replace the necrotic tissue, producing an ulcer.

Acute phlegmonous inflammation (cellulitis) of subcutaneous fat tissue (Fig 9–11). Diffuse leukocytic inflammation of the skin has developed mainly in the loose subcutaneous fat tissue, in which it can easily spread. Histologically, there is a diffuse, dense, streaklike infiltration of polymorphonuclear leukocytes that surround islands of remaining fat cells. Streptococci are the usual causative agent.

Anaphylactoid purpura (Henoch-Schönlein, Fig 9–12) *is an inflammatory vasculitis of the skin of infectious, drug allergy, or, not uncommonly, an unknown origin, manifested by skin hemorrhages (petechiae and ecchymoses) and frequently also by involvement of internal organs (intestine, kidney, joints).* Histologically in a **fresh nodule** the vascular endothelial cells are swollen, the vessel walls are necrotic, and there are dense collections of neutrophils (occasionally eosinophils or lymphocytes) surrounding them (→). Typically there are nuclear fragments derived from destruction of neutrophils. Older lesions are recognized by the appearance of erythrocytes.

Purpura occurs in several infectious bacterial diseases (e.g., meningococcal meningitis, subacute bacterial endocarditis). Purpura caused by drug allergy shows the same histologic picture as anaphylactoid purpura.

Rheumatoid nodule (Fig 9–13). *In both acute rheumatic fever (see chap. 1) and chronic rheumatoid arthritis (see chap. 13) skin nodules may develop with central zones of fibrinoid necrosis and a palisade-like arrangement of histiocytes.* In a hematoxylin-eosin–stained section (Fig 9–13, top) it is easy to see the central zone of eosinophilic, anuclear necrosis surrounded by a wall-like arrangement of histiocytes with elongated nuclei. The fibrinoid necrosis characteristically stains red with azan (Fig 9–3, bottom).

Rheumatic skin nodules occur preferentially at the elbow, knee joint, and ankle. They may attain a diameter of 2 cm or more. Rheumatic nodules develop usually in the deeper layers of the skin, i.e., in the panniculus adiposus. Granuloma annulare occurs in the corium, but otherwise there is much similarity in the histologic picture of the two diseases.

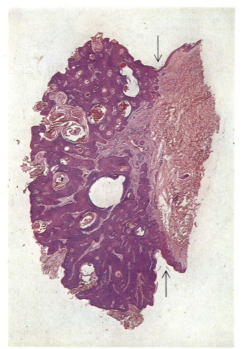

Fig 9–14.—Seborrheic keratosis (hematoxylin-eosin; 5×).

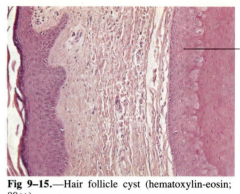

Fig 9–15.—Hair follicle cyst (hematoxylin-eosin; 80×).

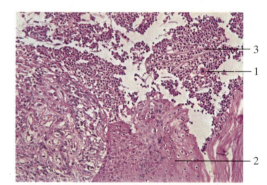

Fig 9–16.—Ruptured epidermal cyst (hematoxylin-eosin; 80×).

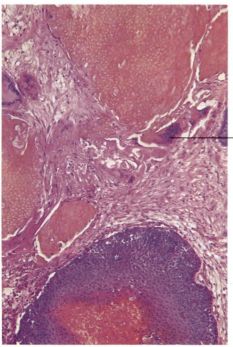

Fig 9–17.—Benign calcifying epithelioma of Malherbe (trichoepithelioma) (hematoxylin-eosin; 80×).

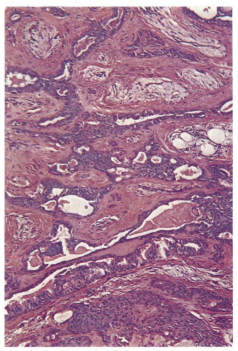

Fig 9–18.—Sweat gland adenoma (hematoxylin-eosin; 80×).

Seborrheic keratosis (basal cell papilloma, verruca senilis, senile wart, Fig 9–14). *This is a common benign neoplasm which develops most often in areas of nonexposed skin in older people* and is manifested by proliferation of the cells of the basal layer and horny keratosis. Histologically there is a caplike tumor, located on the surface of the skin (→ ←), that is composed of proliferated basal cells (hence the marked basophilia). Superficially and between the cells there is cornification which is derived from the granular cell layer. The basal portion of the tumor shows marked melanin pigmentation. The stroma of chronically irritated lesions show inflammatory cellular infiltration.

Seborrheic warts are one of the commonest of skin neoplasms. In younger men there are often engulfed islands of prickle cells (baso-prickle cell acanthoma). Basal cell carcinoma is seldom cornified and invades more deeply than seborrheic wart, from which it must be differentiated.

Dermal cysts are of two types: (1) **Hair follicle cysts** (Fig 9–15), derived from the epithelial sheath of hair follicle. Histologically the cyst is lined by multilayered epithelium (→ 1) and shows amorphous, acidophilic, frequently centrally calcified masses containing cholesterin crystals. 2. **Epidermal cysts** (Fig 9–16), in contrast to hair follicle cysts, are lined by keratotic, cornified epithelium and contain layered horny lamellae. When a dermal cyst ruptures a *foreign body reaction* develops with accumulation of inflammatory and giant cells (→ 1) about the remaining epithelium (→ 2) and the cornified lamellae (→ 3).

Dermal cysts are among the commonest tumors of the skin. True dermoid cysts are uncommon—apart from *pilonidal sinus* or *sacral dermoid,* which is a dermal foreign body reaction caused by broken and impacted hairs in corium.

Benign calcifying epithelioma of Malherbe (Fig 9–17) *is a benign tumor of squamous epithelium of the matrix of the hair follicle.* Histologically the tumor consists in part of bands of intact basophilic epithelium (bottom of Fig 9–17) and in part of necrotic epithelium without nuclei (so-called shadow cells: top of Fig 9–17). The necrotic parts may calcify or occasionally even ossify. A foreign body reaction in the stroma with multinucleated giant cells (→) is typical.

Sweat gland tumors can show a variety of architectural patterns. **Syringoma** (Fig 9–18) serves as an example. There is a double layer of epithelium and a fibrous stroma. In general the cells have a uniform appearance.

There are numerous variants of *benign sweat gland tumors* which can only be mentioned here: papillary syringoma, eccrine spiradenoma (myoepithelioma), eccrine acrospiroma (clear cell myoepithelioma), chondroid syringoma with cartilaginous stroma, eccrine dermal cylindroma, and hidradenoma. Mucinous adenocarcinoma of the skin is a special, malignant variant of sweat gland tumors.

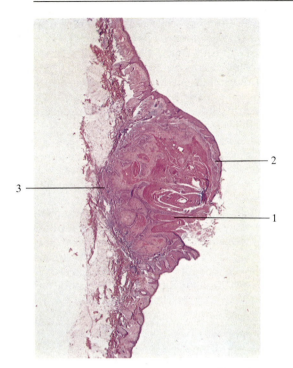

Fig 9–19.—Keratoacanthoma (hematoxylin-eosin; 8×).

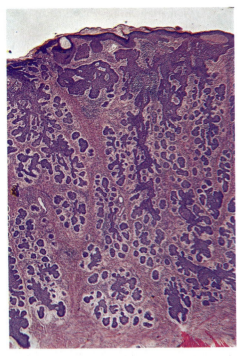

Fig 9–20.—Basel cell carcinoma (hematoxylin-eosin; 25×).

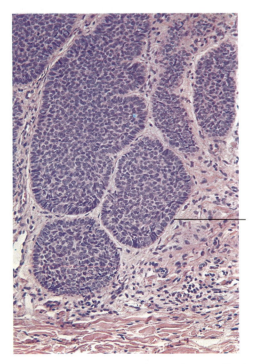

Fig 9–21.—Basal cell carcinoma (hematoxylin-eosin; 80×).

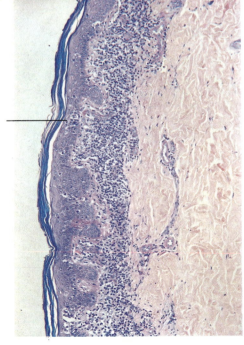

Fig 9–22.—Mycosis fungoides (hematoxylin-eosin; 80×).

Keratoacanthoma (molluscum sebaceum, Fig 9–19) *is a benign, rapidly growing skin tumor, probably virus produced, which develops on the face of elderly people. Most are self-healing in a few months.* The histologic picture is very characteristic. The tumor is a sharply defined, superficial plaque composed of proliferating squamous epithelium. The surface is depressed, bowl shaped (→ 1), markedly hyperkeratotic, and partially covered by overlapping contiguous epidermis (→ 2). Deeper portions of a keratoacanthoma show distinct stromal invasion (→ 3).

Keratoacanthoma is usually a solitary lesion, developing within a few months and then regressing spontaneously. If only a part of the tumor is examined histologically it may be very difficult to differentiate from a well-differentiated squamous cell carcinoma.

Basal cell carcinoma (Figs 9–20, 9–21, synonyms: rodent ulcer, basal cell epithelioma) *is a locally destructive, expanding skin tumor composed of basal cells. It very rarely metastasizes.* Histologically it is chiefly located beneath the level of the skin and shows a decidedly deep pattern of growth (Fig 9–20). Under **high magnification** (Fig 9–21) there are solid nests of tumor composed of dark cells (scanty cytoplasm). In the periphery of the nests the cells show a typical palisade arrangement reminiscent of the basal layer of the epidermis (→). The surrounding stroma is fibrotic and infiltrated by inflammatory cells.

Basal cell carcinoma occurs chiefly in elderly persons in areas of the skin exposed to light and the weather. They are also seen in younger persons in chronic arsenic intoxication, xeroderma pigmentosum, and the nevoid basal cell carcinoma syndrome (Gorlin-Goltz syndrome: multiple pigmented basal cell carcinomas in squamous epithelial-lined maxillary cysts and other incidental anomalies or malformations). *Histologic variants of basal cell carcinomas:* there are solid, cystic, fibroepithelial (Pinkus tumor) and superficial multicentric forms. Clinically it is important to differentiate the sclerosing type (morphea type), which should not be irradiated. Basal cell carcinoma showing disorderly cell growth, squamous differentiation, and cornification (basosquamous carcinoma) is considered to be a separate tumor since it occasionally metastasizes.

Mycosis fungoides (Fig 9–22) *is a lymphohistiocytic disease of the skin with an intermittent course that is thought to be a non-Hodgkin type of lymphoma of low-grade malignancy and thus a true neoplasm.* In the first or erythematous or premycosis stage the disease, both clinically and histologically, is not characteristic. Only the appearance of an infiltrate in the deeper layers of the corium gives a hint of the diagnosis. In the second or plaque stage (Fig 9–22) typical tissue changes occur. The epidermis is thick, acanthotic, and hyperkeratotic and contains small collections of lymphohistiocytic cells (→), or *microabscesses.* In the subepidermis (corium) pleomorphic and atypical lymphoid cells form a bandlike layer. These so-called *mycosis fungoides cells* have hyperchromatic nuclei of various sizes (see also Fig 41, section on General Pathology).

Mysosis fungoides occurs after the 40th year. After a long course of 5–10 years the disease progresses from the second or plaque stage to the third or tumor stage in which there are an increased number of atypical cells, mitoses, and deeper invasion of corium and subcutis. In about 60%–80% of cases not only are subcutaneous lymph nodes involved, but also internal organs (liver, lung, spleen, kidney).

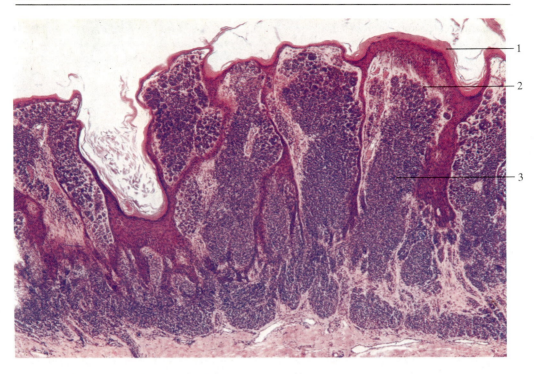

Fig 9–23.—Pigmented intradermal nevus (hematoxylin-eosin; 50×).

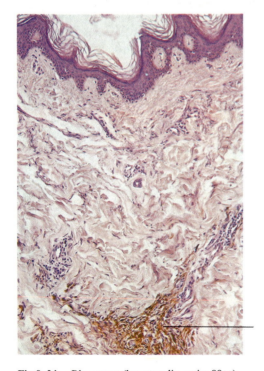

Fig 9–24.—Blue nevus (hematoxylin-eosin; 80×).

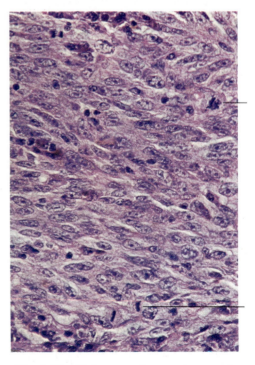

Fig 9–25.—Malignant melanoma (hematoxylin-eosin; 350×).

Pigmented Tumors

Introductory remarks. The term nevus (mole) describes a number of tumor-like malformations (hamartomas) of the skin that may arise either from newly formed capillaries *(vascular nevus)*, hyperplastic sebaceous glands *(sebaceous nevus)*, papillomatous and hyperplastic epidermis *(verrucous nevus)*, or melanin-producing cells *(pigmented nevus)*. Nontumorous disorders of pigmentation that are concerned with increase in numbers of the pigment-producing cells include *lentigo* (infantile and senile forms) and *mongoloid spots*. Among the benign tumors are *pigmented nevi* and *blue nevi*, while *malignant melanomas* belong to the group of malignant pigmented tumors.

Pigmented intradermal nevus (Fig 9–23) *consists of ball-shaped collections of nevus cells localized in the dermal papillae. As they are derived from melanoblasts they are of neuroectodermal orgin.* Histologically (Fig 9–23) they have a papillary structure and show marked cornification of the superficial epidermis ($\rightarrow$ 1). Between the elongated rete pegs can be seen the dark blue-staining nevus cells ($\rightarrow$ 3). Beneath the epidermis there is a zone of connective tissue ($\rightarrow$ 2) containing no tumor cells. The nevus cells show distinct melanin pigmentation.

Different sorts of pigmented nevi are recognized—nevi with *proliferative activity at the junction between dermis and epidermis (junctional nevus)* occurring most commonly in children and able to convert to a compound nevus. A *compound nevus* is a pigmented intradermal nevus that simultaneously shows border activity. Pure pigmented *intradermal or corium nevi* correspond to the type described above. They can be flat, raised, or verrucous.

Blue nevus (Fig 9–24) *is a round, circumscribed skin nodule of dark blue color comprised of elongated, markedly melanin-pigmented cells* (melanocytes of mesodermal origin). Histologically, beneath a normal epidermis and in the region of the midcorium there are elongated cells containing granular brown pigment ($\rightarrow$). This pigment is iron-negative and when stained by **Masson's silver stain** shows black, intracytoplasmic desposits (Fig 9–24,A).

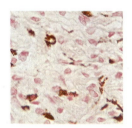

Fig 9–24.—A, blue nevus (Masson silver stain; 320 ×).

Malignant melanoma (Fig 9–25) *is the malignant variant of pigmented tumors and biologically is characterized by the frequency with which it metastasizes.* Histologically it is formed of cells that resemble in part carcinoma and in part sarcoma. This part sarcoma-like and part carcinoma-like structure is absolutely typical of malignant melanoma (sarcomatous-like carcinomas also occur in thyroid and renal carcinomas). The cytologic evidences of malignancy are present: cell atypia (cells of different sizes), mitoses ($\rightarrow$) and invasion of epidermis. The stroma shows an inflammatory reaction as well. About 10% of malignant melanomas are not pigmented (amelanotic melanoma).

Malignant melanoma occurs most frequently after 40 years of age. It is especially frequent in white people in the tropics. The commonest sites are skin (face, extremities), genitalia, eye, oral cavity, and colon. Among melanomas of the skin it is important to distinguish *superficial spreading melanoma* (intraepidermal metastasis), *the infiltrating, nodular type* and melanoma in the base of *malignant lentigo* (diffuse infiltration of the epidermis by pigment cells without infiltration of the *corium* = melanoma in situ = *melanosis praeblastomatosa circumscripta of Dubreuilh*).

For the most part malignant melanoma develops after puberty. Occasionally in small children pigmented tumors are seen that have marked cellular polymorphism and sometimes invasive growth. These pigmented tumors are benign and are referred to as *benign juvenile melanomas* or *Spitz-Allen tumors*.

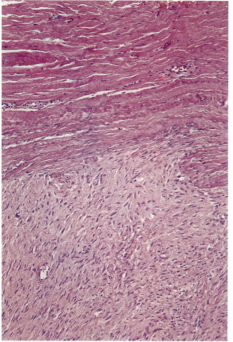

Fig 9–26.—Palmar fibromatosis (Dupuytren's contracture) (hematoxylin-eosin; 100×).

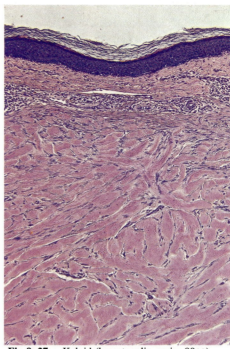

Fig 9–27.—Keloid (hematoxylin-eosin; 90×).

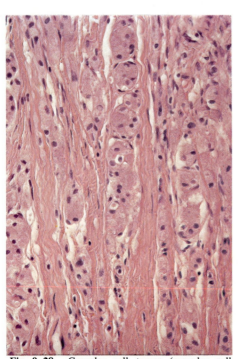

Fig 9–28.—Granular cell tumor (granular cell myeloblastoma) (hematoxylin-eosin; 200×).

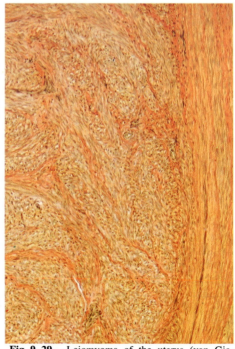

Fig 9–29.—Leiomyoma of the uterus (van Gieson's stain; 90×).

250

Fibromatoses

Introductory remarks: Fibromatoses are diffuse proliferations of connective tissue composed of fibroblasts and newly formed collagen. Such lesions can occur in any organ and at all ages. The term fibromatosis includes 12 different conditions: (1) fibrous scarring, (2) radiation fibromatosis, (3) fibromatosis of the penis, (4) palmar fibromatosis, (5) plantar fibromatosis, (6) and (7) abdominal and extra-abdominal fibromatoses, (8) nodular fasciitis, (9) keloid, (10) fibromatosis of the neck, (11) nasopharyngeal fibroma, and (12) generalized congenital fibromatosis. Fibromatoses manifest locally invasive growth that may last for years. Recurrences are frequent but there are no metastases.

Palmar fibromatosis (Dupuytren's contracture, Fig 9–26). This is a benign proliferation of fibrous tissue, partly diffuse, partly nodular, in the palmar aponeurosis that produces a flexion contracture of the fingers. Figure 9–26 shows a taut, collagen-rich connective tissue (upper half of the picture) as well as groups of fibrocytes situated in looser stroma (lower half of picture).

The disease affects mainly men between 50 and 60 years old. It runs in stages, the last of which is retraction of the palmar fascia.

Keloid (Fig 9–27) is not a true tumor but an excessive, superficial nodular scar. Histo logically, there is a circumscribed, but not encapsulated, nodule composed of broad, glassy, eosinophilic bundles of collagen, between which nuclei of a few fibroblasts and inflammatory cells may be seen. Atrophic epidermis covers the surface (no rete pegs).

Keloids commonly develop in postoperative abdominal scars and in the face after trauma. They tend to recur after excision.

Mesenchymal Tumors

Both benign and malignant mesenchymal tumors are encountered. They are classified histogenetically, taking into consideration the parent tissues of the tumors. **Benign mesenchymal tumors** show a high degree of tissue maturity, as well as slow, expansive growth, but do not metastasize. **Malignant mesenchymal tumors** are grouped under the general heading of sarcoma. They may be undifferentiated or may show a high degree of cellular and tissue differentiation, corresponding to their histogenetic origin (e.g., myosarcoma, liposarcoma, or osteosarcoma).

Granular cell tumor (granular cell myoblastoma, Fig 9–28) is a benign mesenchymal tumor composed of cells in a strandlike arrangement, central, round nuclei, and finely granular cytoplasm. The cytoplasmic granules are PAS positive.

Granular cell tumors occur in many organs, especially the tongue and larynx. Their pathogenesis is controversial. Because the tumor cells show a similarity to Schwann cells under the electron microscope, they are probably of neurogenic origin.

Leiomyoma (Fig 9–29). This is a benign tumor of smooth muscle, particularly common in the myometrium. Histologically it is composed of interlacing smooth muscle fibers with elongated, cylindrical, blunt-ended nuclei, and with cytoplasm that stains yellow by van Gieson's method. Interspersed between groups of muscle fibers is a dense collagenous network that is stained red by van Gieson's stain.

Leiomyomas grow by expansion and may show hyalinization, calcification, and ossification, which are signs of regressive changes. Malignant transformation is rare. Retroperitoneal leiomyomas (e.g., arising from blood vessel walls), however, are potentially malignant.

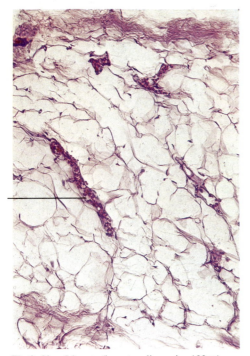

Fig 9–30.—Lipoma (hematoxylin-eosin; 100×).

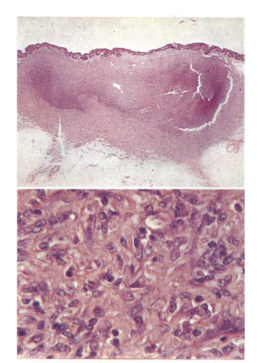

Fig 9–31.—Histiocytoma (**top,** low magnification; 8×; **bottom,** high magnification, hematoxylin-eosin; 200×).

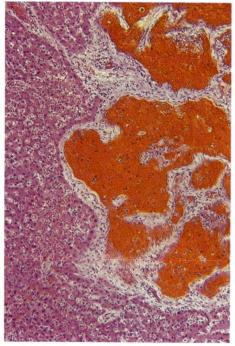

Fig 9–32.—Cavernous hemangioma of the liver (hematoxylin-eosin; 60×).

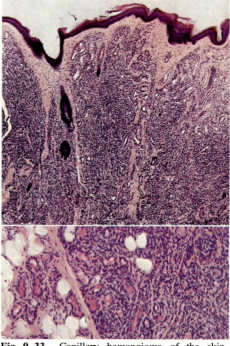

Fig 9–33.—Capillary hemangioma of the skin (**top,** low magnification, 30×; **bottom,** higher magnification, hematoxylin-eosin; 60×).

Lipoma—Histiocytoma—Hemangioma

Lipoma (Fig 9–30). *A benign, lobulated tumor derived from mature fat tissue.* Histologically it is composed of cells that deviate from normal fat cells only in their variation in size. They have distinct cell borders, rounded nuclei situated at the periphery, and optically empty cytoplasm; the fat is dissolved by paraffin embedding. A fibrous capsule covers the surface. Many capillaries ($\rightarrow$) are seen lying between the fat cells.

Lipomas develop in subcutaneous fat tissue and occasionally retroperitoneally or in other organs. They grow slowly. *Hibernoma* is a special variant of lipoma that arises from fetal fat cells (small, cuboidal cells with finely vacuolated cytoplasm).

Histiocytoma (Fig 9–31, sclerosing hemangioma of Wolbach). *This is a circumscribed but not encapsulated tumor located in the subepidermal corium and composed of proliferating histiocytes.* Under low magnification (Fig 9–31, top) the tumor appears bluish and is covered with intact epidermis. With higher magnification (Fig 9–31, bottom) the bizarre nuclei of the histiocytes can be identified and the partly whorled arrangement of the newly formed collagen fibers seen. There are also solitary macrophages containing fat or hemosiderin. The surface epidermis shows in part pseudoepitheliomatous thickening and in part atrophic shrinkage and is separated from the histiocytoma by a narrow band of acellular corium.

Angiomas *are benign vascular tumors that in most cases are hamartomas, i.e., tumor-like malformations of local tissue.* They may arise from blood vessels *(hemangioma)*, from lymph vessels *(lymphangioma)*, or from neuromyoepithelial tissue *(angiomyoma or glomus tumor)*.

Cavernous hemangioma (Fig 9–32) develops most frequently in the liver. It consists of many large spaces tightly packed with erythrocytes, traversed by connective tissue septa, and lined with endothelial cells. The neighboring liver parenchyma may show pressure atrophy.

Capillary hemangioma (Fig 9–33) is the commonest type of vascular tumor. Under low magnification (Fig 9–33, top) it appears as an ill-defined, lobulated, and very cellular new growth, extending from the subepidermal corium to the subcutis. Medium magnification (Fig 9–33, bottom) shows fissured or oval spaces bordered by endothelial cells and containing occasional erythrocytes. The newly formed capillaries enclose fat cells. Because this is a tumor-like malformation that develops in the local fat tissue there is no true invasion.

253

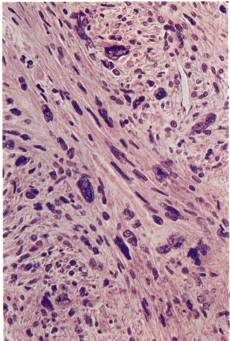

Fig 9–34.—Leiomyosarcoma (hematoxylin-eosin; 450×).

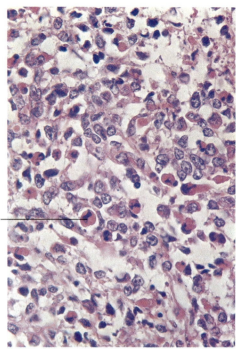

Fig 9–35.—Embryonal rhabdomyosarcoma (hematoxylin-eosin; 320×).

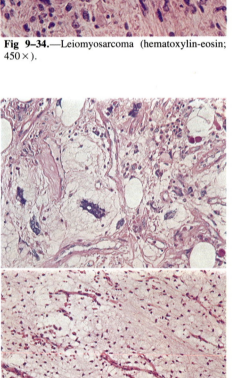

Fig 9–36.—Liposarcoma. **Top,** pleomorphic liposarcoma with lipoblasts (200×). **Bottom,** myxoid liposarcoma (hematoxylin-eosin; 80×).

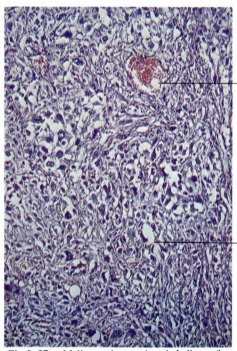

Fig 9–37.—Malignant hemangioendothelioma (hematoxylin-eosin; 120×).

Leiomyosarcoma—Liposarcoma—Rhabdomyosarcoma—Malignant Hemangioendothelioma

Leiomyosarcoma (Fig 9–34) *is a malignant tumor of smooth muscle.* Histologically it is a spindle cell sarcoma with bundles of elongated tumor cells which in the figure are seen partly in longitudinal section (middle of picture) and partly in cross section. The cells have abundant cytoplasm and are very pleomorphic with variably large, hyperchromatic nuclei. The presence of mitoses is of diagnostic significance since cellular atypia also occurs in uterine leiomyomas.

Leiomyomas of the uterus seldom undergo malignant change. Leiomyosarcomas are seen especially in the extremities and intestinal and blood vessel walls (retroperitoneal). They produce distant metastases early and thus are particularly malignant, in this respect standing in contrast to the well-differentiated fibrosarcoma. *Leiomyoblastomas* are benign neoplasms that occur in the gastrointestinal tract as well as the mesentery and retroperitoneal region. They consist of polygonal cells with clear cytoplasm.

Rhabdomyosarcoma (Fig 9–35) *is a malignant tumor of striped muscle.* In most cases it is a polymorphocellular sarcoma. The recognition of cross-striations in the cytoplasms of these tumors is pathognomonic, but they are not often visible on light microscopy. Brick-red tumor cells with centrally placed, hyperchromatic, contracted nuclei ($\rightarrow$) are quite typical of **embryonal rhabdomyosarcoma.**

Rhabdomyosarcoma belongs to the most malignant tumors of striated muscle. A special variant is *sarcoma botryoides,* which occurs in the genital tract of young women. The diagnosis of rhabdomyosarcoma in the last analysis can be made only by finding rhabdomyofibrils. Usually these can only be demonstrated by electron microscopy as rudimentary sarcomeres. *Rhabdomyomas* are benign, very rare tumors of striated muscle, especially of myocardium. The cells have perinuclear glycogen vacuoles, spindle-shaped, drawn-out nuclei, and cytoplasmic cross-striations.

Liposarcoma (Fig 9–36) *is a malignant tumor of fat tissue.* A typical liposarcoma shows large, polymorphous tumor cells (lipoblasts, Fig 9–36, top) with bizarre, hyperchromatic nuclei and many cytoplasmic vacuoles containing fat. In addition there are large, mature fat cells as well as cells with finely vacuolated cytoplasm (immature or "fetal" fat cells). A **myxoid variant** (Fig 9–36, bottom) is the most common liposarcoma. It consists of a myxoid ground substance enclosing star-shaped cells or nuclei. Since mitoses and lipoblasts are rare, a myxoid liposarcoma sometimes is mistaken for a benign lipoma. All variants of liposarcoma are malignant. In most cases they arise de novo, that is, they do not as a rule arise from a preexisting lipoma. Common sites are the gluteal region, thigh, mesentery, and retroperitoneum.

Malignant hemangioendothelioma (Fig 9–37) *is a relatively rare malignant tumor arising from the vascular system.* Histologically it has a polymorphocellular, sarcomatous structure with small slitlike spaces lined by very atypical tumor cells and occasionally containing blood ($\rightarrow$). The larger tumor cells often contain phagocytosed erythrocytes (*erythrophagocytosis* occurs commonly in hemangioendotheliomas).

Hemangioendotheliomas occur particularly in the liver (e.g., following chronic arsenic poisoning or storage of thorotrast) and in the thyroid. It is a malignant tumor with a high incidence of metastasis. Together with chorionepithelioma and malignant hepatoma it is the bloodiest of tumors. The malignant counterpart of the lymphatic vascular system is *lymphangiosarcoma* and may give rise to the Stewart-Treves syndrome: sarcoma arising in the setting of chronic edema of the arm after total mastectomy and axillary lymph node extirpation for mammary carcinoma.

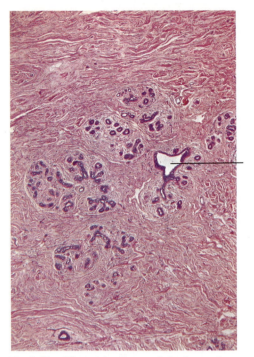

Fig 9–38.—Fibrocystic disease of the breast (hematoxylin-eosin; 32×).

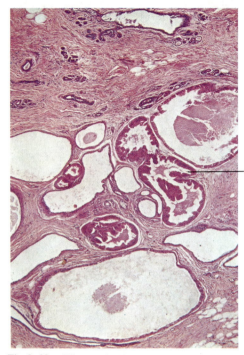

Fig 9–39.—Fibrocystic disease of the breast (hematoxylin-eosin; 32×).

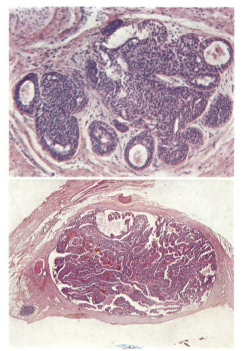

Fig 9–40.—Top, dysplasia with epitheliosis (hematoxylin-eosin; 80×). **Bottom,** dysplasia with intraductal proliferation (hematoxylin-eosin; 10×).

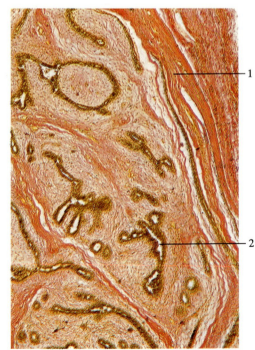

Fig 9–41.—Intracanalicular fibroadenoma (van Gieson's stain; 50×).

Breast

Fibrocystic disease of the breast (cyclomastopathy) is a disorder of the female breast in which there are simultaneously atrophy, hyperplasia, and metaplasia as well as various clinical signs. It is due to dysfunction of sex hormones, but the pathogenesis is still unknown. For prognostic and therapeutic reasons a distinction is made between *simple mastopathy* and *proliferative mastopathy*.

In *simple mammary mastopathy* proliferation of intralobular and perilobular fibrous connective tissue predominates, hence the name **fibrous dysplasia** (Fig 9–38). The mammary lobules are encased by collagenous stroma and the acini are pressed together. The arrow points to a dilated excretory duct. In **fibrocystic dysplasia** (fibrocystic disease, Fig 9–39) cysts lined by flattened epithelium dominate the histologic picture. In part they are dilated preexisting excretory ducts and in part newly formed cysts lined with tall eosinophilic epithelium showing apocrine secretion and reminiscent of sweat glands (therefore the designation **sweat gland metaplasia,** →). The fibrous component of the dysplasia is seen in the upper third of the picture.

The myoepithelial cells (basket cells) are also hypertrophied in simple dysplasia of the breast. They are large cells, seen in the region of the acinar epithelium, with distended vesicular cytoplasm and distinct dark nuclei. Frequently they form a discrete, solid nodule, the center of which may be sclerotic. Such lesions are described as *adenosis* or *sclerosing adenosis*. They are of diagnostic significance since they can be mistaken for a scirrhous carcinoma when seen under low magnification or in frozen sections.

In **proliferative dysplasia** (Fig 9–40) *there is marked intraductal epithelial proliferation with formation of solid, adenomatous, or papillary structures.* In **epitheliosis** (Fig 9–40, top) small excretory ducts are filled with proliferated epithelium, which may show a **papillary structure,** i.e., they consist of branching stroma covered by epithelium (*pseudopapillary growth,* in contrast, consists only of epithelium). Of particular prognostic significance is the presence of cell atypia (polymorphic cells with hyperchromatic nuclei, increased mitoses) which is found in *atypical proliferating breast dysplasia.*

Simple fibrocystic disease of the breast is common and develops in practically every breast after age 25 and should not be considered precancerous. On the other hand *atypical proliferative breast dysplasia* has an increased risk of cancer. Women with this lesion have up to 30 times the chance of developing breast cancer than do "normal women." Other cancer risk factors are early menarche, late menopause, childlessness, non-breast-fed infants, prolonged estrogen therapy, and mammary carcinoma in sisters.

Fibroadenoma of the breast (Fig 9–41) *is a benign, true mixed tumor with both epithelial and mesenchymal components that occurs preferentially in younger women.* Figure 9–41 shows an **intracanalicular fibroadenoma** with branching, tubelike structures lined by deeply stained epithelium and having slitlike lumens (→ 2). The connective tissue in the immediate neighborhood of the epithelium is myxomatous and does not stain as intensely with van Gieson's stain as normal connective tissue (→ 1). In some fibroadenomas the connective tissue surrounds in concentric fashion differentiated tubules showing epithelial proliferation (*pericanalicular fibroadenoma*).

Fibroadenomas are solid, greyish white, coarsely lobulated nodules of firm consistency. They are easily enucleated. Rarely there is marked atypical cellular proliferation, particularly of the mesenchymal component. Such tumors can reach considerable size and are then called *cystosarcoma phylloides.* They are usually only locally malignant and seldom have distant metastases.

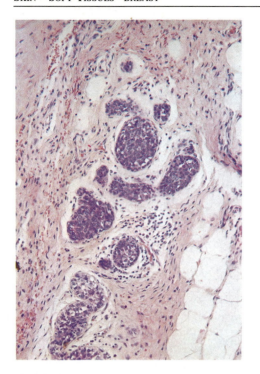

Fig 9–42.—Lobular carcinoma in situ of the breast (hematoxylin-eosin; 100×).

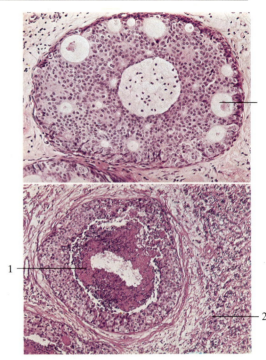

Fig 9–43.—**Top,** cribriform carcinoma of the breast (hematoxylin-eosin; 50×). **Bottom,** comedocarcinoma (hematoxylin-eosin; 50×).

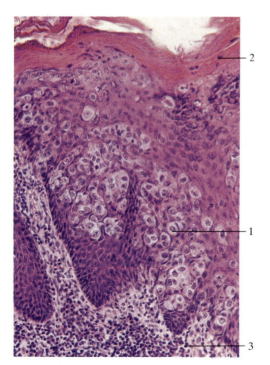

Fig 9–44.—Paget's disease of breast (hematoxylin-eosin; 200×).

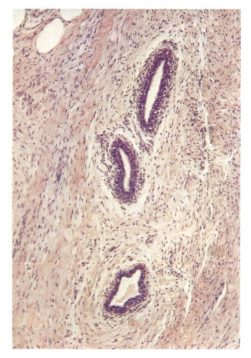

Fig 9–45.—Gynecomastia (hematoxylin-eosin; 80×).

Mammary Carcinoma—Gynecomastia

In women, carcinoma of the breast is the chief cause of death from malignant tumors (about 26% of malignant neoplasms in women in the U.S.). The average age of those women is 60 years. The WHO international classification of carcinoma of the breast contains the following groups. Group I: noninfiltrating intraduct and lobular carcinoma. Group II: infiltrating duct–derived carcinoma (scirrhous, solid carcinoma simplex, medullary carcinoma). Group III: special types of carcinoma (papillary, cribriform, mucinous, medullary carcinoma with lymphoid infiltration of stroma, squamous carcinoma, Paget's disease, carcinoma arising in a fibroadenoma). Carcinomas of Group II make up about 92% of breast cancers, and the other 2 groups, 8%.

Lobular carcinoma in situ (Fig 9–42) as a rule is discovered by chance on histologic examination of the breast. The figure shows solid islands of atypical cells replacing and filling the lobule. The basement membrane is preserved which is an indication of lack of stromal invasion.

Most authors are of the opinion that *lobular carcinoma in situ* of the breast is a precancerous lesion and not a true carcinoma growing in situ (see p. 52).

Other breast tumors with an intraductal pattern of growth are papillary, cribriform, and comedocarcinomas. In **cribriform carcinoma** (Fig 9–43) the tumor cells fill large and medium-sized excretory ducts, producing multiple small lumina (→ "glands within glands") thus giving the tumor a characteristic sievelike appearance. In **comedocarcinoma** (Fig 9–43, bottom), the ducts are also distended by the solid growth of the carcinoma. Typical of this carcinoma are eosinophilic, central areas of necrosis (→ 1)—often with granular calcium deposits—and marked polymorphism of the tumor cells. Comedocarcinoma usually shows invasion of the stroma (→ 2).

Paget's disease of the breast (Fig 9–44) *refers to intradermal spread of an intraduct carcinoma and is manifested clinically by an eczematous lesion of the nipple.* Figure 9–44 shows the large, clear carcinoma cells (→ 1), which are to be found in all layers of the epidermis. The cells are distinctly polymorphic and there are many mitoses. The overlying surface epidermis is hyperkeratotic (→ 2) and the underlying stroma contains chronic inflammatory cells (→ 3).

The pathobiologic prognosis of mammary carcinoma: The prognosis of various malignant tumors (in particular mammary carcinoma) depends decisively on the pathologic anatomical findings. The final fate of a woman with mammary carcinoma is not determined by the primary tumor itself, but rather by the development of lymphogenous (axillary, supraclavicular) and hematogenous (lung, liver, bones) distant metastases. If lymph node metastasis is already present, then only a small percentage survive beyond 5 years. Lymph node metastases occur chiefly with primary tumors of infiltrative type (Group II) having a diameter greater than 2 cm. In contrast, the 5- and 10-year survival rate is relatively high for mucinous carcinoma, medullary carcinoma with lymphocytic stroma, and noninfiltrating carcinomas of Group I.

Gynecomastia (Fig 9–45) *is a hormonally conditioned hyperplasia of the ducts and stroma in the male breast.* Histologically there is mild proliferation of duct epithelium. The connective tissue is increased and in the region of the excretory ducts shows a concentric and myxomatous arrangement. There is practically no formation or differentiation of acini. In *pseudogynecomastia* enlargement of the breast is attributable to overgrowth of fat.

Gynecomastia is seen regularly at the onset of puberty and regresses spontaneously. Otherwise it occurs in men with liver cirrhosis and following prolonged estrogen therapy (e.g., for prostatic carcinoma). *Carcinoma of the breast in males* is a rarity (less than 1% of all breast carcinomas). It is usually observed after estrogen therapy and in the Klinefelter syndrome.

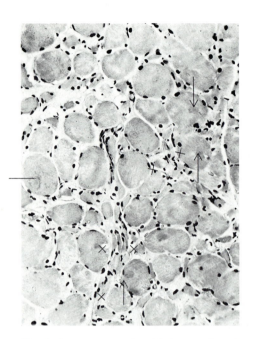

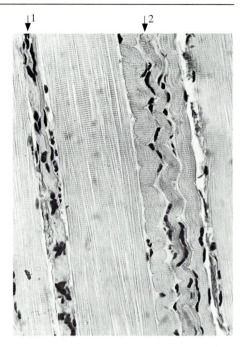

Fig 10–1.—Recent atrophy with degeneration of muscle fibers occurring in acute polyneuritis (hematoxylin-eosin; 170×).

Fig 10–2.—Chronic neurogenic muscular atrophy in polyneuritis (hematoxylin-eosin; 320×).

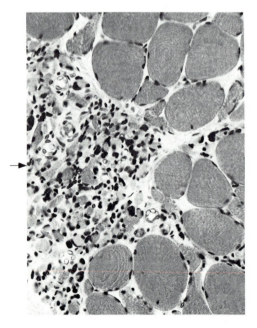

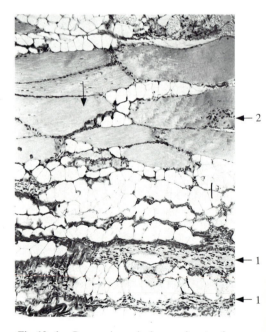

Fig 10–3.—Progressive spinal muscular atrophy (infantile form) (hematoxylin-eosin; 233×).

Fig 10–4.—Progressive spinal muscular atrophy (pseudomyogenic form) (van Gieson's stain; 60×).

10. Muscles

Skeletal muscles can be affected in *generalized disease states* or they can be *affected independently*. In both cases, the result is either *degeneration of the muscle fibers* themselves or secondary involvement of the muscle from extension of primary disease of the *interstitial tissues*. In primary degenerative muscle disease, acute degenerative changes occur and lead to necrosis. They must, of course, be differentiated from chronic atrophies of muscle fibers.

Muscular atrophies are the result of neurogenic or of myogenic disease. The basis of *neurogenic atrophies* is peripheral denervation, due either to a primary lesion in the anterior horn cells *(spinal muscular atrophy)* or to a lesion along the course of *peripheral motor nerves*.

The early stages of **neurogenic muscular atrophy** are well seen in cases of polyneuritis. Figure 10–1 **(recent muscular atrophy in acute polyneuritis)** illustrates the atrophy of individual muscle fibers in cross section (between the crosses). The fibers are smaller and the nuclei lie closer together. Although the other muscle fibers seem unchanged in size, they already show early degeneration, as evidenced by the loss of their regular fibrillary cytoplasmic structure (compare this with Fig 10–3) and the very characteristic localized clumps of contractile material, the so-called target fibers (→).

If neurogenic atrophy develops slowly, the histologic picture will consist of groups of markedly atrophic muscle fibers intermixed with essentially intact fibers. The former represent areas innervated by affected motor axons or their branches **(chronic neurogenic muscular atrophy in polyneuritis).** Figure 10–2 is a longitudinal section showing typical groups of atrophic muscle fibers. It can be seen that the fibers about → 1 are more severely atrophied than those about → 2. The atrophy in this case affects only small groups, corresponding to the so-called subunits of a motor unit.

Motor unit = anterior horn cell with its corresponding peripheral motor axon, its collaterals, the motor end-plates, and the muscle fibers. Depending on the type of muscle involved, a motor unit is composed of 800–1,700 or more muscle fibers.

Spinal muscular atrophy, as a result of destruction of anterior horn cells of the spinal cord, always involves entire motor units and not just subunits, leading to atrophy of all the muscle fibers supplied by a particular unit. Figure 10–3 **(the infantile form of progressive spinal muscular atrophy)** shows more widespread involvement of larger groups of muscle fibers (→). The cross-sectional view reveals the very thin fibers and closely placed nuclei so that they seem to have multiplied (frustrated regeneration). The other muscle fibers are unaffected and have retained the integrity of their intracytoplasmic structure.

Spinal progressive muscular atrophy of adults (pseudomyogenic type) (Fig 10–4). This lesion progresses very slowly so that adaptation and regeneration are prominent. The figure shows a longitudinal section of a muscle bundle (→ 1) surrounded by tongues of connective tissue and proliferated lipomatous tissue. The groups of intact muscle fibers undergo compensatory hypertrophy as a result of increased demand. There are increased numbers of nuclei centrally located in muscle cells (→ 2). This fibroadipose transformation and replacement of muscle is a nonspecific manifestation of chronic, progressive wasting of muscles. Similar changes to these are also seen in chronic muscular atrophy having an inflammatory or degenerative basis (Fig 10–5).

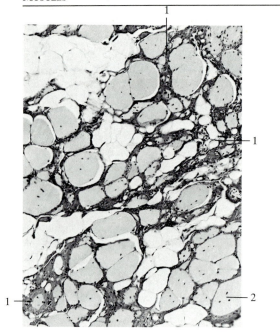

Fig 10–5.—Progressive muscular dystrophy (Erb) (van Gieson's stain; 80×).

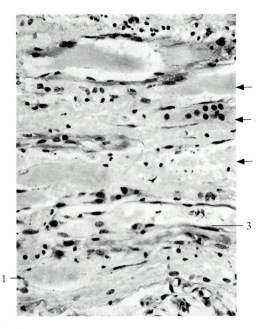

Fig 10–6.—Early muscular necrosis in acute polymyositis (hematoxylin-eosin; 200×).

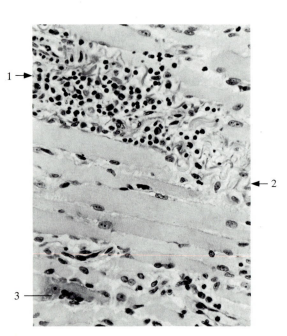

Fig 10–7.—Dermatomyositis (hematoxylin-eosin; 250×).

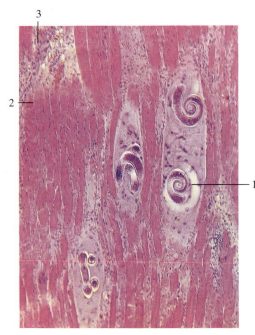

Fig 10–8.—Trichinosis (hematoxylin-eosin; 78×).

Progressive muscular dystrophy (Erb) (Fig 10–5). In contrast to spinal progressive muscular atrophy, *the primary disturbance in progressive muscular dystrophy (myogenic atrophy) resides in the muscle cells themselves* (hereditary metabolic disorder of unknown origin). Thus, the atrophic manifestations do not correspond to a motor unit distribution. Instead, they represent disseminated atrophy of individual fibers without regular distribution.

The section shows atrophic fibers (→ 1) adjoining numerous normal as well as hypertrophic fibers. Many have central nuclei (→ 2). In addition, the muscle fibers are surrounded by connective tissue and the degenerated and atrophic fibers have been replaced by fat tissue (*fibroadipose replacement*). The scarring can produce secondarily a lobular arrangement of muscle bundles, giving a cirrhosis-like appearance.

Dystrophic muscles frequently show early stages of muscle fiber degeneration, such as occur in systemic diseases, e.g., the progressive degeneration of the abdominal musculature in typhoid. Figure 10–6 (**early muscular necrosis in acute polymyositis**) show several types of degeneration that may lead to necrosis. The first change is often waxy degeneration (→ 1) leading to dissolution of the fibrous proteins and cross-striations. Gradually, as the nuclei degenerate, lumpy aggregates (→ 2) become evident, and as the sarcoplasm comes apart and vanishes, only empty sarcolemmal sheaths are left behind (→ 3) (compare Figs 1–15, 1–16). Focal groups of muscle nuclei can be seen, indicating a regenerative activity (→ 4).

Acute muscular degeneration of such severity often results in development of the so-called *crush syndrome* in the kidney (p. 139). It occurs not only with necrotizing myositis but also with *intoxications* (e.g., CO poisoning) and in severe muscle trauma.

Dermatomyositis (Fig 10–7) is a *necrotizing panmyositis with dermatitis* which in the acute stages prominently displays the degenerative and necrotizing changes described above. In addition, the tissues are densely infiltrated with lymphocytes and plasma cells. In the subacute and chronic stages of this intermittently progressive disease, there is mainly interstitial infiltration (→ 1), scarring (→ 2), and tissue replacement. Additionally, there may be marked regeneration of the muscle fibers themselves (→ 3).

The clinical course of *necrotizing polymyositis* consists of extensive paralysis of the peripheral muscles, which, because of its resemblance to the muscular paralysis of trichinosis, is at times referred to as pseudotrichinosis.

Trichinosis of muscle (Fig 10–8). *The embryos of* Trichinella spiralis *pass through the lacteals of the intestine into the bloodstream and so reach striated muscle, where they develop into spiral-shaped larvae.* Sexually mature worms live in the small intestine (man, swine, dogs, etc.). When the infected muscle (meat) reaches the stomach larvae are freed and can develop into sexually mature worms. In massive trichinal infestation intestinal manifestations are prominent (diarrhea) and are followed by muscle pains (myolysis). Later, prolonged complaints of muscular rheumatism may develop. Histologically, the cross-cut or tangentially cut, spiral-shaped trichinellae are surrounded by a hyaline capsule (→ 1) and can be easily seen even at low power. Adjoining muscle fibers show considerable alteration, e.g., granular and waxy degeneration (→ 2). The interstitial tissue contains aggregations of eosinophils and chronic inflammatory cells.

Macroscopic: Small white nodules.

Nonspecific Lymphadenitis

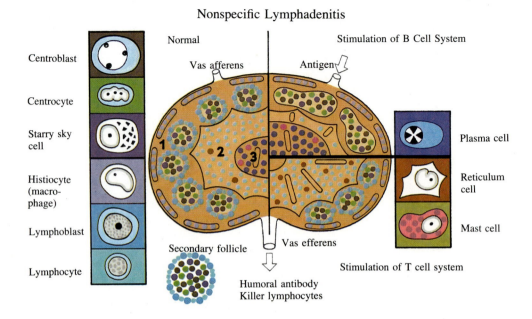

Centroblast

Centrocyte

Starry sky cell

Histiocyte (macro-phage)

Lymphoblast

Lymphocyte

Normal

Vas afferens

Secondary follicle

Vas efferens

Humoral antibody
Killer lymphocytes

Stimulation of B Cell System

Antigen

Plasma cell

Reticulum cell

Mast cell

Stimulation of T cell system

Malignant Lymphoma

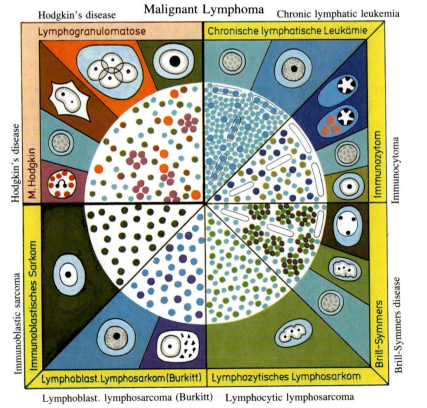

Hodgkin's disease

Lymphogranulomatose

Chronic lymphatic leukemia

Chronische lymphatische Leukämie

Hodgkin's disease

M. Hodgkin

Immunoblastic sarcoma

Immunoblastisches Sarkom

Immunozytom

Immunocytoma

Brill-Symmers

Brill-Symmers disease

Lymphoblast.Lymphosarkom(Burkitt)

Lymphozytisches Lymphosarkom

Lymphoblast. lymphosarcoma (Burkitt)   Lymphocytic lymphosarcoma

Fig 11–1.—Schematic illustration of normal lymph nodes, nonspecific lymphadenitis, and malignant lymphomas.

11. Lymph Nodes—Spleen

Lymph nodes: Recent advances in immunology have made clear that the immunologic responses of lymph nodes must be assigned to different components (Fig 11–1, top). When an antigen reaches lymph nodes by way of the vas afferens, it may stimulate either *humoral antibody production* (**B cell system** = bone marrow–dependent system) or the *cell-bound immune system* (**T cells** = thymus-dependent system). The B cell system is represented by the secondary follicles with germinal centers in the cortex (1 in Fig 11–1, top) and medulla (3 in Fig 11–1, top) of lymph nodes. The T cell system is represented by the paracortical zone (lying between medulla and cortex: 2 in Fig 11–1, top). Experimentally, after thymectomy in newborn animals there is no paracortical zone.

On **stimulation of the B cell system** (Fig 11–1, top right) the antigen causes an intensified reaction, especially of the germinal centers of the secondary follicles, which may become enormously enlarged and contain increased numbers of centroblasts and centrocytes as well as phagocytes containing nuclear fragments (so-called starry sky cells). It is assumed that the antigen is taken up and processed by cells of the germinal center. Production of humoral antibody takes place in the plasma cells of the medulla of lymph nodes. The medulla then increases in width because of the numerous plasma cells. How the immunologic message of the cortex is transmitted to the medulla is not known (cellular, lymphogenous?). If the **T cell system** (Fig 11–1, top right) is stimulated by antigen then the paracortical zone increases, as do the T lymphocytes, reticulum cells, and mast cells. In the spleen the follicles correspond to the B cell system and the pulp to the T cell system. These different sorts of reaction in lymph nodes have been shown to have practical significance: in the area of drainage of a carcinoma (breast, uterine cervix) if stimulation of T cells (paracortical zone) is observed, the patient's prognosis is better than if activity in the B cell region or no lymph node reaction at all occurs.

In **nonspecific lymphadenitis** there is an increase in sinus histiocytes, which are probably the first site of uptake of antigen. The lymphatic tissue may respond by follicular hyperplasia (enlarged reaction centers) and an increase in the medulla (B cell stimulation) or by lymphoid hyperplasia (increase of the paracortical zone). Both of these reactions may occur simultaneously.

Special sorts of lymph node reactions. Focal epithelioid cell reaction (Piringer): small nodules of clustered epithelioid cells in the cortex with sinus histiocytosis accompanying nonspecific lymphadenitis occur in toxoplasmosis and also are seen with carcinomas and in the very early stages of Hodgkin's disease. *Sarcoid:* an epithelioid cell granuloma. *Caseous tuberculosis:* caseation (necrosis surrounded by epithelioid cells and Langhans' giant cells). *Pseudotuberculosis:* (1) *Pasteurella pseudotuberculosis* (pseudotuberculosis of Masshoff), chiefly in mesenteric lymph nodes. (2) *Tularemia (Pasteurella tularensis)* contracted from wild game (pelt and game handlers). (3) *Cat scratch fever* (viruses of the Miyagawanella group). All these forms have a similar appearance. At first there is focal overgrowth of reticulum cells, then central necrosis, then demarkation by epithelioid cells or reticulum cells.

Tumors of lymph nodes (Fig 11–1; bottom): Primary tumors of lymph nodes as a rule are malignant (exception: *benign lymphocytoma of Castleman,* arising preferentially in the mediastinum and showing germinal centers with onion layer-like arrangement of lymphocytes) and are classified under the general heading of **malignant lymphomas.** Among such tumors **Hodgkin's disease** has been separated as a distinct disease process and the remaining tumors have been classified as **non-Hodgkin's lymphomas** (see Fig 11–1, bottom).

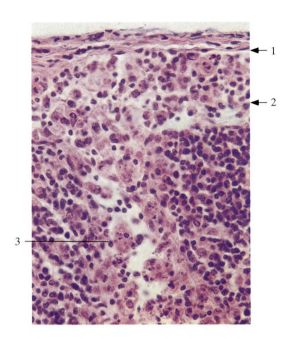

Fig 11–2.—Acute nonspecific lymphadenitis (sinus catarrh) (hematoxylin-eosin; 360 ×).

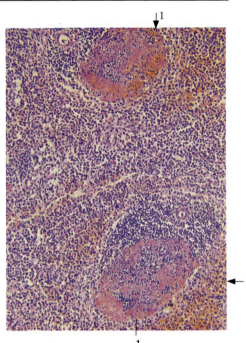

Fig 11–3.—Follicular necrosis in diphtheria (hematoxylin-eosin; 108 ×).

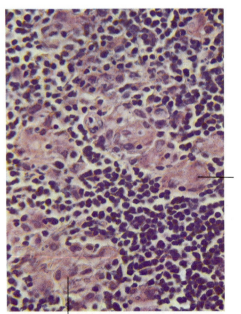

Fig 11–4.—Piringer's lymphadenitis (focal small epithelioid reaction) (hematoxylin-eosin; 420 ×).

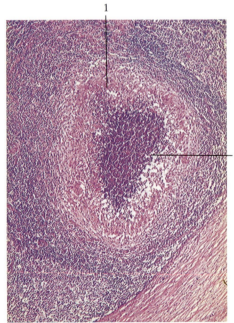

Fig 11–5.—Suppurative reticulocytic lymphadenitis (hematoxylin-eosin; 80 ×).

Forms of Lymph Node Reactions

Acute nonspecific lymphadenitis (sinus catarrh) (Fig 11–2) is one histologic form of lymph-adenitis (see Fig 11–1, top). This histologic feature of sinus catarrh is proliferation of the reticulum cells (histiocytes) of the sinus due to their exposure to increasing amounts of resorbable substances (protein breakdown products, as from nearby cancers, bacteria, toxins, etc.). The proliferating reticuloendothelial cells become detached in large numbers and lie in the lumen of the sinus as isolated, round or oval histiocytes with a pale eccentric nucleus: *sinus histiocytosis*. Figure 11–2 shows the cortical sinus of a lymph node with nonspecific lymphadenitis. The sinuses are wide (→1 and →2: border of the sinus) and filled with large cells with abundant cytoplasm which are detached reticulum cells containing cytoplasmic nuclear fragments (→3). Single lymphocytes and leukocytes are also present.

Follicular necrosis is diphtheria (Fig 11–3). A particularly pronounced lymphadenitis with necrosis of the germinal centers of the secondary follicles occurs in diphtheria (direct toxic effect). Histologically, the reactive centers of the follicles are changed into necrotic eosinophilic masses (→1) in which nuclear debris can still be seen. A narrow margin of lymphocytes is preserved at the periphery of the follicles. The remainder of the lymph node is acutely inflamed and frequently hemorrhagic (→2). Also seen in the mesenteric lymph nodes of small children with acute enteritis (nondiphtheritic).

Piringer's lymphadenitis (Fig 11–4). In most cases, Piringer's lymphadenitis is most commonly due to toxoplasmosis and occurs preferentially in the lymph nodes of the neck (75%). The characteristic histologic changes are small focal collections of epithelioid cells, proliferation of immature histiocytes in the sinuses, hyperplasia of lymphoid follicles having large germinal centers, and perilymphadenitis. Figure 11–4 shows several groups of 4–8 large epithelioid cells with abundant pale eosinophilic cytoplasm (→). The nuclei of these cells are oval or shaped like a cat's tongue and possess a loose chromatin structure.

Similar foci of small epithelioid cells may be found in lymph nodes in the early stages of Hodgkin's disease, in infectious mononucleosis, and in lymph nodes draining degenerating tumors.

Suppurative reticulocytic lymphadenitis (Fig 11–5). This type of lymphadenitis occurs in various infections: *Yersinia* or *Pasteurella* pseudotuberculosis infection of mesenteric and ileocecal lymph nodes which, in children, mimics the clinical picture of appendicitis; infection with *Pasteurella tularensis* and the agent of cat scratch fever which attack the regional lymph nodes draining the infection (primary complex), especially in juveniles.

All these infections of lymph nodes show a similar histologic picture. In the fully developed stages, there is extensive focal reticulum cell proliferation (→1) with areas of destruction of tissue (abscess, →2) surrounded by polymorphonuclear granulocytes. Next to the abscess and the cuff of reticulum cells there is a secondary follicle with a distinct reaction center (→3) and several so-called stellate cells (→4), phagocytes containing nuclear fragments. Other changes seen in this disease—not represented in the illustration–are considerable perilymphadenitis, endophlebitis, and endarteritis of neighboring blood vessels.

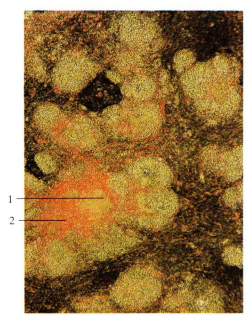

Fig 11–6.—Hyperplastic (epithelioid cell) tuberculous lymphadenitis (van Gieson's stain; 44×).

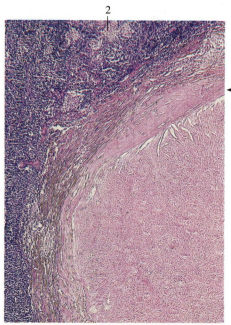

Fig 11–7.—Caseous tuberculous lymphadenitis (hematoxylin-eosin; 20×).

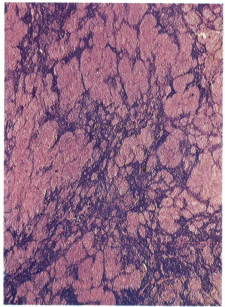

Fig 11–8.—Sarcoidosis of hilar pulmonary lymph node (hematoxylin-eosin; 40×).

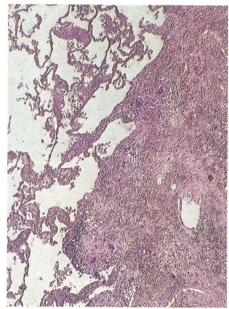

Fig 11–9.—Sarcoid scar in the lung (hematoxylin-eosin; 100×).

Specific Inflammation of Lymph Nodes

In hyperplastic tuberculous lymphadenitis (Fig 11–6), the microscopic section shows numerous, closely packed tubercles containing chiefly epithelioid cells. The rounded, frequently confluent lesions are conspicuous under low-power magnification. Higher magnification reveals typical epithelioid cells and solitary Langhans'-type giant cells. There can be secondary central necrosis (→1). In older lesions, a good deal of hyaline connective tissue may appear (→2) and finally lead to scar formation.

In caseating tuberculosis of lymph nodes (Fig 11–7), necrosis completely dominates the histologic picture, and the specific granulation tissue is visible only as a narrow border or, as in this illustration, is for the most part replaced by a fibrous capsule (→1). With the unaided eye, large homogeneous eosinophilic masses (caseation) are seen to have replaced the lymphoid tissue. Higher magnification shows extensive finely granular areas of necrosis without remnants of the original tissues. Peripheral to the focus of caseation there are noncaseating granulomas of epithelioid cells (→2).

Macroscopic: Compartmented cut surface with focal or maplike dry yellow areas.

Sarcoidosis (Boeck's sarcoid, Besnier-Boeck-Schaumann disease, Figs 11–8, 11–9, and 11–10) is a disease entity that arises sui generis. The morphological substrate is an epithelioid cell tubercle without caseation. Practically any organ can be affected; lymph nodes in the pulmonary hilus are involved at the beginning of the disease (clinical stage I, 40% heal).

Figure 11–8 shows a pulmonary hilar lymph node at low magnification. There are numerous epithelioid cell granulomas which in part are confluent. Higher magnification shows the same histologic picture as Figure 3–41: a thick layer, chiefly of plump epithelioid cells with oval or cat's tongue shaped nuclei as well as Langhans' giant cells. In contrast to tuberculosis there is no caseation and the granulomas tend to fibrose from the periphery toward the center. Frequently the epithelioid cells contain small conchoid-shaped calcified bodies (Fig 11–10), so-called *conchoid* bodies or Schaumann bodies (cell inclusions: calcified lysosomes? are detected in 80% of sarcoidosis cases and in only 6% of tuberculosis cases). Figure 11–10 shows these small bodies with doubly refractive centers in polarized light.

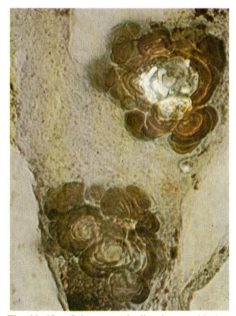

From the lymph nodes in the pulmonary hilus the granulomas spread by lymphatics to the lungs (inter- and intra-alveolar, perivascular, and in the bronchial wall). Stage II, 40% heal. Figure 11–9 shows the beginning of stage III (fibrosis of lung, death from dyspnea) with scarring of the granuloma and solitary giant cells of Langhans type. The surrounding tissue shows emphysema (scar emphysema). Distant organs may be involved (hematogenous dissemination?)

Note: epithelioid cell granulomas occur in tuberculosis, sarcoidosis, after beryllium exposure, accumulation of plastic materials, in lymph nodes draining malignant tumors, in terminal ileitis, toxoplasmosis, etc. The granulomas are thus a relatively nonspecific tissue reaction to the most varied agents. The diagnosis of sarcoidosis must be clinically confirmed.

Young women are chiefly affected. Frequency 1:1,000

Fig 11–10.—Schaumann bodies in sarcoidosis (polarized light) (hematoxylin; 700×).

269

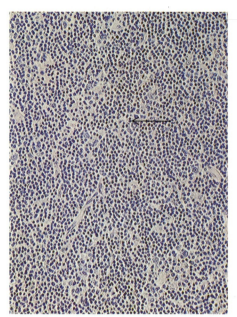

Fig 11–11.—Hodgkin's disease, lymphocytic predominance (hematoxylin-eosin; 250×).

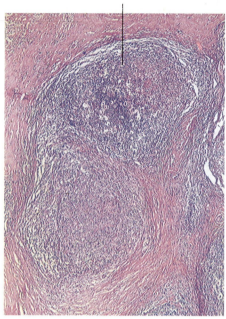

Fig 11–12.—Hodgkin's disease, nodular sclerosis (hematoxylin-eosin; 100×).

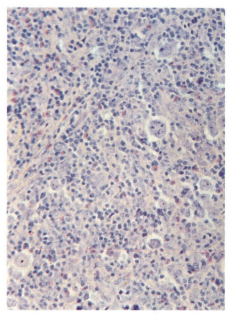

Fig 11–13.—Hodgkin's disease, mixed form (Giemsa stain; 200×).

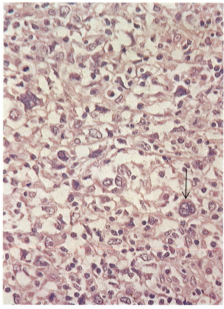

Fig 11–14.—Hodgkin's disease, sarcoma form (hematoxylin-eosin; 200×).

Hodgkin's Disease (Hodgkin's Lymphoma)

Hodgkin's disease (malignant lymphoma of Hodgkin, Figs 11–11 through 11–15) *is the most frequent of all malignant diseases of lymph nodes* (50% of primary lymph node tumors). *It has a proliferative, granulomatous type of growth that possesses specific tissue characteristics.* The typical histologic appearance shows the following: destruction of the normal structure of lymph nodes by granulomatous tissue comprised of atypical reticulum cells (possibly epithelioid cells), lymphocytes, eosinophilic granulocytes, and Reed-Sternberg cells (Fig 11–15). The characteristic cell type of the disease is the Reed-Sternberg cell which arises either from reticulum cells or lymphoblasts (× and →1 in Fig 11–15). In one form, the Hodgkin cell has a striking, pale, vesicular nucleus with a distinct nuclear membrane surrounded by a narrow margin of poorly defined, basophilic cytoplasm (Giemsa stain). From these cells are derived the multinucleated Reed-Sternberg cells. Their nuclei are likewise vesicular and partially overlap and they have abundant cytoplasm (Fig 11–15, →2). Different forms of Hodgkin's disease, each with a different prognosis, are recognized:

1. Lymphocytic predominance (diffuse or nodular): previously called paragranuloma. Figure 11–11 shows the predominance of lymphocytes whereas only a few atypical reticulum cells and Hodgkin cells (→) are seen.

Eosinophilic leukocytes for the most part are lacking. Mostly affects young men (30–40 years). Good prognosis (50–60% live longer than 6 years). Transition to mixed form or sarcoma forms is possible.

2. Nodular sclerotic form: a special form that seldom changes to another type of Hodgkin's disease. Figure 11–12 shows the typical findings. The lymph nodes are traversed by broad bands of collagenous connective tissue (doubly refractive in polarized light) having a ringlike arrangement. The granuloma tissue consists chiefly of lymphocytes, solitary atypical reticulum cells, and so-called lacunar cells (histiocytes with finely granular cytoplasm) which appear as small, round clear cells (→) in Figure 11–12. There are many Reed-Sternberg cells. Chiefly affects young women. Sixty percent live longer than 6 years.

3. Mixed form (Fig 11–13): There are typical granulomatous tissue as described above and atypical reticulum cells, lymphocytes, eosinophilic leukocytes, Reed-Sternberg giant cells, and Hodgkin cells. Survival rate: 25% live longer than 6 years. Occurs about equally in men and women.

4. Lymphocytic depletion:

(a) Diffuse fibrosis: Collagenous scar tissue with little granulomatous tissue. Scanty lymphocytes; abundant atypical reticulum cells and Reed-Sternberg giant cells.

(b) Reticular form (Hodgkin's sarcoma): Figure 11–14 shows that the cellular growth consists chiefly of reticulum cells and Hodgkin cells, especially Reed-Sternberg giant cells (→), while lymphocytes are almost completely lacking. Hematogenous metastases. Both sexes are equally affected. Course: only 20% live longer than 2 years.

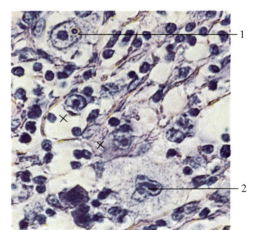

Fig 11–15.—Hodgkin's disease, Reed-Sternberg giant cells (Giemsa stain; 400×).

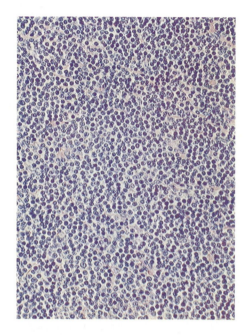

Fig 11–16.—Chronic lymphatic leukemia (hematoxylin-eosin; 300×).

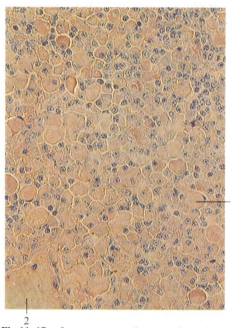

Fig 11–17.—Immunocytoma (hematoxylin-eosin; 300×).

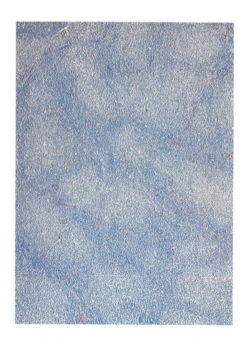

Fig 11–18.—Brill-Symmers disease (Giemsa stain; 40×).

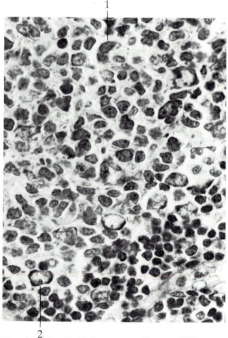

Fig 11–19.—Brill-Symmers disease (Giemsa stain; 500×). (Stein)

Non-Hodgkin's Lymphomas

Malignant lymphoma (non-Hodgkin's lymphoma, see Fig 11–1). By the coordinated use of subtle investigative techniques (Giemsa stain, electron microscopy) and recent advances in immunology and of retrospective clinical studies, it has been possible to devise a prognostically signifcant classification of malignant lymphomas. Unfortunately there is still no uniformly agreed on nomenclature. As of today we distinguish between *lymphomas with low-grade malignancy* (average course, 5–15 years; chronic lymphatic leukemia, immunocytoma, lymphocytic lymphosarcoma, Brill-Symmers disease) and *lymphomas with higher-grade malignancy* (course up to 3 years: immunoblastic sarcoma, lymphoblastic lymphosarcoma).

Chronic lymphatic leukemia (CLL, Fig 11–16) may occur with an aleukemic (so-called lymph-adenosis), subleukemic, or leukemic blood picture. Histologically (Fig 11–16) there is characteristically diffuse proliferation of typical lymphocytes with only a few lymphoblasts (→). Lymph node sinuses are mostly preserved. Splenic follicles and hepatic periportal fields are infiltrated with leukemic cells. Bone marrow is also involved.

Most frequent of all leukemias. Age 60–70 years. Male/female ratio, 2:1. Course: 3–10 years. Immunoglobulin (IgM) can be detected in the tissue.

Immunocytoma *(lymphocytoid-plasma cell immunocytoma, Fig 11–17).* These cases were formerly called *Waldenström's macroglobulinemia,* which showed a somewhat different tissue pattern (lymphocytoid plasma cells, mast cells, protein lakes) and a consistently present increase of blood IgM. Figure 11–17 shows the typical increase of plasma cells containing cytoplasmic Russell bodies (→ 1, storage of secreted immunoglobulin). In addition there are lymphoid elements that resemble in part lymphoid plasma cells. Immunoblasts are also seen, similar to those shown in Figure 11–21. At →2 there is a portion of a protein lake. IgM and IgG can be detected in tissue but not always in blood.

Higher age groups: men attacked more frequently than women. Longer course. Corticoid therapy.

Giant follicular lymphoma (synonyms: germinoblastoma, centrocytic or centroblastic lymphoma). **Brill-Symmers disease,** giant follicular lymphoblastoma, Figs 11–18 and 11–19). Figure 11–18 shows the lymph nodes to contain numerous pale germinal centers which for the most part are smaller than in nonspecific lymphadenitis. With higher magnification (Fig 11–19) it is possible to identify the cells in the germinal centers: germinocytes with oval nuclei (→1) and germinoblasts with marginal nucleoli and basophilic cytoplasm (→2). Absent are macrophages containing nuclear debris such as are seen in nonspecific lymphadenitis.

Age: 20–30 years and 60 years. Men are chiefly affected; 60% live longer than 5 years. Fifty percent of cases progress to sarcoma (germinoblastic sarcoma). Tissue IgM or IgG increased.

Lymphocytic lymphosarcoma (well-differentiated or small cell lymphosarcoma): diffuse proliferation of lymphocyte-like cells but having paler nuclei than lymphocytes, appearing more square than round and without distinct cytoplasm. According to Lennert, these should be considered germinocytes (diffuse germinocytoma). May have leukemic manifestations. Occurs at all ages. Prognosis variable (months to years). Tissue IgM present.

Lymphoblastic lymphosarcoma (Fig 11–20): The best-known representative of this group is the *Burkitt tumor,* which occurs mostly in central Africa but has been observed also in other places. There is proliferation of large lymphoblasts derived from B lymphocytes, with round nuclei, 1–2 nucleoli, and basophilic cytoplasm. Numerous histiocytes containing nuclear debris (→) are very characteristic.

Children are chiefly affected. Male/female ratio, 3:1. Epstein-Barr virus or its genome is present, as it is in nasopharyngeal carcinomas in Chinese.

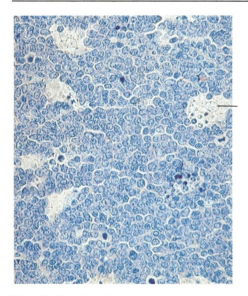

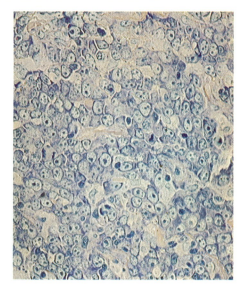

Fig 11–20.—Lymphoblastic lymphosarcoma (Giemsa stain; 300×).

Fig 11–21.—Immunoblastic sarcoma (Giemsa stain; 400×).

Immunoblastic sarcoma (histiocytic lymphoma, formerly reticulum cell sarcoma). Figure 11–21 shows diffuse proliferation of large cells with basophilic cytoplasm and round or ovoid nuclei with a distinct nuclear membrane and a large nucleolus. With electronmicroscopy the cytoplasm is seen to be rich in polysomes and ribosomes. The network of reticulin fibers, formerly considered typical of reticulum cell sarcoma, is often conspicuous. IgM can almost always be demonstrated in the tumor tissue. Age: 60–70 years. Course: ½–1 year.

Immunologic Considerations.

As shown in Figure 11–1, there are B and T cell regions in lymph nodes. The immunologic response of an organism can involve **B cells** (bone marrow lymphocytes) with stimulation of B lymphocyte precursors (Fig 11–23: enlargement and loosening of nuclear chromatin, increase in the width of the cytoplasm with abundant rough endoplasmic reticulum and microvilli on the cell membrane), or **immunoblasts** (increase of all organelles, above all, ribosomes) or differentiation to **plasma cells** (formation of humoral antibody-immunoglobulin). Simultaneously cells increase by mitosis.

If the **T cell system** (thymus-dependent lymphocytes) is stimulated the same cellular processes result (stimulated lymphocytes, immunoblasts). Further differentiation, however, leads to production of lymphocytes designated "killer lymphocytes" since they have the capability of recognizing foreign cells not belonging to the organism and destroying them with lymphotoxin (e.g., destruction of tumor cells). In autoimmune diseases also there may be destruction of body specific cells. Other kinds of T cells are the T helper cells and T suppressor cells (see textbooks of immunology). Morphologically, killer lymphocytes cannot be differentiated from resting lymphocytes that have not yet come into contact with the antigen, and from so-called memory cells. Memory cells or their precursors have at one time already come in contact with antigen and possess an immunologic memory for the specific antigen so that on further contact they give rise to cells that produce antibody. Current opinion is that antigen is first taken up by macrophages and further processed by them and that a specific immunologic message is transferred to lymphocytes. Figure 11–22 shows that specific antigen receptors (immunoglobulin) are located on the surface of lymphocytes, which thus can bind antigen (sheep erythrocytes in Fig 11–22) by immunoadherence.

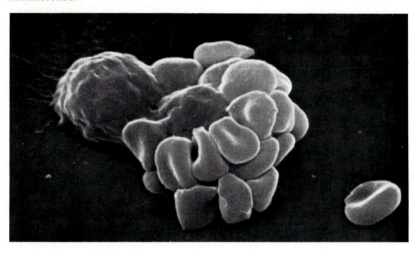

Fig 11–22.—Antigen binding by lymphocytes (mouse): scanning electron microscopy. Absorption of antigen by immunoadherence (sheep erythrocytes) to a lymphocyte with antigen-specific surface receptors, immunoglobulin receptors (rosette test of Biozzi) (4,700×). (Brücher, Gudat, and Villiger)

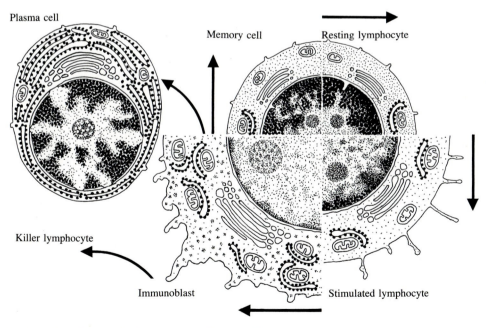

Plasma cell

Memory cell   Resting lymphocyte

Killer lymphocyte

Immunoblast   Stimulated lymphocyte

Fig 11–23.—Scheme of the development of B and T cells.

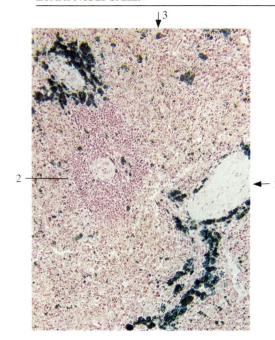

Fig 11–24.—Hemosiderin in the spleen (Prussian blue reaction; 100×).

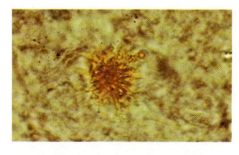

Fig 11–25.—Hematoidin crystals in a splenic infarct (hematoxylin-eosin; 380×).

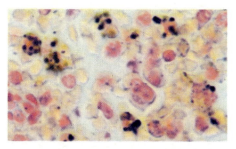

Fig 11–26.—Formalin pigment in the spleen (nuclear fast red stain; 950×).

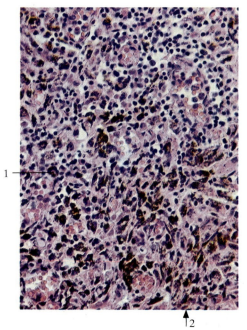

Fig 11–27.—Anthracosis of lymph nodes (hematoxylin-eosin; 300×).

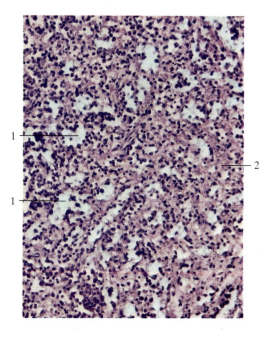

Fig 11–28.—Spleen in chronic portal hypertension (hematoxylin-eosin; 180×).

Spleen

Pathologic changes occurring in the spleen are considered with respect to the trabecular architecture, the sinuses of the red pulp and the white pulp. Special attention should be paid to blood content, the fibrous framework, the number of cells, and any foreign deposits.

Siderosis of spleen (Fig 11–24). In increased erythrocytic destruction (hemolytic anemia, repeated blood transfusions) and after large parenteral iron supplements, iron pigment is stored in the reticulum cells of the spleen (see Table 2, section on general pathology). Histologically, low-power examination of sections stained with Prussian blue shows foci of blue, layered masses in the red pulp and trabeculae (→1), (→2: follicles). High power shows that the siderin, which is stained blue by the Prussian blue reaction, lies within the cytoplasm of reticulum cells. To see this clearly, look for a part of the section in which the pigment is not so thick and where individual cells can be recognized (→3).

Hematoidin crystals in a splenic infarct (Fig 11–25). These consist of crystals of bilirubin in the form of red or orange needles or rhomboid plates. When blood is broken down and not removed by cellular resorption, for example, as may occur in the center of a hematoma or splenic infarct, iron-free pigment is formed from the hemoglobin freed from the erythrocytes (compare Table 2, section on general pathology).

Formalin pigment (Fig 11–26) is an artifact. The dark brown, granular, doubly refractile deposits are grouped together. They arise from the reaction of formaldehyde with unbound hemoglobin (probably protoporphyrin). The pigment gives a positive benzidine test and is soluble in weak acid.

Macroscopic: With Formalin fixation, the blood apears brown or brownish black.

Anthracosis of lymph node (Fig 11–27): Inhaled carbon pigment leaves the lung by way of the lymph channels and travels to the hilar lymph nodes, whence it can be carried even farther to the para-aortic lymph nodes. Rupture of markedly anthracotic lymph nodes into blood vessels in the hilus of the lung can result in spread via the bloodstream and thus give rise to so-called pigment metastases in various organs.

In the hilar lymph nodes, the granular carbon pigment is first phagocytized by the sinus histiocytes. With further accumulation, pigment is also found in histiocytes in the cortical and medullary pulp, especially around the lymphoid follicles. Higher magnification shows the carbon granules to be in individual histiocyte cells and to surround and compress the nucleus (→1). Progressive atrophy of lymphoid tissue occurs, and finally fibrosis of the node. Figure 11–27 shows the atrophy of the lymphocytes→2.

Macroscopic: Early, there is diffuse or mottled gray discoloration of the lymph nodes; later, they are homogeneous black (the cut surface is moist, in contrast to silicosis).

Fibrosis of spleen in portal hypertension (Fig 11–28): This term is used to describe chronic congestive induration of the spleen in portal hypertension; for example, in cirrhosis of the liver. Following dilation of the sinusoids from acute congestion, hyperplasia of reticulum cells and reticular fibers develops between the sinusoids and increases with the duration of the stasis. Collagenization of the reticular fibrils ensues. The sinusoids, which are largely free of erythrocytes in the illustration (→1), become surrounded by thick, rigid walls (→2). Simultaneously, the white pulp atrophies.

Macroscopic: Marked splenic enlargement. The spleen frequently weighs more than 500 gm. The splenic capsule is thickened by fibrosis and often hyalinized. The spleen has a tough, elastic consistency. The cut surface is dark red. After hemorrhage, for example from esophageal varices, the organ is light red, firm but elastic.

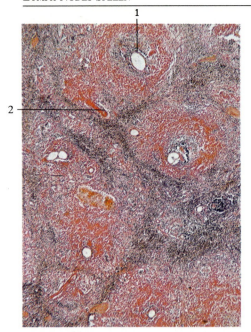

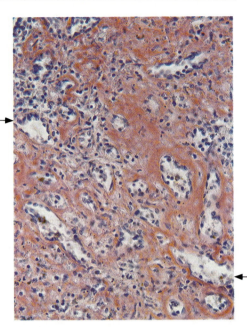

Fig 11–29.—Follicular amyloidosis in the spleen (Congo red stain; 25×).

Fig 11–30.—Amyloidosis of the splenic pulp (Congo red stain; 263×).

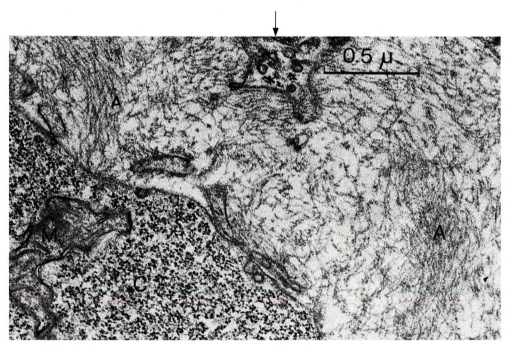

Fig 11–31.—Experimental amyloidosis of the mouse after administration of sodium caseinate. *A,* fibrous amyloid outside the cytoplasm *(C)* of a reticulum cell of the spleen. In the cytoplasm, there are numerous aggregates of ribosomes (polysomes), an indication of high protein synthesis. *M,* mitochondria (giant mitochondria); →, part of a neighboring cell (49,000×). (Caesar)

Amyloidosis

Amyloid is a glassy, translucent, homogeneous substance of firm consistency which stains red with eosin and positively with Congo red (see Fig 10,A, section on General Pathology). The composition of amyloid is 90% protein (by amino acid analysis this may be derived from variable fragments of light chain molecules of antibody) and carbohydrates (chondroitin sulfate and neuraminic acid). The binding of Congo red probably takes place with the carbohydrate component of amyloid in which a distance of 10 Å of the reactive groups of the stain is required (similar to cellulose). The fact that after staining with Congo red the amyloid is doubly refractile is proof of direct deposition of the stain on the amyloid fiber. In the majority of cases, amyloid is not related to immunoglobulin light chains. The composition of such amyloid protein can vary considerably. Congo red birefringence (green birefringence after staining with Congo red) is due to the "β-pleated sheet structure" of the various amyloid proteins. Typically, amyloid is an extracellular deposit. Electron microscopically, amyloid shows fibers about 80 Å (50–150 Å) thick (Figs 11–31, 11–32), which, with the usual techniques, show no internal structure. However, with special techniques, it has been observed that these fibers consist of 2 fibrils, each 25 Å in diameter.

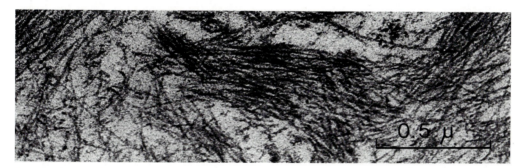

Fig 11–32.—Amyloid fibers without distinct internal structures in experimental amyloidosis in a mouse (63,000 ×). (Caesar)

Several types of amyloidosis are recognized morphologically: (1) **Typical amyloidosis:** spleen, kidney, liver, adrenal, intestinal mucosa (rectal biopsy for confirmation of diagnosis). (2) **Atypical amyloidosis:** any organ in addition to those mentioned above may be affected. *Amyloidosis in the aged* particularly involves the heart; 3% of cases occur in persons over 70 years old. (3) **Tumor-like amyloidosis:** nodules of amyloid infiltrated by plasma cells may occur, e.g., in the tongue. Tumor-like deposits may also occur in pancreatic islets and in C-cell thyroid tumors (calcitonin-producing cells). *Etiological classification:* (1) **Primary hereditary amyloidosis, e.g.,** familial Mediterranean fever (typical amyloidosis), neuropathic amyloidosis (atypical amyloidosis). (2) **Secondary acquired amyloidosis:** (typical amyloidosis) in chronic inflammation (tuberculosis is present in 50% of cases of amyloidosis, osteomyelitis in 12%, chronic lung infection in 10%, other chronic infections in 12% (hyperimmunization). In rheumatoid arthritis 20% of cases show amyloidosis. *Experimental:* repeated doses of foreign protein.

Follicular amyloidosis (Fig 11–29). Low magnification of a section stained with Congo red demonstrates the red-colored follicles which are seen as red circles or little disks, sometimes with a central artery (→1). →2, amyloid in an artery in the pulp. The follicles contan no lymphocytes; the pulp is poor in cells.

Macroscopic: Multiple small glassy nodules = Sago spleen.

Pulp amyloidosis (Fig 11–30): Low magnification shows red homogeneous tissue and focal round pale areas corresponding to the follicles. Higher magnification shows the amyloid lying between dilated sinuses lined by large endothelial cells (→1).

Macroscopic: Enlarged, firm spleen of wooden consistency and lardaceous glassy cut surfaces.

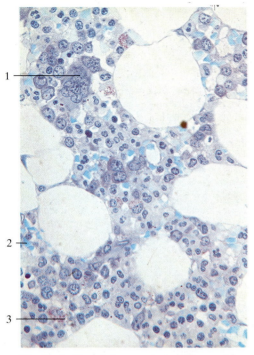

Fig 12–1.–Normal bone marrow (Giemsa stain; 320×).

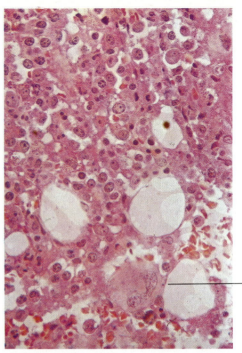

Fig 12–2.—Polycythemia vera (Ladewig stain; 320×).

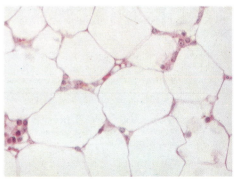

Fig 12–4.—Acute myelogenous leukemia (immature cell) (Giemsa stain; 320×).

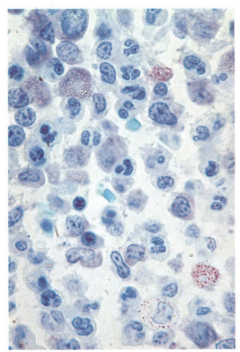

Fig 12–3.—Chronic myelogenous leukemia (Giemsa stain; 600×).

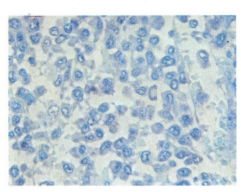

Fig 12–5.—Aplasia of bone marrow (Ladewig stain; 200×).

12. Blood—Bone Marrow

Definitive diagnosis of diseases of the blood depends on examination of a peripheral blood smear and a bone marrow biopsy. With the introduction of bone marrow biopsy and the use of pathologic anatomical methods of investigation (paraffin embedding, histologic staining, histochemical reactions, and electron microscopy) the pathologist is frequently confronted with the collection and interpretation of hematologic data. A bone marrow biopsy (pelvic crest) has distinct advantages over a bone marrow smear but does not replace it. The cells can be studied as a tissue rather than as isolated cells and in relation to the other components of the bone marrow, e.g., bone trabeculae, osteoblasts, osteoclasts, and blood vessels. A biopsy rather than a smear is especially advantageous in evaluating a *cellularly depleted* bone marrow with replacement by fat cells (e.g., *bone marrow aplasia,* Fig 12–5) or by fibrous tissue (in *osteomyelofibrosis*). The greatest difficulty of bone marrow biopsy heretofore has been the difficulty of cytomorphological cell differentiation in paraffin sections over 5 μ thick. This difficulty has now been overcome by the introduction of other embedding materials. Today with material embedded in methacrylate it is possible to prepare semithin sections of 0.1–2 μ thickness with which the routine staining (hematoxylin-eosin, Giemsa, Ladewig, Gomori) or histochemical (PAS, Prussian blue) procedures can be carried out without disturbance of cellular and nuclear relationships.

Normal bone marrow (Fig 12–1) is cellular and very variegated in its composition. In semithin sections it is possible to differentiate the first stages of myelopoiesis. Especially clearly shown are the multinucleated megakaryocytes (→1), the dark blue erythrocytes (→2), and the granules of the eosinophiles (→3). Large fat cells are present in the marrow (optically empty spaces).

In **polycythemia vera** (Fig 12–2) *all blood forming elements are increased: there are polycythemia leukocytosis, and thrombocytosis.* An increase in megakaryocytes (→) which lie chiefly in the marrow sinuses is very characteristic.

Polycythemia vera commonly occurs in persons aged 50–60 years and after a long course progresses to osteosclerosis or chronic myeloid leukemia (about 10% of cases). Pure erythropoietic hyperplasia, in which the peripheral erythrocyte count may be over 10 million/cu mm, is referred to as *polycythemia.* In addition to the *idiopathic form* there is *secondary polycythemia,* resulting from other causes (chronic lung diseases, hypernephroma [due to increased production of erythropoietin]).

Leukemia (or leukosis) *is a neoplastic disease in which the blood-forming cells of the hematopoietic system show abnormal, autonomous proliferation that may develop either quickly or slowly.* Any series of the hematopoietic system may be involved *(myelocytic, lymphocytic, monocytic, erythrocytic, megakaryocytic, or plasma cell leukemias).* Depending on the maturity of the cells and the duration of the disease, we distinguish *chronic* (relatively mature cells) and *acute* (immature cells) *leukemias.* Chronic leukemias as a rule are accompanied by the appearance of the abnormal cells in peripheral blood, so that there may be a leukocytosis of 500,000 to over 1,000,000 cells. In acute leukemias the leukocyte count more often may be normal or even subnormal *(aleukemic leukemia).* As a consequence of the increased number of leukemic cells the appearance of the bone marrow is altered by displacement of normal cells, leading to reduced erythropoiesis (→ anemia) and reduced thrombocytopoiesis (→ thrombocytopenia → hemorrhagic diathesis).

In **chronic myeloid or myelogenous leukemia,** also called granulocytic leukemia, (Fig 12–3) semithin sections stained with Giemsa stain have a variegated and richly cellular appearance. Besides mature polymorphonuclear granulocytes there are immature cells, especially pro- and metamyelocytes. In **acute myeloid leukemia,** by contrast, the cellular picture is monotonous. Chiefly there are paramyeloblasts, (Fig 12–4). Smears of peripheral blood usually show segmented leukocytes as well as paramyeloblasts, but no intermediate forms *(leukemic hiatus).*

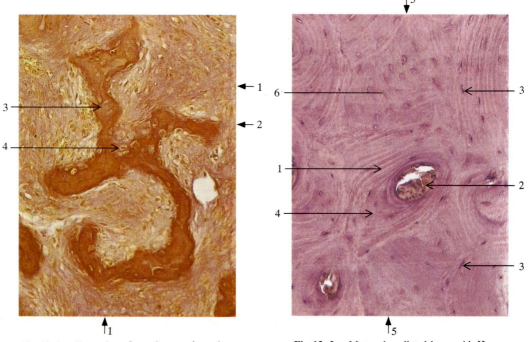

Fig 13–1.—Formation of membranous bone (van Gieson's stain; 82×).

Fig 13–2.—Mature lamellated bone with Haversian osteons (hematoxylin-eosin; 200×).

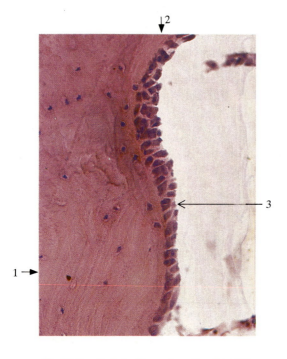

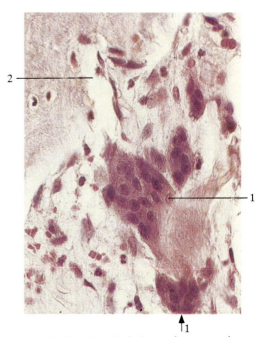

Fig 13–3.—Endosteal bone formation (hematoxylin-eosin; 200×).

Fig 13–4.—Osteoclastic lacunar bone resorption (hematoxylin-eosin; 160×).

13. Bones—Joints

Microscopic study of bone sections necessitates knowledge of the *type of bony tissue* being examined (whether compact bone with Haversian systems or spongy bone without Haversian systems). The *quantitative relation between cancelous part and marrow space* must be evaluated (e.g., in the rarefaction due to osteoporosis or the reduction of marrow spaces in osteosclerosis) as well as the *types of cells appearing in the marrow spaces* (active hematopoietic, fatty or fibrous marrow, inflammatory infiltrates, etc.). It is important to see if the osteocytes in the *trabeculae* are stained (in bone necrosis the nuclei do not stain. Care must be exercised, however, for severe decalcification causes negative nuclear staining). The number of osteoblasts, the width of the osteoid margins, the degree of calcification of newly formed bone, and the number of osteoclasts serve as an *indication of bone formation or resorption.*

The reactions of bony tissue under abnormal circumstances consist in formation of new bone or bone resorption. It is of decisive significance whether damage occurs while the skeleton is immature or after it is fully mature.

Formation of new bone occurs by means of cells that have the capacity to proliferate and to differentiate. Thus, undifferentiated mesenchyme gives rise to preosteoblasts that later become osteoblasts. While preosteoblasts can proliferate through cell division, osteoblasts cannot do so. Osteoblasts have a high content of alkaline phosphatase, which is necessary for calcification of bone. Osteoblasts have three main functions: (1) formation of mucopolysaccharide-protein complexes, (2) synthesis of collagen fibers, and (3) participation in mineralization. Collagen synthesis begins as an intracellular process, but its final stage—formation of osteoid—occurs outside of cells. Inactive osteoblasts are fusiform; active osteoblasts resemble epithelial cells. An active osteoblast daily produces a layer of osteoid measuring approximately 1 μ in width. On average, the width of osteoid margins of bony trabeculae is 6 μ. Seventy percent of newly formed osteoid is calcified in 3–4 days, the remainder within 6 weeks. Darker-staining cement lines (Fig 13–2 → 1) indicate that mineralization of osteoid occurs in stages.

There are several forms of new bone formation: (1) *Periosteal new bone formation,* proceeding from periosteal osteoblasts. Pathologically this occurs in periostitis ossificans, osteomyelitis, and formation of bony spicules in bone tumors. (2) *Endosteal new bone formation,* which proceeds from endosteal osteoblasts. Pathologically this occurs in the callus of a healing fracture, osteomyelitis, and Paget's disease (osteitis deformans). (3) *Formation of new bone in Haversian osteons,* proceeding from perivascular osteoblasts. Pathologically this occurs in fracture callus, osteomyelitis, and osteoid osteoma. (4) *Formation of spongy bone through differentiation of connective tissue cells* into bone cells. Pathologically this occurs in fibrous dysplasia and ossifying fibromas. Figure 13–1 shows typical **formation of spongy (membranous) bone.** Within a cellular collagen connective tissue (→1) fibroblasts differentiate into osteoblasts and intercellular collagen is formed, which later is mineralized (→2). Thus, a network of bony trabeculae is formed (i.e., membranous bone, →3). The collagenous fibers of the trabeculae continue into the surrounding connective tissue. Osteoblasts may be present or absent, but the bony trabeculae contain large osteocytes (→4).

The cortex of long bones is composed of **lamellated bone.** During the second year of life Haversian osteons develop and spread through the bone. Through resorption of old and formation of new osteons there develops a pattern of complete and incomplete osteons in compact bone (compacta). This architecture is shown in Figure 13–2. Layers of bony tissue surround Haversian canals (→2), through which run capillaries. The bony layers are demarcated by cement lines (→1). Within the compact bone there are osteocytes (→3) which give bone its vital capacity. These osteocytes have elongated nuclei and are situated in tiny lacunae. One can recognize almost completed, newly formed osteons (→4) and older, incomplete osteons (→5). At →6 there is an interposed lamella.

Endosteal formation of new bone is seen in Figure 13–3, which shows lamellae in a trabecula of spongy bone (→1) in which osteocytes are enclosed. The outer layer (→2) shows a seam of osteoid on which there are active osteoblasts (→3). This osteoid is undergoing mineralization and thus the trabecula becomes broader.

Resorption of bone is accomplished by multinucleated osteoclasts that have a ruffled border which is rich in acid phosphatase. These cells elaborate proteolytic enzymes by means of which bone resorption occurs. There are several ways of resorption: (1) *Lacunar resorption,* as shown in Figure 13–4; groups of multinucleated osteoclasts (→1) are apposed to calcified bone and have produced Howship's lacunae (→2). This has given the trabeculae wavy borders. (2) *Smooth resorption.* This is a gradual resorption by cells with single nuclei, resulting in diminution of trabeculae. Howship's lacunae are absent. (3) *Perforating resorption.* Calcified bone is "tunneled" by osteoclasts possessing one or more nuclei. The osteoclasts originate in Haversian canals.

283

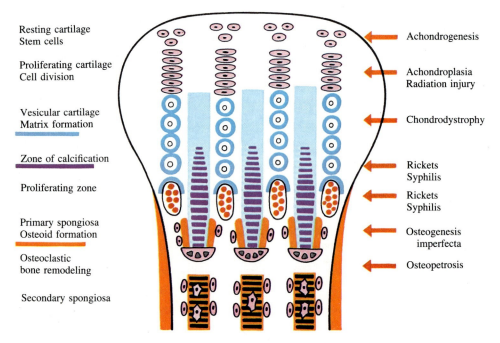

Resting cartilage
Stem cells

Proliferating cartilage
Cell division

Vesicular cartilage
Matrix formation

Zone of calcification

Proliferating zone

Primary spongiosa
Osteoid formation

Osteoclastic
bone remodeling

Secondary spongiosa

Achondrogenesis

Achondroplasia
Radiation injury

Chondrodystrophy

Rickets
Syphilis

Rickets
Syphilis

Osteogenesis
imperfecta

Osteopetrosis

Fig 13–5.—Schematic representation of endochondral ossification and its disorders.

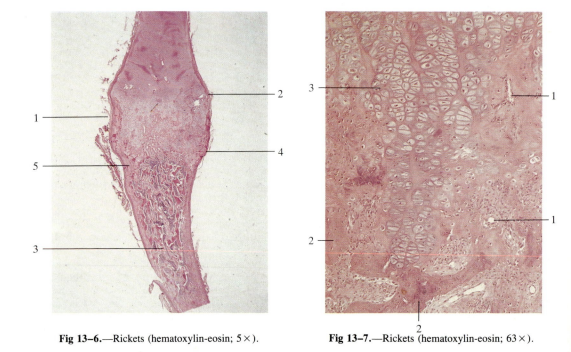

Fig 13–6.—Rickets (hematoxylin-eosin; 5×).

Fig 13–7.—Rickets (hematoxylin-eosin; 63×).

Disturbances of Bone Development

Disturbances of skeletal development occur in childhood and adolescence. Figure 13–5 is a diagram of endochondral ossification and its disturbances. On the left side the various zones of normal ossification are listed: resting cartilage, columnar cartilage, vesicular cartilage, provisional zone of calcification, primary and secondary spongiosa. Disturbances can occur at each step of the complex process. If there is no differentiation of stem cells in the resting zone, achondrogenesis results. In achondroplasia there is inadequate proliferation of cartilage cells. Defective or absent growth of columnar cartilage gives rise to chondrodystrophy. If calcification in the zone is deficient, rickets results. Deficient osteoid formation leads to osteogenesis imperfecta. If remodeling of lamellar bone is disturbed, the result is osteopetrosis.

Rickets (Figs 13–6, 13–7) results from a disturbance of endochondral ossification in the growing skeleton in consequence of deficient calcification, particularly in the provisional zone of calcification, where the uncalcified osteoid accumulates. Causes of rickets are vitamin D deficiency and malfunction of kidney tubules (renal rickets). Figure 13–6 shows a rachitic junction of bone and cartilage in a rib (costochondral junction). The junctional zone is widened and swollen (part of a "rickety rosary"→). Above this zone there is normal cartilage (→2), below it normal spongiosa (→3). The cartilage in the widened zone of ossification is elongated (→4) and poor in blood vessels. In place of the zone of provisional calcification, normally adjacent to vesicular cartilage, there is a zone of cartilaginous osteoid (→5). Neither osteoid nor cartilage matrix is calcified. **Higher magnification** (Fig 13–7) reveals irregular bands of cartilage between the penetrating vessels of the primary spongiosa (→1) and there are broad, unmineralized trabeculae of osteoid. Above this region one sees the zone of columnar cartilage (→3) whose ground substance is also unmineralized. The osteoid cannot be resorbed by osteoclasts, and this leads to a delayed formation of secondary spongiosa. The result of this is a broadening of the metaphysis. Since perichondrial and intramembranous ossification is also disturbed (Table 13–1), the primary calcified bone of the calvarium is resorbed and replaced by uncalcified osteoid; the parietal bones remain soft and the posterior fontanelle does not close (craniotabes). Increased deposition of poorly calcified bony tissue in the frontal and parietal bones leads to caput quadratum. There are marked deformations of thorax and pelvis ("chicken breast," rachitic pelvis). The lower extremities are curved (bowlegs, knock-knees). Because of vitamin D prophylaxis, fully developed rickets is rarely encountered nowadays.

TABLE 13–1.—DISTURBANCES IN OSSIFICATION IN THE OSTEODYSTROPHIES

	CHONDRO-DYSTROPHY	RICKETS	SYPHILITIC OSTEOCHON-DRITIS	OSTEOGENE-SIS IMPER-FECTA	OSTEOPE-TROSIS

Compensatory bone formation
  Enchondral ø.
    Epiphyseal ø.
	▇	▇	▇	▇	▇

Metaphyseal ø.	▇	▇	▇	▇	▇
Perichondral ø.		▇		▇	▇
Periosteal bone formation		▇		▇	▇

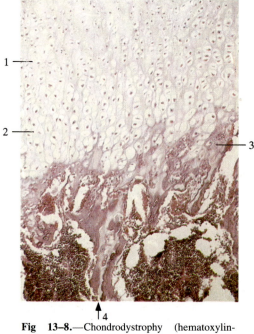

Fig 13–8.—Chondrodystrophy (hematoxylin-eosin; 63 ×).

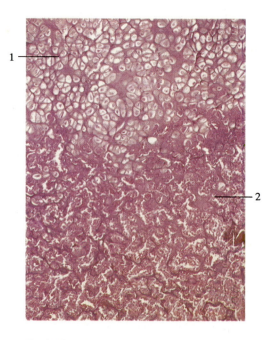

Fig 13–9.—Osteogenesis imperfecta (hematoxylin-eosin; 63 ×).

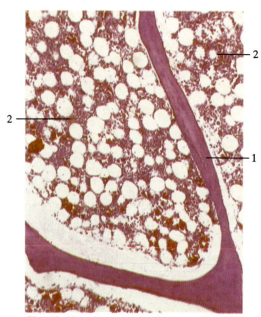

Fig 13–10.—Osteoporosis (hematoxylin-eosin; 63 ×).

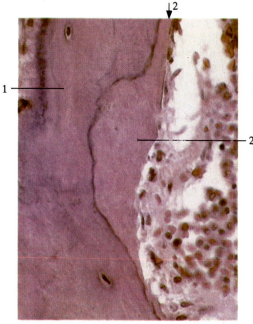

Fig 13–11.—Osteomalacia (hematoxylin-eosin; 250 ×).

Chondrodystrophy (Fig 13–8). In chondrodystrophy endochondral ossification stops early. Since the formation of columnar cartilage is impeded, the longitudinal growth of bone is diminished. However, periosteal bone formation is undisturbed, so that the bones are relatively thicker. Thus develops the chondrodystrophic dwarf (short, thick extremities with normally developed axial skeleton). The large head of such a dwarf somewhat resembles an inverted pear, a result of the disturbed growth of the base of the skull (the intramembraneous bone formation of the skull is unaffected). The disturbance affects bones with metaphyses. As can be seen in Fig 13–8, there is little proliferation of chondrocytes, which are small ($\rightarrow$1) and have small round nuclei. The cartilaginous columns ($\rightarrow$2) possess only 6–8 chondrocytes instead of the normal 20. Provisional calcification and the formation of osteoid are also reduced. The zone of osteoid bordering the provisional zone of calcification is barely developed ($\rightarrow$3). The lower portion of Figure 13–8 shows components of secondary spongiosa ($\rightarrow$4).

Osteogenesis imperfecta (Fig 13–9). Osteogenesis imperfecta is an inheritable disease of the skeleton characterized by marked fragility of the bones. This is due to defective collagen synthesis and insufficient formation of bone. *Osteogenesis imperfecta congenita* leads to intrauterine death. *Osteogenesis imperfecta tarda* is associated with multiple bone fractures, but the patients have a normal life expectancy. As can be seen in Figure 13–9, endochondral proliferation of cells into columnar cartilage ($\rightarrow$1) is normal. However, there are fewer osteoblasts and osteoclasts in the provisional zone of calcification than is normal. Formation of osteoid along the spicules of calcified cartilage is markedly diminished. The primary spongiosa consists merely of a tight mesh of cartilaginous matrix ($\rightarrow$2). Thus, the primary and secondary spongiosa cannot be fully developed. The result is a high-grade osteoporosis and strong susceptibility to fractures.

Osteoporoses and Osteopathies

Osteoporosis with bony atrophy (Fig 13–10). In this condition there is atrophy of bony tissue, which is diminished and radiographically less dense than normal. Osteoporosis is the most frequent alteration in the adult skeleton. It is the result of negative bone metabolism (increased resorption with decreased formation of bone). Figure 13–10 shows markedly thinned bony trabeculae which, though possessing lamellar structure, have tiny osteocytes ($\rightarrow$1). Since there are no osteoclasts or resorption lacunae, this may be called *smooth* resorption of bone. The regressive remodeling of bone is accompanied by enlargement of marrow spaces filled with fatty and hematopoietic marrow ($\rightarrow$2). The Haversian canals of the bony cortex are widened (not shown in picture).

Osteomalacia (Fig 13–11). Osteomalacia represents a disturbance of calcification of bone in adults and is comparable to childhood rickets. Among causes may be listed vitamin D deficiency, calcium deficiency, and certain kidney diseases. The osteoid in the bones is increased, while there is insufficient calcification. Histologically (Fig 13–11) one sees reduction in mineralization of bony trabeculae ($\rightarrow$1) that are lined by abnormally wide seams of osteoid ($\rightarrow$2; wider than 10 μ), upon which there are scattered osteoblasts. The broad seams of osteoid appear as homogeneous, pale red bands that are distinct from the calcified bone. Roentgenograms show an indistinct bony structure. The bones are soft and deformable. Among the resulting deformations are kyphosis, coxa vara, and deformed pelvis.

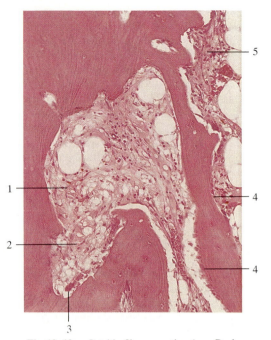

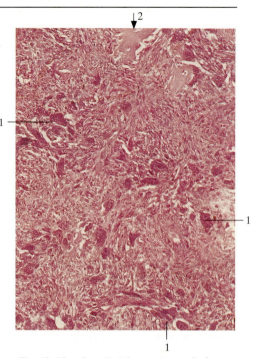

Fig 13–12.—Osteitis fibrosa cystica (von Recklinghausen) (hematoxylin-eosin; 180×).

Fig 13–13.—So-called brown tumor in hyperparathyroidism (hematoxylin-eosin; 180×).

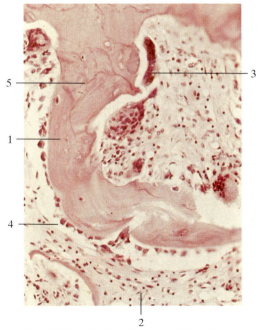

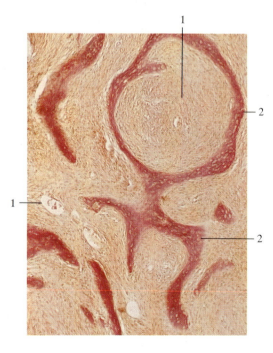

Fig 13–14.—Osteitis deformans (Paget) (hematoxylin-eosin; 150×).

Fig 13–15.—Fibrous dysplasia of bone (Jaffé-
Lichtenstein) (van Gieson's stain; 60×).

Osteitis fibrosa cystica of von Recklinghausen (Fig 13–12). This is a focally distributed but generalized osteoporotic disease of the skeleton due to increased secretion of parathormone. The increased levels of parathormone may be due to adenomas, hyperplasia, or carcinomas of the parathyroid glands. Osteoclasts, osteoblasts, and fibroblasts in the bones become activated. Histologically (Fig 13–12) the bony trabeculae have irregular borders with deep resorption lacunae. The recesses are invaded by cellular and collagenous tissue resembling granulation tissue (→1). The recesses produced by resorption are filled by loose vascular connective tissue with prominent fibroblasts (→2). The adjacent bony tissue has a wavy border on which there are multinucleated osteoclasts (→3). Besides these, there are also rows of osteoblasts (→4) on bony trabeculae. Where bony trabeculae adjoin the marrow, there may be endosteal fibrosis (→5). This histologic picture is typical for primary hyperparathyroidism.

The so-called **brown tumor** (Fig 13–13) is not a neoplasm of bone but a resorptive granuloma with giant cells which develops in advanced hyperparathyroidism. The osteolysis induced by the hormonal excess diminishes the strength of the skeleton and leads to spontaneous fractures with intraosseous bleeding. Activated osteoclasts tend to produce a focally prominent osteolysis that may be mistaken for bone tumor on x-ray films. Histologically (Fig 13–13) there is loose vascular connective tissue with hemorrhages and deposits of hemosiderin. Osteoclastic giant cells (→1) are irregularly and prominently distributed in the fibrous tissue. The osseous tissue of the spongiosa is largely destroyed. Only remnants of trabeculae remain (→2), and these are undergoing osteoclastic resorption. Morphologically, there is a great similarity to osteoclastoma (see Fig 13–29), from which the giant cell granuloma must be distinguished.

Osteitis deformans (Paget's disease of bone, Fig 13–14). This disease is an osteodystrophy of unknown etiology which occurs only in older people. In 81% the skull, vertebral column, pelvis, femurs, and tibiae are involved. Histologically there is a marked remodeling of bones. Figure 13–14 shows a coarsely deformed bony trabecula (→1). The marrow space is occupied by loose connective tissue with many capillaries (→2). Sometimes such connective tissue also shows serous inflammation. On one side the trabecula has been eroded by multinucleated osteoclasts (→3). On the opposite side new bone is being formed by osteoblasts (→4). The incessant resorption of bone, along with disorderly formation of bone, produces new cement lines (→5) which are short and interrupted, producing a mosaic. This remodeling of bone leads to deformities and an increased tendency to fracture.

Fibrous dysplasia of bone (Jaffé-Lichtenstein, Fig 13–15) represents a faulty development of bone-forming mesenchyme in which bone marrow is replaced by connective tissue. Also, bone formed in connective tissue is not transformed into lamellar bone. This leads to bone cysts that are visible on roentgenograms. Figure 13–15 shows a region of fibrous dysplasia in which fibrous connective tissue has replaced normal spongiosa. The fibrous tissue is seen as strands and whorls (→1). Note also the numerous thin bony trabeculae that are hooked or horseshoe-shaped (→2); these are not lined by osteoblasts. This dysplasia of bone, which is relatively frequent, results in skeletal deformities and pathologic fractures.

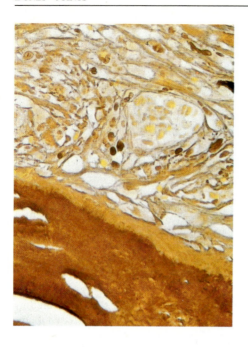

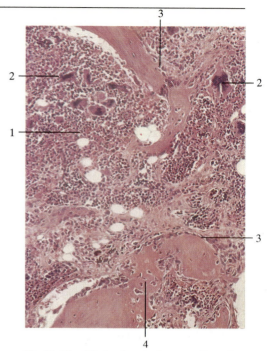

Fig 13–16.—Myelofibrosis (van Gieson's stain; 200×).

Fig 13–17.—Myelosclerosis (hematoxylin-eosin; 100×).

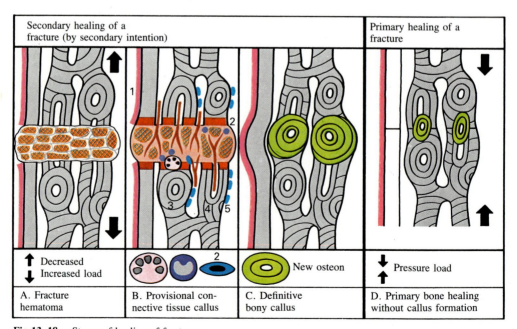

Secondary healing of a fracture (by secondary intention)			Primary healing of a fracture
↑ Decreased ↓ Increased load		New osteon	↓ Pressure load ↑
A. Fracture hematoma	B. Provisional connective tissue callus	C. Definitive bony callus	D. Primary bone healing without callus formation

Fig 13–18.—Stages of healing of fractures.

Myelosclerosis (Figs 13–16, 13–17). In myelosclerosis the bone marrow is gradually but generally replaced by connective tissue, some of which in turn becomes ossified. This results in replacement of bone marrow and marrow insufficiency. Then extramedullary hematopoiesis develops in spleen, liver, lymph nodes, and other organs, and eventually there is aplastic anemia. In the initial phase of this disease (fibro-osteoclastic phase) there is focal transformation of bone marrow into reticular connective tissue. This is followed by the development of an irregular network of collagen fibers in which there are numerous capillaries. This stage, which may be called **myelofibrosis,** can be seen in Figure 13–16. There the marrow between bony trabeculae with lamellar structure has been replaced by loose connective tissue that is mainly composed of thick, long, disorderly collagen fibers (→2). Between the collagen fibers there are dilated capillaries and a few lymphocytes. In the process of fibrosis bony trabeculae are resorbed by osteoclasts and become jagged or wavy (→3). In an intermediate phase a network of osteoid is formed in the connective tissue and is later transformed into bone. Figure 13–17 shows the fully developed picture of **myelosclerosis.** The marrow spaces are filled by partly loose, partly dense, connective tissue in which immature erythroid and myeloid cells are situated (→1). Note also the numerous giant cells with dense, bizarre nuclei (→2); these are atypical megakaryocytes. During the stage of myelofibrosis, bone resorption due to osteoclasts predominates, but in myelosclerosis rows of osteoblasts that cover the bony trabeculae (→3) produce new bone. One can also see newly formed, branching nonlamellar bone (→4) that borders on lamellar bone. The etiology of myelosclerosis is unknown, but toxic damage of bone marrow may be one cause.

Bone Fracture

In a fracture there is a complete or incomplete interruption of the continuity of a bone which is due to direct or indirect force. The result is an orderly tissue reaction that is designed to restore bony continuity. Figure 13–18 shows the sequence of events. At first a hematoma forms at the two ends of a fracture. On the second day granulation tissue that is rich in capillaries grows into the hematoma. Then fibroblasts form a bridge, thus giving rise to the provisional connective tissue callus. Between the seventh and ninth day mesenchymal cells become transformed into osteoblasts that produce osteoid. A series of chemical reactions leads to production of a supersaturated solution of calcium and phosphate ions from which hydroxyapatite precipitates. Then bony trabeculae are formed in the connective tissue and unite the ends of the fracture. This represents a **provisional bony callus** that cannot yet bear a load. After 4–5 weeks a definitive callus is formed, in which the intrafibrous bony trabeculae are gradually replaced by lamellar bone. Bone provisionally formed by the periosteum and endosteum is resorbed. New bone in the cortex becomes oriented in accord with weight-bearing. The fracture is now fully healed.

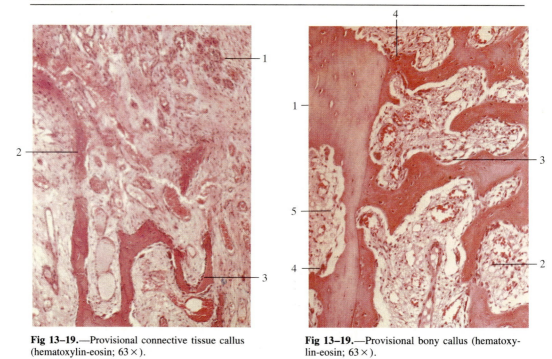

Fig 13–19.—Provisional connective tissue callus (hematoxylin-eosin; 63 ×).

Fig 13–19.—Provisional bony callus (hematoxylin-eosin; 63 ×).

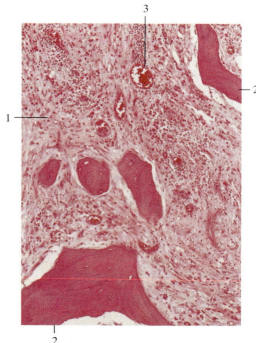

Fig 13–21.—Acute suppurative osteomyelitis (hematoxylin-eosin; 100 ×).

Fig 13–22.—Chronic osteomyelitis (hematoxylin-eosin; 63 ×).

Provisional connective tissue callus (Fig 13–19). Figure 13–19 shows loose connective tissue between the ends of a fracture. This is partly granulation tissue containing numerous capillaries and capillary sprouts as well as some infiltrating lymphocytes, plasma cells, and histiocytes (→1). Thin bony trabeculae have formed within this connective tissue (→2). These branching trabeculae contain many osteocytes. Elsewhere the trabeculae are more mineralized and are adjoined by osteoclasts with single nuclei (→3). (Healing fractures of ribs and the zygoma develop, in addition, a cartilaginous callus under the influence of motion, e.g., breathing, chewing.)

Provisional bony callus (Fig 13–20). Situated in the left half of Figure 13–20 is original lamellar bone (→1) that contains few osteocytes. Irregular bony trabeculae have formed in the granulation tissue of the fracture (→2). These trabeculae, though devoid of lamellae, are well-calcified, and on one side are covered by rows of osteoblasts (→3) that are forming osteoid. On the other side of the new trabeculae, osteoclasts are resorbing bone (→4). One also can see lacunar resorption of original bone (→5): this has progressed far and is characterized by the presence of osteoclasts.

Inflammation of Bones

Acute suppurative osteomyelitis (Fig 13–21). Osteomyelitis is an inflammation of bone, usually caused by bacteria. The condition is primary in the marrow and secondarily involves the bony structures. Many sorts of bacteria can produce osteomyelitis, but some give rise to characteristic histologic alterations: specific forms of osteomyelitis are associated with tuberculosis, typhoid, syphilis, and various mycoses, but histologically nonspecific osteomyelitis occurs most frequently and is commonly caused by *Staphylococcus aureus*. The organisms can reach the bone directly in an open fracture but in most cases they do so by the hematogenous route, and often no portal of entry is demonstrable. Figure 13–21 is a typical picture of *suppurative osteomyelitis*. The marrow seen in this picture is filled with highly cellular inflammatory tissue and is permeated by edema fluid (→1). Note the large collection of segmented leukocytes (granulocytes) that have replaced the original marrow. The trabeculae of spongiosa are necrotic (→2). The bony lamellae are in the process of disappearing. The lacunae are empty, without osteocytes. This is a sequestrum of spongiosa (→2). Sequestra maintain the inflammatory process within the bone marrow and must therefore be removed. Sometimes true abscesses are formed in bone marrow.

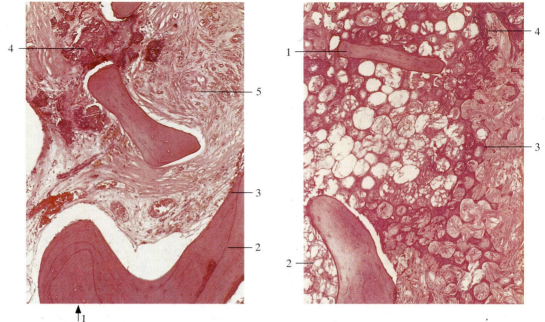

Fig 13–23.—Primary ischemic necrosis of head of femur (hematoxylin-eosin; 63 ×).

Fig 13–24.—Anemic infarct of bone (hematoxylin-eosin).

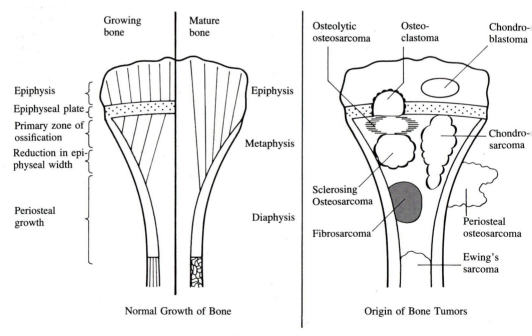

Growing bone

Mature bone

Epiphysis

Epiphyseal plate

Primary zone of ossification

Reduction in epiphyseal width

Periosteal growth

Epiphysis

Metaphysis

Diaphysis

Normal Growth of Bone

Osteolytic osteosarcoma

Osteoclastoma

Chondroblastoma

Chondrosarcoma

Sclerosing Osteosarcoma

Fibrosarcoma

Periosteal osteosarcoma

Ewing's sarcoma

Origin of Bone Tumors

Fig 13–25.—**Left,** topographic and functional differentiation of normally growing and of mature bone. **Right,** topographic localization of several bone tumors.

Chronic Osteomyelitis (Fig 13–22). *Acute suppurative osteomyelitis can last a long time, with extensive healing, but without cessation of the progressive inflammatory process. The combination of continued inflammation, destruction of bone, and fibrosis of the marrow is termed chronic osteomyelitis.* Figure 13–22 shows complete replacement of marrow by scar tissue (→1). Instead of the original bony trabeculae of the spongiosa there are irregular thick trabeculae (→2), situated within the fibrous scar tissue. Here and there the connective tissue appears looser and is penetrated by capillaries (→3). In these areas there are collections of plasma cells, lymphocytes, and histiocytes as well as a few segmented granulocytes that bear witness to the smoldering inflammatory process. In this condition fistulas through the bony cortex and the soft tissues may develop, and the chronic inflammation may be associated with amyloidosis elsewhere in the body.

Necrosis of Bone

Necrosis of bone represents intravital death of ossified tissue. It may be due to (1) disturbed circulation in the bone, (2) osteomyelitis, (3) effects of ionizing radiation, (4) trauma (e.g., fractures), or (5) hormonal disturbances (e.g., Cushing's disease). Histologically the necrosis is characterized by the absence of osteocytes and indistinct lamellar markings in the affected trabeculae. The adjacent marrow usually shows inflammatory reactions.

Ischemic necrosis of the head of the femur (Fig 13–23). Aseptic necrosis in the head of the femur occurs in adolescents and adults and is thought to be due to a circulatory disturbance in the bone. This, in turn, is often due to traumatic luxation or to fracture of the neck of the femur. Figure 13–23 shows an old aseptic necrosis in which bony trabeculae have become widened in consequence of reparative processes (→1). The lamellar structure is indistinct, and the osteocytes have disappeared. Attenuated cement lines (→2) are clearly visible. These represent former sites of repair. In places there are also seams of osteoid (→3). The marrow contains amorphous, necrotic, and calcified material (→4), as well as collagenous connective tissue (→5). Elsewhere (not shown in the picture) there are resorption lacunae with osteoclasts.

Bone infarct (Fig 13–24). This is a circumscribed zone of necrosis with a hemorrhagic margin and is situated within a bone. It occurs most commonly under the influence of increased glucocorticoid levels (adrenocortical hyperplasias, tumors, corticosteroid therapy). Figure 13–24 shows a markedly narrowed bony trabecula (→1) with a wavy border but without adjoining osteoclasts. Only portions of the fatty marrow have become necrotic (→3). At →4, scar tissue may be seen, which adjoins an older area of necrosis. At the borders of such infarcts "calcium soaps" may be deposited, creating jagged lines on roentgenograms.

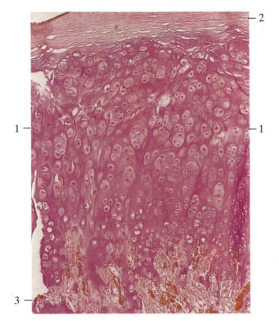

Fig 13–26.—Osteochondroma (hematoxylin-eosin; 40×).

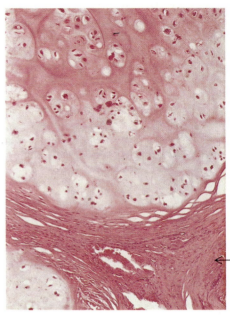

Fig 13–27.—Enchondroma (hematoxylin-eosin; 63×).

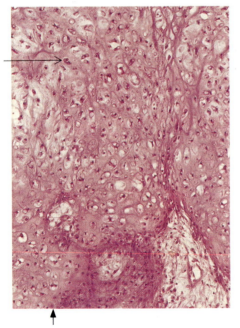

Fig 13–28.—Chondrosarcoma (hematoxylin-eosin; 100×).

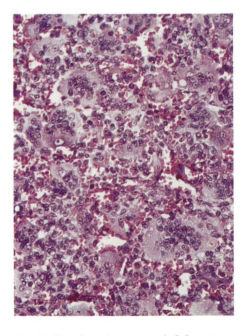

Fig 13–29.—Osteoclastoma, grade I (hematoxylin-eosin; 160×).

Tumors of Bones

Osteochondroma (Fig 13–26). This is a bony neoplasm that is covered by a cap of hyaline cartilage and protrudes, mushroom-like, into the surrounding soft tissues. Figure 13–26 shows a cartilaginous cap (→1) that grossly measured 1–3 cm and is covered by periosteal connective tissue (→2). The hyaline cartilage contains groups or rows of cartilage cells resembling those in normal epiphyses. The cartilaginous tissue extends finger-like projections into the subjacent, newly formed bony tissue (→3). Within this ossified zone there may be islands of cartilaginous tissue that can become calcified. Osteochondromas may also contain adipose and fibrous tissue or foci of hematopoiesis. The structure of the cartilaginous component is the decisive factor in judging whether a tumor is an osteochondroma (benign tumor). These are the most common benign tumors of bone; however, when multiple osteochondromas are present, malignant change may occur in 10% of cases.

Enchondroma (Fig 13–27) is a neoplasm that is located centrally in the marrow spaces of a bone and is composed of mature hyaline cartilage. It probably represents a hamartoma of heterotopic nests of cartilage cells. Figure 13–27 shows a lobular formation of hyaline cartilage cells. These have rather uniform, round nuclei and are situated in lightly stained hollows. Some cells have two nuclei. The cells are irregularly distributed and lack mitoses. Sometimes there are degenerative changes in such tumors (pyknotic nuclei, mucinous degeneration, calcification). After hematoxylin-eosin staining the ground substance appears blue or pale red (acid mucopolysaccharide). The tumor is delimited by connective tissue or newly formed bone (→). The location of these tumors determines their behavior. Enchondromas of fingers and toes are benign, those in ribs or long bones can show malignant features, those in the pelvic bones almost always behave as malignant tumors.

Chondrosarcoma (Fig 13–28). Malignant tumors of cartilage can develop directly in orthotopic cartilage (primary chondrosarcoma) or in a benign tumor of cartilage (secondary chondrosarcoma). Most develop in the interior of a bone and retain their essentially cartilaginous character. Figure 13–28 shows lobulated, hyaline cartilaginous tissue in which there are irregularly distributed cartilage cells that are situated in clear spaces of varying size. The cells themselves vary in size and some have abnormally large, coarse, hyperchromatic nuclei (→). Multinucleated cells and giant cells are frequent and there may be abnormal mitoses. The matrix usually stains pale blue and may show areas of calcification or ossification. However, the tumor cells do not form osteoid. In contrast to osteosarcoma, chondrosarcoma grows relatively slowly and metastasizes late.

Osteoclastoma (Fig 13–29). Tumors of bone in which osteoclasts are the neoplastic cells are called osteoclastomas. They are to be distinguished from so-called brown tumors (see Fig 13–13). Osteoclastomas are considered semimalignant tumors, of questionable behavior, with a strong tendency to become malignant. In Figure 13–29 there are many multinucleated osteoclastic giant cells in a loose vascular stroma that also contains rather uniform spindle cells. The giant cells are relatively evenly distributed through the tumor. There is no osteoid, no bony or cartilaginous tissue. There can be hemorrhages, areas of necrosis, and foam cells in these tumors.

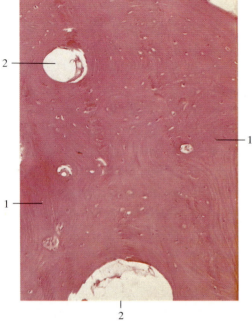

Fig 13–30.—Eburnating osteoma (hematoxylin-eosin; 63×).

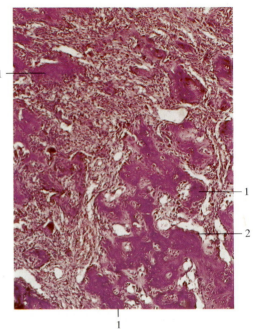

Fig 13–31.—Osteoid osteoma (hematoxylin-eosin; 80×).

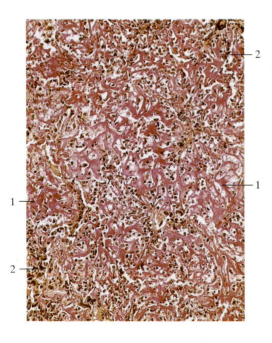

Fig 13–32.—Osteosarcoma (van Gieson's stain; 100×).

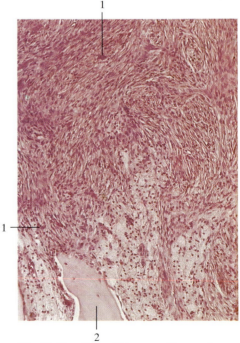

Fig 13–33.—Nonossifying osteofibroma (hematoxylin-eosin; 63×).

Osteoma (Fig 13–30). Osteoma is a circumscribed tumor of mature bony tissue that is formed either in periosteal connective tissue or by bone-forming cells in membranous bone. Osteomas are most frequently encountered in the skull, especially in the sinuses. If the tumor is composed of dense lamellar bone, it is an **eburnating osteoma;** if cancellous bone predominates, it is a **cancellous osteoma.** Figure 13–30 shows mature lamellar bone containing well-formed osteocytes (→1). The Haversian canals in the tumor (→2) are narrow and have smooth lining. This is an eburnating osteoma with a smooth external border. Roentgenograms of such tumors show circular shadows.

Osteoid osteoma (Fig 13–31). This is a benign tumor of bone occurring most frequently in short and long tubular bones. Radiographically it reveals itself by a less dense central area and a more dense periphery. Figure 13–31 shows the interior of the tumor to be an irregular mesh of osteoid trabeculae (→1) that are unevenly mineralized, of varying thickness, and partly covered with osteoblasts (→2). Between the trabeculae there is a vascular stroma with thin-walled capillaries and scattered plasma cells and lymphocytes. The inner portion of the tumor (the "nidus") is surrounded by sclerotic bone.

Osteosarcoma (Fig 13–32). This is a malignant neoplasm that displays the manifold potential of osteoblasts with respect to osteogenesis and osteolysis. Characteristically, these tumors are mosaics of sarcomatous stroma, cartilaginous foci, calcified tissue, mucinous material, osseous tumor, islets of giant cells, and neoplastic osteoid. The tumor osteoid is formed by sarcomatous connective tissue. Figure 13–32 shows polymorphic neoplastic tissue that has formed a network of thin and broader trabeculae of osteoid (→1) that are partly covered by dark-staining pleomorphic nuclei (→2). Between the osteoid structures there is a stroma, composed of spindle cells with pleomorphic nuclei and containing many capillaries. Elsewhere there may be foci of atypical cartilage. The neoplastic tissue has destroyed the original bony trabeculae. Some osteosarcomas contain many multinucleated giant cells. In *osteoplastic osteosarcoma* neoplastic osteoid and bone predominate; in *osteolytic osteosarcoma* giant cells with few nuclei, pleomorphic spindle cells, and blood vessels dominate the picture. Osteosarcoma occurs mainly in adolescents, near the knee joint, and has a bad prognosis.

Nonossifying osteofibroma of bone (Fig 13–33). This is a common benign tumor of bone that occurs in the metaphyses of long tubular bones in adolescents. Radiographically it is recognized by the presence of botryoid (grapelike) osteolysis surrounded by a dense border. This neoplasm is frequently discovered accidentally and its radiographic appearance is diagnostic. Figure 13–33 shows that the neoplastic tissue is composed of richly collagenous connective tissue that forms whorls and contains many elongated fibrocytes without mitoses. Relatively small giant cells (→1) and groups of foam cells are scattered through the tumor. The tissue is poor in blood vessels and has not formed bone. It is bordered by mature lamellar bone (→2).

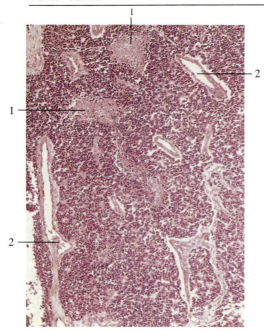

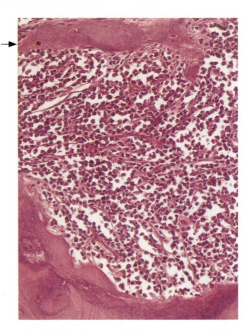

Fig 13–34.—Ewing's sarcoma (hematoxylin-eosin; 63×).

Fig 13–35.—Immunoblastic sarcoma (non-Hodgkin's lymphoma of bone) (hematoxylin-eosin; 100×).

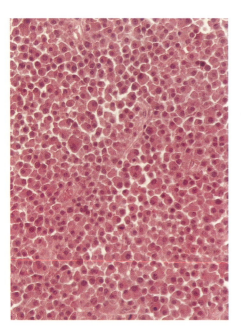

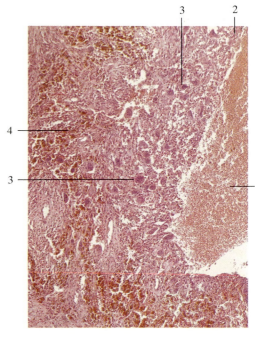

Fig 13–36.—Medullary plasmacytoma (hematoxylin-eosin; 180×).

Fig 13–37.—Aneurysmal bone cyst (hematoxylin-eosin; 63×).

Ewing's sarcoma (Fig 13–34). This is a highly malignant neoplasm of bone occurring in childhood and adolescence. It is said to originate in immature reticulum cells of bone and its diagnosis is often difficult because it possesses no pathognomonic structures. Figure 13–34 shows richly cellular neoplastic tissue containing small round cells and bands of necrosis (→1). Cells with pyknotic nuclei border the areas of necrosis. The tumor cells are best preserved around blood vessels, and the tissue has thereby acquired pseudorosettes (→2). The small, round, uniform tumor cells seem to possess almost no cytoplasm; but they are 2–3 times the size of lymphocytes. Occasionally one may encounter stellate cells with abundant cytoplasm that may produce a "starry sky" picture in sections. This tumor lacks intercellular matrix. The spherical nuclei have a loose chromatin structure and 1–2 dense nucleoli. Mitoses are rare. PAS-positive granules may be demonstrable in the cytoplasm. There is no intercellular reticulin. Clinically the tumor may mimic osteomyelitis.

Immunoblastic sarcoma (non-Hodgkin's lymphoma, Fig 13–35). This is a malignant tumor of bone which may be related to Ewing's sarcoma. It occurs mainly in the third through seventh decades. Figure 13–35 shows a rather uniform colony of polygonal cells that are larger than those in Ewing's sarcoma. Necrotic areas are usually lacking. Many tumor cells are connected by cytoplasmic processes and many are lined up on delicate reticulin fibers that have formed a network. The nuclei are indented and often vesicular. Mitoses occur frequently. The tumor cells are PAS-negative but may be associated with a reactive production of new bone (→).

Medullary plasmacytoma (Fig 13–36). This is the most frequent malignant tumor of bone and occurs either singly or multiply in bone marrow. It is characterized by proliferation of atypical (neoplastic) plasma cells. The blood plasma of affected individuals contains abnormally increased immunoglobulins (IgG, IgA, IgD, IgM, or, more rarely, IgE) which usually are monoclonal. Heavy and/or light chains are also secreted by plasmacytomas. The urine often contains Bence Jones protein (light chain protein), and hyalin droplets appear in the proximal tubular epithelial cells. Bone marrow smears reveal atypical plasma cells with eccentric nuclei, whose chromatin may resemble that of plasma cells. Multinucleated and giant tumor cells also occur. Plasmacytomas occur almost exclusively after age 50 and produce characteristic foci of osteolysis (e.g., in the calvarium). The prognosis is poor.

Aneurysmal bone cyst (Fig 13–37). This is a benign tumor-like lesion of bone that is composed of a focus of osteolysis within bone and an adjoining cystic part that resembles an aneurysm and is situated outside the bone. This lesion occurs in the second decade of life. Histologically (Fig 13–37) the focus of osteolysis consists of large cystic spaces that are lined by flat cells and filled with blood (→1). The walls of the cysts are composed of an inner layer of spindle cells (fibrocytes, fibroblasts:→2) and an outer layer containing numerous osteoclasts (→3). Outside of this there is loose connective tissue containing many capillaries, some lymphocytes and plasma cells, and hemosiderin-laden macrophages (→4).

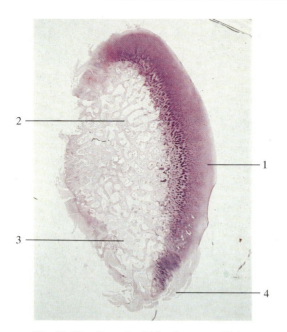

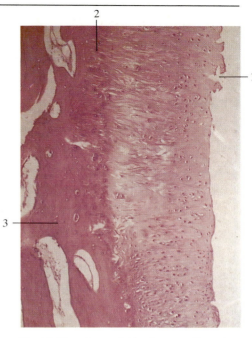

Fig 13–38.—Osteochondritis dissecans (''joint mouse'') (hematoxylin-eosin; 8 ×).

Fig 13–39.—Osteoarthritis (hematoxylin-eosin; 63 ×).

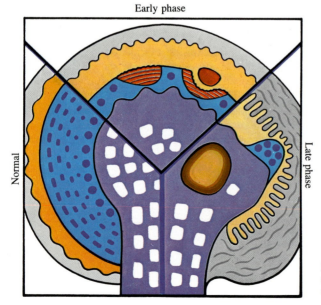

Early phase

Normal

Late phase

Results of chronic changes in joints in arthritis deformans
1. Normal joint
2. Early phase:
   fibrillation of joint cartilage, osteochondritis dissecans, and subchondral spongiosa hypertrophy
3. Late phase:
   hyperplastic fibrosis of joint capsule, subchondral involuted cysts, and capsular regeneration

Fig 13–40.—Development of the bony changes resulting from degenerative injury of the joint cartilage.

Degenerative Joint Diseases

Osteochondritis dissecans (Fig 13–38). In this condition there is circumscribed sub-chondral osteonecrosis. It usually occurs in large joints of adolescents and can cause considerable reduction in the function of an affected joint. Local trauma and diminished vascular perfusion are among the causative factors. A convex segment of the joint (e.g., hip joint, knee joint) becomes necrotic and is set free, forming a "joint mouse." This leads to an **arthrosis** that limits the motion of the joint. Figure 13–38 shows a bone fragment that is covered by cartilage ($\rightarrow$1). The subchondral bony tissue is avascular and necrotic ($\rightarrow$2). The marrow between the osteocyte-free bony trabeculae is also necrotic and has formed detritus ($\rightarrow$3). Part of the joint capsule (necrotic connective tissue) can be seen at $\rightarrow$4.

Degenerative joint disease or osteoarthritis (Fig 13–39). This is a common degenerative disease of joints in which primary lesions develop in cartilages of joints. These are followed by secondary reactive changes and deformities of joints. Metabolic (chemical) changes in joint cartilage as well as wear and tear are thought to be causes of the primary lesions. The secondary lesions are due to several sorts of damage in joint cartilage. Figure 13–39 shows a fissured cartilaginous joint surface in which collagenous fibrils have become "unmasked." The surface shows some clefts ($\rightarrow$1) that are probably due to friction. At $\rightarrow$2 groups of ballooned chondrocytes are situated between zones of degeneration and necrosis. The necrotic cartilage is removed after capillaries have grown into it. The bone underneath the cartilage shows osteosclerotic thickening ($\rightarrow$3). The neighboring marrow contains collagenous fibrous tissue. The trabecular bone may develop microscopic fractures that give rise to cystic spaces. The ultimate result is the development of nodular irregularities of the joint surface, narrowing of the joint space, and an irregular periarticular osteosclerosis.

The development of **degenerative joint disease** (osteoarthritis) is depicted schematically in Figure 13–40. In the earliest stage there is mucoid degeneration of joint cartilage. This is followed by the unmasking of collagen fibrils in the cartilage. At first the chondrocytes are preserved, but later they also perish and the lesion is then described as **fibrillation of cartilage.** This occurs most commonly in costochondral cartilage. Acellular cysts develop in such cartilage and may be invaded by granulation tissue that later becomes ossified. Destruction of cartilaginous tissue weakens hyaline joint cartilage and diminishes its resistance to shearing forces. These forces are then more readily transmitted to the underlying bone, which protects itself by a reactive subchondral osteosclerosis. The latter process may virtually transform spongiosa into compact bone. Marginal hyaline cartilage that bears less weight develops regions of cell proliferation with ossified centers. This in turn results in characteristic bulging joint deformities. The joint capsule also becomes thickened by fibrous tissue and increasingly rigid. The secondary changes in osteoarthritis greatly reduce joint motion, but the joint space is not obliterated.

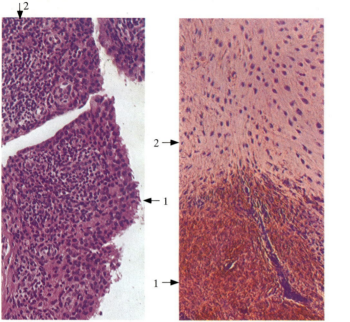

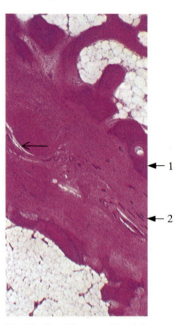

Fig 13–41.—Rheumatoid arthritis (inflammation of the joint capsule) (hematoxylin-eosin; 200×).

Fig 13–42.—Rheumatoid arthritis (destruction of cartilage by granulation tissue) (hematoxylin-eosin; 300×).

Fig 13–43.—Rheumatoid arthritis (fibrous ankylosis in a finger joint)(hematoxylin-eosin; 100×).

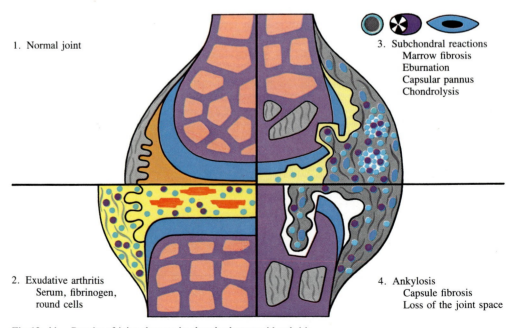

1. Normal joint

3. Subchondral reactions
   Marrow fibrosis
   Eburnation
   Capsular pannus
   Chondrolysis

2. Exudative arthritis
   Serum, fibrinogen,
   round cells

4. Ankylosis
   Capsule fibrosis
   Loss of the joint space

Fig 13–44.—Results of joint changes in chronic rheumatoid arthritis.

Inflammatory Diseases of Joints

In **rheumatic fever** there are genuine Aschoff bodies in the loose connective tissue of affected joint capsules, particularly in large joints and principally in children and adolescents (see also Figures 1–28, 1–29, and 1–30).

Ankylosing spondylitis (Marie-Strümpell's disease) begins with slight inflammation in which lymphocytes infiltrate capsules and ligaments of the small vertebral joints. Later there is deposition of new bone that causes ankylosis in the vertebral column.

Rheumatoid arthritis is associated with variable chronic inflammation (Figs 13–41 through 13–43). Small joints (fingers, toes) are most frequently involved. Severe destructive changes lead to ankylosis and fixation of joints.

The disease begins in the joint capsule and secondarily involves the articular cartilage and subchondral bone. There may be several causes, either infectious or noninfectious. In the course of the disease, which may involve large as well as small joints, lesions develop in the joints that resemble those associated with rheumatic fever. **Rheumatoid arthritis** is a *collective term* that is based on morphologically similar lesions in joints and does not necessarily imply a common etiology (Fig 13–44). As shown in Fig 13–41, the disease begins with inflammation of the joint capsule. An exudate forms in the joint, consisting of blood plasma and cells (granulocytes with cytoplasmic inclusions that contain rheumatoid factor, synovial cells, lymphocytes, plasma cells). Synovial cells lining the joint capsule are focally destroyed and replaced by fibrin. Elsewhere there is proliferation of synovial cells (→1 in Fig 13–41). The synovial connective tissue contains packed infiltrates of plasma cells and lymphocytes (→2 in Fig 13–41) that may form small follicles. There is also focal fibrinoid necrosis.

Figure 13–42 depicts replacement of cartilage (→2) by highly vascular granulation tissue (→1) that has grown in from the synovia and from the marrow. Thus the articular cartilage is attacked from two sides: through the joint space, by a fibrous and vascular **pannus,** and from the bone marrow by other granulation tissue. The result is destruction of the cartilage.

Figure 13–43 shows the final stage of rheumatoid arthritis, **fibrous ankylosis.** Bone subjacent to the articular cartilage is preserved (→1), but only a few remnants of the cartilage remain and these show degenerative changes (→2). The joint space is obliterated by pannus (visible on roentgenograms). In this way (as well as in others) rheumatoid arthritis differs from osteoarthritis. Figure 13–43 shows that the two articular (cartilaginous) joint surfaces are bound together by collagenous tissue (→2).

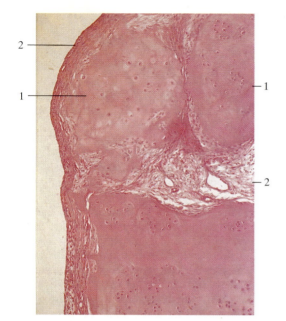

Fig 13–45.—Chondromatosis of joint (hematoxy-lin-eosin; 63 ×).

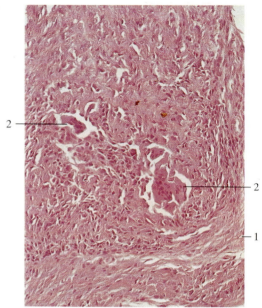

Fig 13–46.—Benign giant cell tumor of synovia (hematoxylin-eosin; 100 ×).

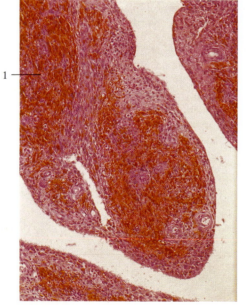

Fig 13–47.—Pigmented villonodular synovitis (hematoxylin-eosin; 80 ×).

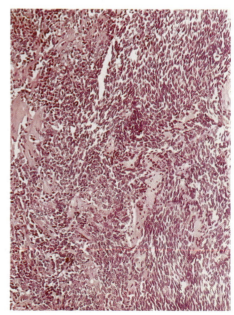

Fig 13–48.—Synovial sarcoma (hematoxylin-eosin; 50 ×).

Tumors of Joints

Chondromatosis of joint (Fig 13–45). This is a benign, tumor-like change in the peri-articular tissue, manifested by metaplastic development of cartilaginous or bony foci in synovia. Occasionally, such changes occur in a tendon sheath or a bursa. The knee joint is involved in more than 50% of cases. Detached bits of cartilage are moving more or less freely in the joint space. Figure 13–45 shows a thickened joint capsule containing relatively large nodules of varying size, composed of proliferating cartilage (→1). Connective tissue surrounds these bodies (→2). They contain ballooned chondrocytes with plump nuclei. There is some calcification; sometimes the cartilage turns into bone.

Benign giant cell tumor of tendon sheath (Fig 13–46). This is a slow-growing prolif-eration of histiocytic cells with accompanying production of collagen and has been classi-fied among the fibrous histiocytomas. This growth can occur in the capsule of the knee joint *(localized nodular synovitis),* but it occurs more frequently in tendon sheaths of fin-gers and toes. Figure 13–46 shows a nodule that is closely apposed to a tendon (→1). The tumor consists of loose connective tissue containing many fibroblasts and histiocytes. Col-lections of foam cells are also frequently found. Note that multinucleated giant cells (→2) are contained within the tumor; these have the appearance of foreign body giant cells. This benign tumor differs from giant cell tumors of bones (Fig 13–29); it has no tendency to become malignant. A bone that adjoins a tendon with this tumor may show an erosion on x-ray films.

Pigmented villonodular synovitis (Fig 13–47). This denotes a diffuse proliferation of synovial epithelium and connective tissue, together with the development of brown villi and nodules. The lesion represents a benign neoplastic counterpart of synovial sarcoma. Figure 13–47 shows broad villi that are covered by flat synovial epithelium. The villi have a loose connective tissue stroma in which there are thin-walled blood vessels. The stroma contains lymphocytes, plasma cells, and macrophages. Many of the latter contain brown hemosiderin pigment (→1), which also can be seen in synovial epithelial cells. Scattered in this tissue are numerous xanthomatous cells that are recognized by their light cytoplasm. Sometimes these lesions also contain giant cells and hyalinized regions.

Synovial sarcoma (Fig 13–48) is virtually the only true primary malignant neoplasm of joints, but it is highly malignant. It usually develops in periarticular tissue and it can invade synovia. On the other hand, it can also arise in a tendon sheath or bursa. It occurs mainly in young adults, and its principal location is the knee joint. It is a highly cellular tumor that is composed of two types of tissue. One component consists of glandlike structures lined by polygonal or cylindrical quasi-epithelial cells, arranged around clefts. These struc-tures suggest adenocarcinoma. The other component is fibrosarcomatous. In Figure 13–48 there are many spindle cells with elongated, dark nuclei and with numerous mitotic figures. Between these cells there is collagen and reticulin. One or the other tissue component can predominate in a synovial sarcoma, making it difficult to distinguish this tumor from fibro-sarcoma, immunoblastic sarcoma, or even from adenocarcinoma.

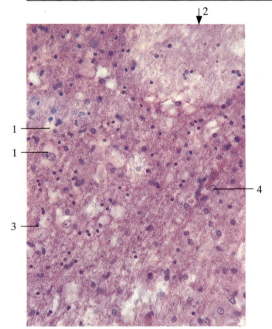

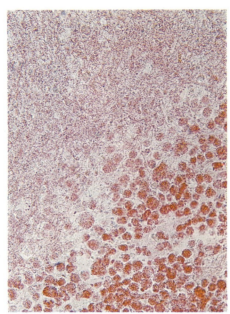

Fig 14–1.—Focal area of recent encephalomalacia or softening of the brain; pallid area (honeycomb area) (hematoxylin-eosin; 248 ×).

Fig 14–2.—Center of an area of encephalomalacia with granular, fat-containing phagocytic cells (gitter cells or compound granular corpuscles) (Sudan stain; 250 ×).

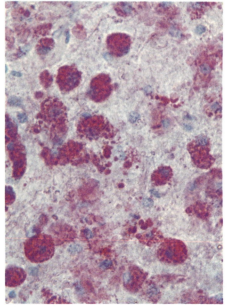

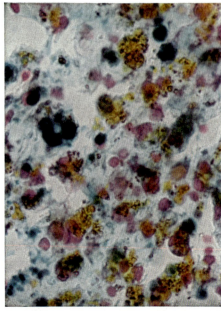

Fig 14–3.—Granular fatty cells (scarlet red–hematoxylin; 512 ×).

Fig 14–4.—Iron-containing phagocytic cells (pigmented granular cells) in encephalomalacia (Prussian blue reaction; 800 ×).

14. Brain—Spinal Cord

Histologic examination of the brain and spinal cord should start with an investigation of the condition of the meninges (cellularity, vascular changes, unusual deposits). The substance of the brain and spinal cord is composed of *neurons with their cytoplasmic processes* (dendrites and axis cylinders or axons surrounded by a myelin sheath—special stains must be used to demonstrate them), *neuroglia* (*astrocytes* with relatively large round nuclei and cytoplasm which is seen well only with special stains, *oligodendroglia* with small round nuclei, and *microglia* with small fusiform nuclei), and *blood vessels*. Both the intact and injured portions of the tissue must be examined (e.g., areas of softening, foci, or demyelinization). Perivascular or tissue infiltrates and the types of cells that compose them should be noted.

Encephalomalacia

This is due to **necrosis** of the brain substance followed by *liquefaction* and *secondary cavitation* (cyst formation) resulting either from occlusion of a nutrient artery (arteriosclerosis, thrombosis, embolization) or from generalized hypoxia. The process has several stages. 1. The stage of *cortical pallor* with ischemic changes in the neurons (shrinkage of both the cell body and nucleus with loss of Nissl substance). There may also be interstitial edema with fiber and nuclear degeneration (so-called honeycomb appearance) and, finally, complete *necrosis* with loss of nuclei. 2. The stage of *softening with granular fatty cells*, also called gitter cells or compound granular corpuscles (stage of resorption). 3. The stage of *cyst formation and glial scarring* (end stage).

Figure 14–1, which shows **focal, recent brain softening,** will serve as an example of the *first stage* (cortical pallor). There is conspicuous edema between fibers and focally around cells (→1), and degeneration of the myelin sheaths, resulting in their complete dissolution (→2). The oligodendrocytes have a shrunken appearance (→3). The nuclei of the macroglia stain weakly (beginning of karyolysis,→4). In the upper portion of the picture (→2) there is a pale red focus in which the process is further advanced. Nuclei are almost totally lacking, the myelin sheaths dissolved.

Macroscopic: The brain tissue is of slightly soft consistency, and the gray substance is pallid.

The *second stage* (stage of *focal softening*) is characterized by resorption of the destroyed myelin substance (lipids). Figure 14–2 shows the center of an area of **brain softening.** Even with the unaided eye, fat stains show a red lesion that stains with Sudan, as well as a loosening of the tissues, which is discernible in the bluish red brain substance. Examination of the lesion with medium high power reveals numerous round cells, the cytoplasm of which is filled with red sudanophilic granules. High power clearly shows (Fig 14–3) these **granular fatty cells** with their eccentrically located nuclei (they are either phagocytic microglial cells or macrophages that have come in via blood vessels). In paraffin sections, the fat droplets are dissolved and the cytoplasm has a vacuolated appearance. In many cases, bleeding into the tissues has occurred in addition to the softening (*hemorrhagic softening*, frequently seen with emboli). The extravasated erythrocytes and hemoglobin are also taken up by phagocytes and broken down to hemosiderin. Such phagocytic cells are called **pigmented granular cells** (Fig 14–4), since the cytoplasm contains brown hemosiderin granules (iron-reaction positive). In addition, granular fatty cells as well as extracellular deposits of brown pigment can be seen (*hematoidin* = bilirubin).

Macroscopic: There is softening and liquefaction of brain tissue. In cases of hemorrhagic softening, there are punctate hemorrhages which show a brown discoloration when the lesion is a little older. In unstained fresh microscopic preparations, numerous granular fatty cells may be seen (granular cytoplasm with glassy granules).

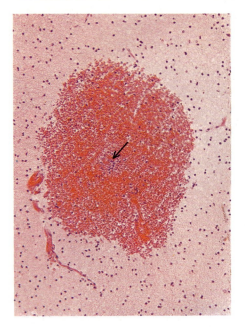

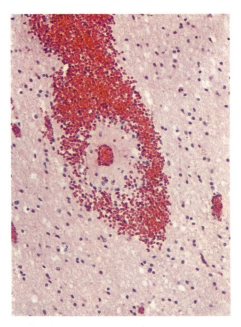

Fig 14–5.—Ball hemorrhage of the brain (hematoxylin-eosin; 120 ×).

Fig 14–6.—Ring hemorrhage of the brain (hematoxylin-eosin; 175 ×).

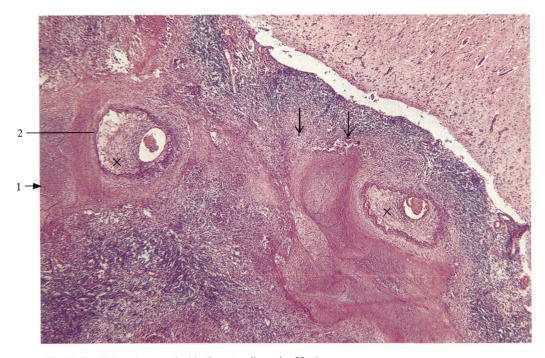

Fig 14–7.—Tuberculous meningitis (hematoxylin-eosin; 33 ×).

Ball and ring hemorrhages of the brain (Figs 14–5, 14–6). *These hemorrhages are due to circulatory disturbances accompanied by necrosis of the vessel wall. Ball hemorrhages* are spherical lesions composed of compactly arranged extravasated erythrocytes, in the center of which can be seen a venule with a necrotic wall (→in Fig 14–5). In **ring hemorrhages** the center of the lesion is occupied by a vessel that is completely plugged with erythrocytes. This is surrounded by a ring of necrotic brain tissue (in this case, homogeneous myelin sheaths and an occasional cell with an intact nucleus). The outer zone consists of a ring of erythrocytes.

Macroscopic: Punctate hemorrhages, which cannot be wiped away, are present on the cut surfaces of the brain. They are common in hypertension, air embolism, sun stroke, and hemorrhagic encephalitis.

Tuberculous meningitis (Fig 14–7). *Tuberculous inflammation of the meninges is hematogenous in origin, affects the base of the brain, and occurs chiefly in children.* In the acute exudative stage there is a rich fibrinous and protein-rich exudate containing polymorphonuclear leukocytes that is especially prominent around blood vessels. Caseation sets in rapidly in the vicinity of the vessels. Figure 14–7 shows the perivascular necrosis and network of fibrin (→1) and the dense cellular infiltration (mainly lymphocytes) of the neighboring tissues. In some areas, the necrosis is already delineated by epithelioid cells. Solitary Langhans' giant cells (→within the picture) are also seen *(subacute proliferative stage)*. Of great importance is the fact that the caseation also affects arteries, causing partial or complete necrosis of the vessel walls (→2). In addition, if the caseation involves the adventitia, an arteritis develops, which, by a process of inward extension, causes marked endarteritis obliterans (×) with intimal proliferation and marked reduction of the lumen. For this reason, secondary foci of encephalomalacia may be seen in the healing stages of tuberculous meningitis. Thus it is especially important to diagnose tuberculous meningitis early. Caution: since it is rare today, typical cases may not be diagnosed.

Macroscopic: Acute: gray granular exudate covers the base of the brain. *Subacute to chronic:* small yellow or grayish white, translucent nodules. In the *end stage*, there is collagenization with grayish white thickening of the meninges.

Purulent meningitis (Fig 14–8). *This inflammation of the leptomeninges arises either from blood-borne infection, from direct spread from suppurative infection of adjacent tissues, or from penetrating wounds.* Microscopic examination with low power reveals a dense cellular exudate in the leptomeninges. Higher magnification shows that the exudate consists of densely packed polymorphonuclear leukocytes intermingled with fibrin strands. Frequently, the inflammation extends into the cortex (→) along blood vessels (meningoencephalitis).

Macroscopic: Sheets of yellow or yellow-green pus cover the gyri underneath the pia meater.

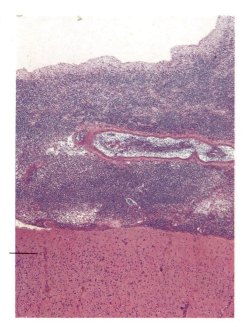

Fig 14–8.—Purulent meningitis (hematoxylin-eosin; 38×).

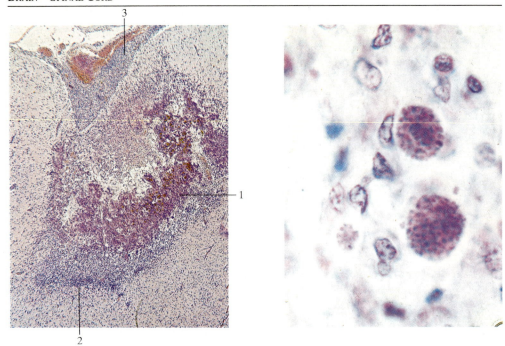

Fig 14–9.—Encephalitis caused by toxoplasmosis (hematoxylin-eosin; 10×).

Fig 14–10.—Pseudocysts of toxoplasmosis in the brain (thionine stain; 1,400×).

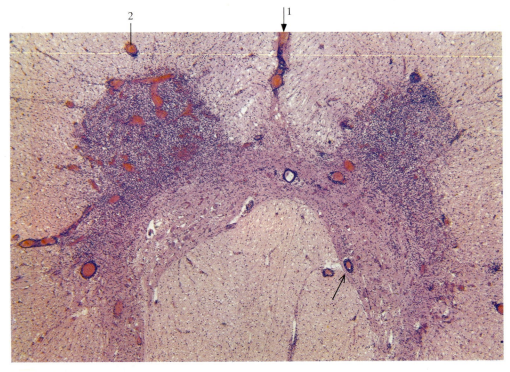

Fig 14–11.—Poliomyelitis (hematoxylin-eosin; 51×).

Encephalitis in toxoplasmosis (Fig 14–9). *This is a granulomatous, necrotizing, and calcifying encephalitis in neonates, caused by* Toxoplasma gondii *(a protozoon)* following infection after the third month of gestation. Examination of the specimen with a scanning lens discloses conspicuous cellular nodules and blue-stained calcified foci in the cortex and white matter. Sometimes there are larger necrotic lesions. Closer inspection shows that the cellular nodules are granulomas consisting of lymphocytes, plasma cells, histiocytes, and glial cells. Figure 14–9 shows such a cortical lesion with a calcified central zone of necrosis (stained violet blue,→1) surrounded by a cellular infiltrate (→2), consisting largely of lymphocytes and histiocytes. The pia-arachnoid (→3) is also infiltrated by lymphocytes.

With oil immersion, **pseudocysts** can often be seen in the granulomas (Fig 14–10) consisting of intracellular colonies of the causative organisms. The infected cells are round and the cytoplasm is filled with bow-shaped toxoplasma containing small, oval inner bodies. There are histiocytes in the surrounding tissues. Toxoplasmosis in adults causes lymphadenopathy with small foci of epitheloid cells (see Forms of Lymph Node Reactions, chap. 11).

Macroscopic: Brown or yellow nodular lesions are seen on the cut surface of the brain.

Poliomyelitis (Figs 14–11, 14–12). *This viral infection affects the motor neurons of the anterior horn of the spinal cord, causing cell destruction and resorption.* Examination of the section with the scanning lens shows dense cellular infiltration of the anterior horns. At the bottom of Figure 14–11 is the anterior median fissure in which may be seen the lymphocytic infiltration of the leptomeninges (→1). The central canal is clearly visible. Dilated vessels (→) in the white matter are also surrounded by cuffs of round cells (→2). The posterior horns are uninvolved.

Under **higher magnification** (Fig 14–12), granulocytes and proliferated glial cells are seen to have replaced the phagocytosed necrotic cells *(neuronophagia)*. In places, the shadowy outlines of nerve cells may be seen in the middle of the exudate (→1: spared neuron;→2:shrunken neuron).

Macroscopic: The anterior horns are indistinct.

Typhus encephalitis (Fig 14–13). *This results from systemic infection with* Rickettsia prowazekii *and is characterized by a nodular form of panencephalitis.* The section shows the olive of the medulla oblongata with two cellular nodules of proliferating microglial cells. These glial cell nodules are situated perivascularly (reaction to rickettsial toxin). The neurons are unchanged. The nodules are not specific for typhus and may occur in other sorts of encephalitis.

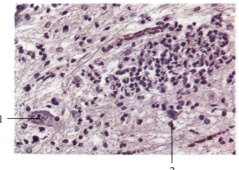

Fig 14–12.—Poliomyelitis (hematoxylin-eosin; 227×).

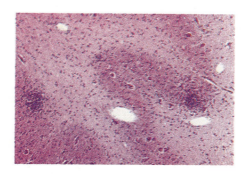

Fig 14–13.—Typhus encephalitis (hematoxylin-eosin; 60×).

313

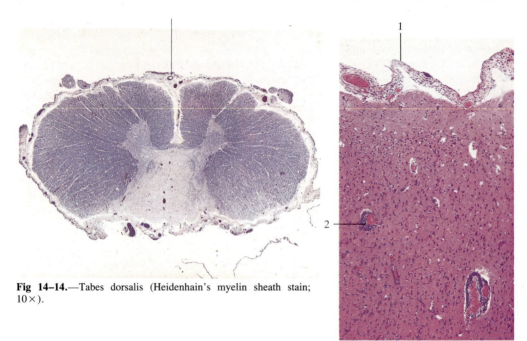

Fig 14–14.—Tabes dorsalis (Heidenhain's myelin sheath stain; 10×).

Fig 14–15.—General paresis (hematoxylin-eosin; 60×).

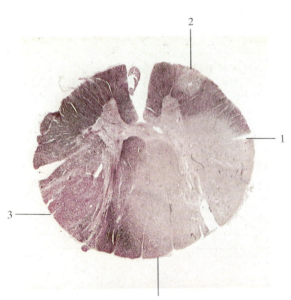

Fig 14–16.—Multiple sclerosis (Sudan stain; 5×).

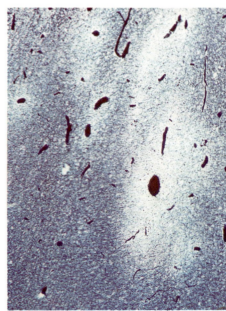

Fig 14–17.—Multiple sclerosis (myelin stain; 60×).

Tabes dorsalis (Fig 14–4). *In the tertiary stage of syphilis, a chronic, slowly progressive meningitis may develop, with injury of the dorsal roots of the spinal cord and secondary degeneration of posterior columns.* The histologic appearance in sections stained for myelin is very typical. With the histologic section oriented according to the deeply indented anterior longitudinal fissure (→), the lack of myelin stain in the region of the posterior columns and dorsal roots is immediately apparent. The gray matter (neurons and unmyelinated fibers of the anterior gray horns) is of almost identical hue. Under higher magnification, individual preserved myelin sheaths or sheaths with clumped degenerated myelin may still be recognized. In the florid stages, sections stained for fat show tissue disintegration and granular fatty cells. The leptomeninges are fibrotic and thickened and infiltrated by lymphocytes.

Macroscopic: The leptomeninges are opaque, especially in the thoracic region, and the spinal cord is shrunken and the posterior columns are discolored gray.

General paresis, also called paralysis of the insane or dementia paralytica (Fig 14–15). This is a *chronic syphilitic encephalitis with frontal lobe atrophy and deposits of iron in the brain tissue.* In contrast to *syphilitic meningoencephalitis,* in which there is a predilection for the *base* of the brain with secondary progression of the inflammation along vascular channels to the cortex, *paresis* affects primarily the *frontal lobes* (insular cortex and temporal lobes) and encephalitis is more marked than is meningitis. The leptomeninges (→1) are thickened by fibrosis and sparsely infiltrated by lymphocytes and plasma cells. The most conspicuous feature is in the cortex, where the adventitia of the small vessels is infiltrated by lymphocytes and plasma cells (→2) which, even under low-power magnification, may be seen as bluish cuffs. In addition, there is a diffuse increase of microglial cells which contain cytoplasmic hemosiderin, as do the macrophages derived from the perivascular tissues.

Macroscopic: Atrophy of the convolutions of the frontal lobe with opaque, thickened leptomeninges.

Multiple sclerosis (Figs 14–16, 14–17). *A chronic, progressive, focally disseminated, demyelinating disease of the brain and spinal cord of unknown etiology.* Myelin stain or Sudan stain (Fig 14–17) demonstrates the demyelinated lesions clearly. A cross section of the spinal cord shows a well-demarcated, pale round lesion located mostly in the vicinity of the dorsal roots (between→ 1in Fig 14–16). However, there are isolated smaller lesions (→ 2) that are not restricted to anatomically distinct fiber tracts (compare this to the picture of tabes dorsalis, Fig 14–14). The spreading of the demyelinating process has been compared to an ink stain on a blotter. An early stage may also be seen in Figure 14–16, in which there is resorption of the myelin substance by granular fatty cells (→3). Even under low power, the light red stain of the neutral fats stored in macrophages is conspicuous, and under higher power these prove to be typical granular fatty cells (see Fig 14–3).

The **myelin stain** (Fig 14–17) shows that the demyelinating process proceeds from the vessels but nevertheless does not correspond to the area of distribution of the vessel. Axons are preserved. A glial scar forms secondarily, consisting of a network of glial fiber and slightly increased numbers of glial cells (sclerosis). The myelin stain colors the erythrocytes in the vessels a deep blue.

Macroscopic: Old lesions appear gray, more recent lesions are salmon colored. *Pathogenesis:* It is now thought to be either a virus infection (slow virus) or an aggressive disease (IgG increased in spinal fluid). Slow virus = viral infection of long duration; occurs in sheep in England, called "scrapie" disease (chronic pruritus). Natives in New Guinea with the slow virus disease, Kuru, show a paralysis agitans.

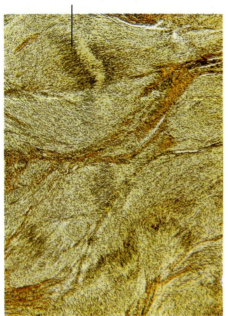

Fig 14–18.—Neurinoma (van Gieson's stain; 47×).

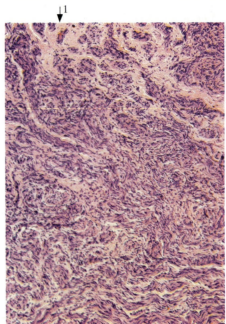

Fig 14–19.—Neurofibroma (hematoxylin-eosin; 90×).

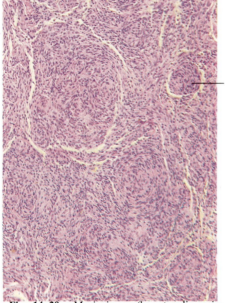

Fig 14–20.—Meningioma (hematoxylin-eosin; 180×).

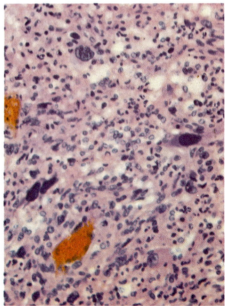

Fig 14–21.—Glioblastoma multiforme (hematoxylin-eosin; 190×).

Tumors of Nerve Tissues

The **neurinomas** (Fig 14–8) present a typical histologic picture, even when examined only at low magnification. There are densely packed spindle-shaped cells and fibers arranged in wide bands. The nuclei are pointed and have an orderly, rhythmic arrangement (so-called palisading of the nuclei:→). Medium magnification of a van Gieson preparation reveals the yellow, drawn-out cytoplasm of the cells which form a syncytium. These cells are derived from the Schwann cells of the nerve sheath ("schwannoma").

Macroscopic: Round, discrete tumors, e.g., in the pontine-cerebellar angle.

Neurofibromas (Fig 14–19) may be solitary or multiple and sometimes are generalized (as part of *von Recklinghausen's neurofibromatosis*). It is only the large amount of collagenous fibrous tissue that distinguishes them from the neurinomas. The tumors are essentially composed of proliferated Schwann cells. The bundles of nerve fibers (yellow with van Gieson's stain) are divided and pressed apart by the proliferating connective tissue (→ 1: red with van Gieson's stain). Figure 14–22 shows a so-called **amputation neuroma** i.e., a club-shaped proliferation of nerve fibers and connective tissue following injury or severance of a nerve. Such a lesion is probably not a true neoplastic condition; rather, it appears to be compensatory regeneration.

Meningioma (Fig 14–20). *Grossly, most meningiomas are spherical tumors situated on the dura and compressing the brain. They derive from the arachnoid fibroblast.* The typical structures can be best located under low magnification. There are spindle-shaped cells in an onion-skin arrangement (→), in the center of which there are hyaline or calcified nodules (necrotic cells) arranged concentrically–the so-called *dural psammoma body*. Scattered between these foci are solid portions containing great numbers of ovoid cells surrounded by collagenous fibrous tissue. Should proliferation of connective tissue predominate, the tumor will resemble a fibroma histologically.

Glioblastoma multiforme (Fig 14–21). The glioblastoma multiforme is the most common malignant brain tumor of adults. Histologically, the tumor is highly cellular with focal areas of necrosis and hemorrhage and has invaded normal brain. A prominent feature is the marked variation of the cells, which have pleomorphic cytoplasm and bizarre, hyperchromatic and pleomorphic nuclei, and frequently are arranged in perivascular fashion. Scattered throughout the tissue there are small round cells. It is not possible to identify any of these cells specifically as either glial cells or astrocytes.

Macroscopic: Variegated cut surface with a mixture of red hemorrhagic portions, yellow areas of necrosis, and gray tumor tissue. Frequently, the surrounding brain tissue is edematous (yellowish gray, gelatinous).

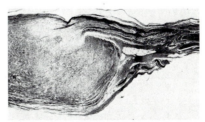

Fig 14–22.—Club-shaped amputation neuroma of a nerve *(right)* (myelin stain; 10×).

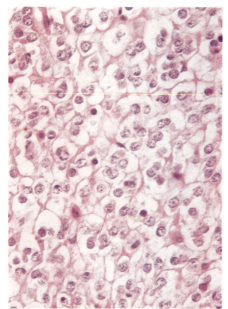

Fig 14–23.—Oligodendroglioma (hematoxylin-eosin; 320×).

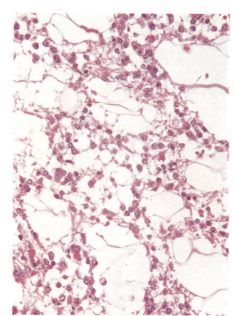

Fig 14–24.—Fibrillary astrocytoma (hematoxylin-eosin; 180×).

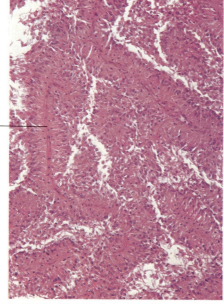

Fig 14–25.—Ependymoma (van Gieson's stain; 180×).

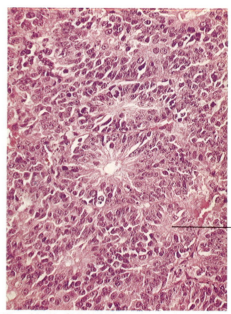

Fig 14–26.—Medulloblastoma (hematoxylin-eosin; 150×).

Oligodendroglioma (Fig 14–23). This is a slowly growing brain tumor which occurs chiefly in the cerebrum. The figure shows that it is composed of relatively uniform cells having round nuclei with compact chromatin structure and optically empty cytoplasm. The cell borders are distinct and resemble those of plants (compare hypernephroma of the kidney). The tumor is poor in blood vessels. Capillaries in the neighborhood of the tumor are frequently calcified (x-ray!)

Mostly 30–50 year olds. Male-female ratio, 3:7.

Fibrillary astrocytoma (Fig 14–24). In adults it occurs in the cerebrum; in children, in the cerebellum or pons. It has an invasive growth pattern and macroscopically is poorly demarcated. There are two types (1) Protoplasmic astrocytoma with plump astrocytes, i.e., large round cells with homogeneous, eosinophilic cytoplasm and eccentrically situated nuclei. These occur only in the cerebrum. (2) Fibrillary astrocytoma (Fig 14–24) composed of bipolar fibrillary astrocytes with round, only moderately polymorphic nuclei. The fibrillary processes of the cells intermingle, forming a loose network. Male-female ratio, 3:2.

Ependymoma (Fig 14–25). Ependymomas arise from the ependymal cells in the ventricles and accordingly occur in the region of the cerebral ventricles (30% of cases, especially young persons), the fourth ventricle (45% of cases), or in the spinal cord (25% of cases). They grow expansively and also into the ventricle and frequently recur. Histologically they have a rosette-like pattern: at the center there is a capillary (→) to the adventitia of which is attached the stretched-out cytoplasm of the ependymal cells. The nuclei lie in the periphery at the opposite end of the cells, thus forming a nucleus-free zone around the central blood vessel.

Medulloblastoma (Fig 14–26). This is the most common brain tumor in childhood (6-14 years) and arises in the cerebellar vermis or cerebellar hemispheres. It is an embryonal tumor and in this respect is similar to embryonal renal tumors. Histologically there are oval, carrot-shaped nuclei which often form pseudorosettes (→) or show a palisade arrangement. If the tumor grows in the fourth ventricle, obstructive hydrocephalus may develop. Metastases may occur within the ventricular system or diffusely in the leptomeninges.

Spongioblastoma also occurs at a young age, especially in girls. These tumors occur in the optic nerves, pons, cerebellum, or hypothalamus. Elongated tumor cells are arranged in fibrous tufts or whorls and produce an abundance of glial fibers. Mostly the tumors are well defined but because of their deep location are difficult to approach surgically.

Brain tumors occupy a special position among malignant tumors because they do not metastasize outside the brain and cerebral symptoms predominate (no cachexia). The commonest intracranial tumor is meningioma (15%–20% of all brain tumors); then follow glioblastoma multiforme with 12%, oligodendroglioma, spongioblastoma, and astrocytoma with 6%–8%, and ependymoma and medulloblastoma with 4%.

Fig 15–1.—Outline of important deep mycoses.*

MORPHOLOGY	MYCOSIS	FUNGUS	TISSUE REACTION	FUNGUS IN TISSUE	SIZE
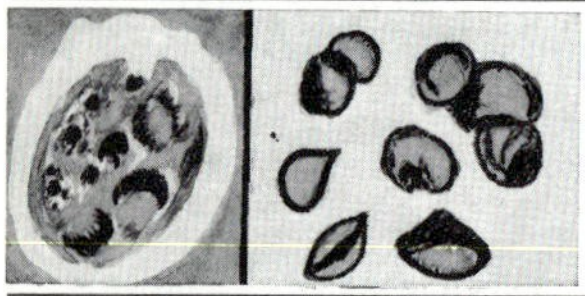	Pneumocy-tosis†	*Pneumocystis carinii*	Interstitial plasma, cell infiltrate; lung; occasionally extrapulmonary	Grocott: round, small Giemsa: cysts with internal bodies	3–4 μm C5–12 μm 10.1–2 μm
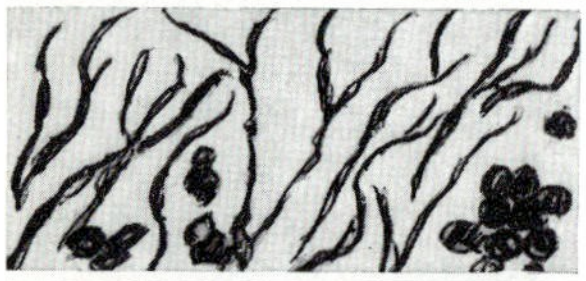	Candidiasis	*Candida albicans, tropicalis,* etc.	Nonspecific granulation tissue	Hyphae and small yeast cells	2–4 μm
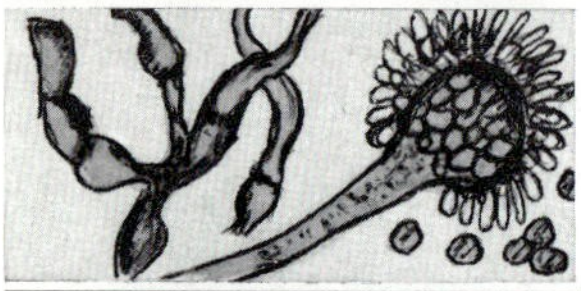	Aspergillosis	*Aspergillus fumigatus*	Nonspecific; usually granulomas with eosinophils and giant cells	Septated hyphae, conidia "fruiting bodies"	Variable
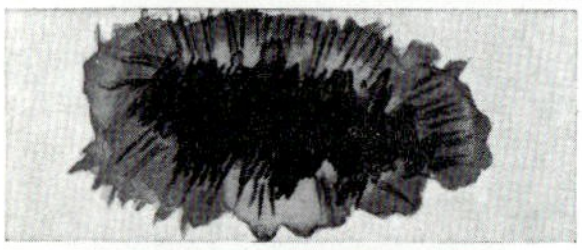	Actinomy-cosis‡	Actinomyces (not a fungus)	Abscesses with foam cells Yellow color Fistulas	Thick bacterial masses; peripherally radiating processes	Variable
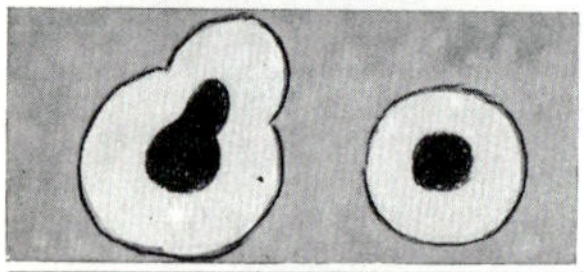	Cryptococ-cosis	*Cryptococcus neoformans*	Increase in histiocytes, granulomas	Thickwalled: solitary buds	4–20 μm
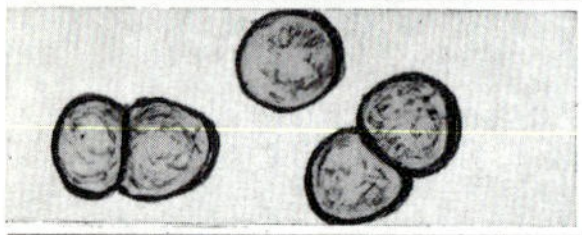	Chromo-mycosis§	*Hormodendrum* and *Phialophora*	Microabscesses and granulomas of the skin	Brown round septated fungal cells	5–12 μm
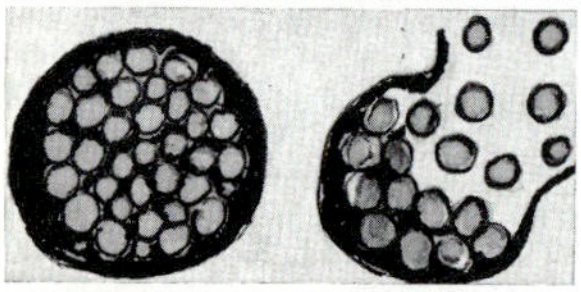	Coccidio-idomycosis	*Coccidioides immitis*	Abscesses, granulomas	Large cysts, endospores	30–60 μm
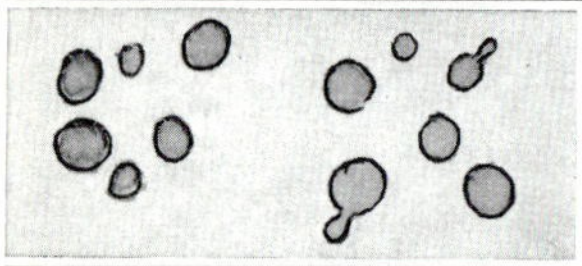	Histoplas-mosis	*Histoplasma capsulatum*	Proliferation of histiocytic tuberculoid granulomas, calcification	Small round yeast-like fungal cells; intracellular solitary buds	2–5 μm
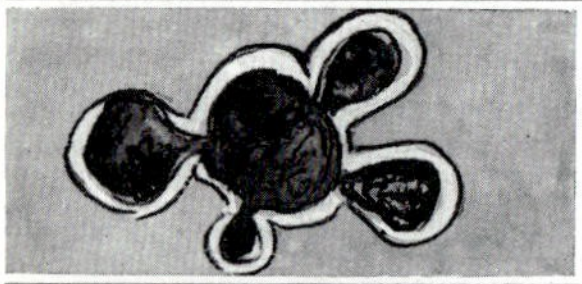	Paracoccid-ioidomyco-sis (South American blastomycosis)	*Paracoccidioides brasiliensis*	Abscesses, granulomas	Yeastlike multiple budding (steering wheel)	5–30 μm
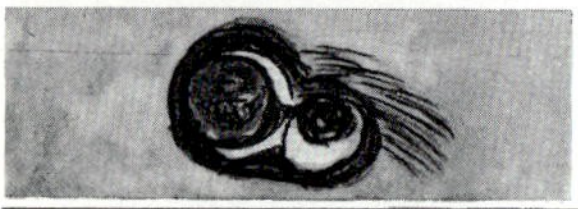	Blastomy-cosis	*Blastomyces dermatitidis*	Abscesses, granulomas	Large yeastlike cells, solitary budding; figure 8 shape	8–15 μm

*Deep mycoses, in contrast to superficial mycoses, show tissue changes beneath the epidermis and mucosa; often generalized.
†Fungal nature not proved.
‡Actinomycetes and nocardes are now considered to be bacteria.
§Chromoblastomycosis.

15. Fungi—Protozoa—Parasites

This chapter has been added in order to facilitate a basic knowledge of these important and frequent diseases. Professor Salfelder* has kindly provided the following pages, which are written from the viewpoint of a pathologist working in a subtropical or tropical region. Nonetheless, this addition to the book is not without importance for physicians in temperate zones for two chief reasons: on the one hand, we are confronted today with an increasing international commerce, and on the other hand, modern therapeutic agents (steroids, antibiotics, cytotoxic drugs, etc.) have changed the pattern of infectious diseases, with the result that overwhelming infections (fungi, protozoa, viruses) are common.

The following introduction gives some suggestions for the identification of fungi and parasites (Table 15–1). For amebae, which are easily confused with large tissue cells, the PAS-reaction is recommended. If parasites of small size are found in routine hematoxylin and eosin slides, or Chagas disease, kala-azar or leishmaniasis is suspected, it is helpful to remember that they are negative with the Gram and Grocott stains for fibrin. For the identification of fungi in tissue, the Grocott stain is superior to all other methods. In tissues, dead fungi retain their structural integrity and staining properties for a long time. The mucicarmine stain is recommended for staining the capsule of *Cryptococcus* in sections. India ink demonstrates the thick capsule of the *Cryptococcus* very well in smears. The capsule remains colorless, bright and shining. In unstained smears, undesired cell and tissue constituents, especially keratin, can be dissolved with 10% potassium hydroxide (10 min), which makes the search for infecting organisms easier. Several species are easily identified with the fluorescent antibody technique (Coons and Kaplan).

TABLE 15–1 METHODS USED FOR IDENTIFICATION OF FUNGI AND PROTOZOA

METHOD	RESULT	REMARKS
Hematoxylin-eosin	Blue	Not all fungal elements stain
Fibrin (Weigert)-Gram	Blue	Fungi only partially stained; protozoa negative
PAS*	Red	Cells of small fungi can be overlooked
Gridley*	Reddish blue	Stains nearly all fungi
Grocott*	Black	Ideal stain, good contrast against light background; also useful for smears; note: coal pigment also stains black, as do erythrocytes and elastic fibers
Mucicarmine*	Red	*Cryptococcus* positive; excludes other fungi
Polarized light	Shining yellowish blue	Shows double refraction and Maltese crosses of yeast-like fungi in paraffin sections of tissue
Fluorescent antibody	Variable	Fungi of many types positive; specificity destroyed by cross reactions
Unstained smear	—	Round forms with doubly contoured capsule: suspect fungi
Smear treated for 10 min with KOH 10%	—	Cell and tissue constituents destroyed; fungi more clearly seen
India ink smear	Black	Wide wall of cryptococcus shines forth against dark background
Giemsa, Wright, May-Grünwald-Giemsa (smear)	Blue	Yeasts and cysts of *Pneumocystis carinii* positive

*Staining of control preparation recommended.

*Director of the Institute of Anatomic Pathology, University of the Andes, Mérida, Venezuela.

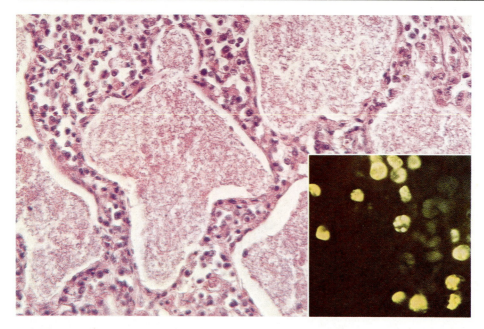

Fig 15–2.—Pneumocystosis with interstitial pneumonia (hematoxylin-eosin; 400×). *Inset: Pneumocystis carinii in smear (rhodamine stain, ultraviolet light; 1,050×).*

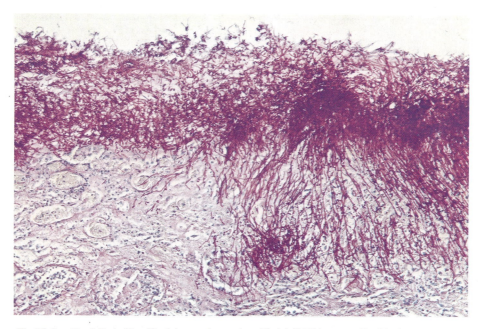

Fig 15–3.—Candidiasis (thrush) of the esophagus (moniliasis) (PAS-hematoxylin; 80×).

Pneumocystosis with interstitial pneumonia (Figs 15–2, 15–4). *Pneumocystosis with interstitial pneumonia occurs frequently in prematurely born infants in the 3rd–6th month of life, but also may occur in older children. When it occurs in adults it is mostly in the end stages of malignant disease (leukemia, sarcoma, carcinoma), particularly after treatment with cytotoxic agents.* **Pneumocystis carinii** is the etiologic agent but whether this is a protozoon or a fungus is still debated. Hematoxylin-eosin–stained sections show finely honeycombed granular material in the alveoli (Fig 15–2). The alveolar lumina are reduced by a thick exudate in alveolar septa. This exudate is composed of lymphocytes, histiocytes, and plasma cells. The appearance, indeed, may lead to confusing this form of interstitial pneumonia with atelectasis. The increased cell content of the alveolar septa and the type of cells should, however, lead to a correct diagnosis. The organisms may be seen in smear preparations stained with Giemsa or rhodamine, in which they appear as cystic forms with internal bodies originating from the honeycombed alveolar contents (see inset in Fig 15–2). With the Grocott stain, numerous yeastlike bodies 3–4 μ in diameter are seen which are often indented and wrinkled (Fig 15–4).

Macroscopic: Liver-like cut surface, gray to red, homogeneous, firm.

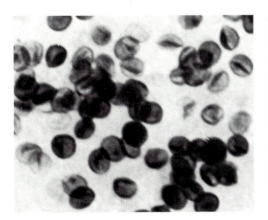

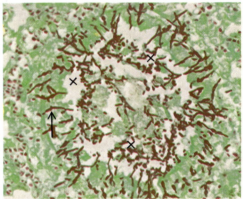

Fig 15–4.—*Pneumocystis* is a smear (Grocott stain; 1,140×).

Fig 15–5.—Hyphae and yeast forms of *Candida albicans* (Grocott stain; 400×).

Candidiasis *(thrush) of the esophagus* (**candidiasis, moniliasis**) (Figs 15–3, 15–5). *Various species of* Candida, *but chiefly* Candida albicans, *cause a mycosis that is localized predominantly in the mucous membranes. Spread to the internal organs occurs infrequently (sepsis), mostly in patients with weakened resistance. Macroscopically,* white plaques or membranes are seen on the mucosa of all the upper alimentary and respiratory tracts. *Microscopically,* numerous fungal filaments forming a mycelium are seen with hematoxylin-eosin, but better with PAS staining (Fig 15–3). The mycelial filaments (hyphae) penetrate between and into the epithelial cells of the mucous membrane, localizing particularly in the zone between the epithelium and tunica propria of the esophagus (see Fig 15–3). They penetrate like the roots of a plant into the upper layers of the connective tissue. The tunica propria is infiltrated by lymphocytes. Figure 15–5 shows the fungal filaments under higher magnification (hyphae,→ in the picture). Yeast forms 2–4 μ in diameter (×) are also present (blastospores) which show budding and pseudohyphae formation. If only yeast forms of *Candida* are present, it may be confused with similar forms of *Histoplasma capsulatum* or small fungus cells of other sorts. The hyphae are thinner than those of aspergilli and some of the phycomycoses.

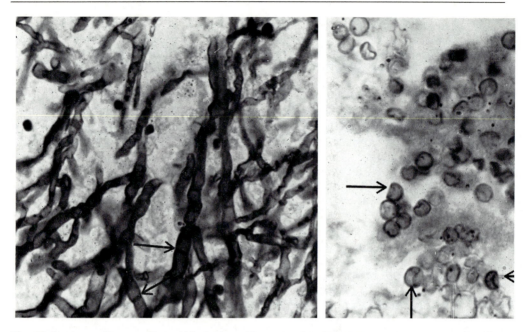

Fig 15–6.—*Aspergillus* mycelium with hyphae (Grocott stain; 800×).

Fig 15–7.—Conidia of *Aspergillus* (Grocott stain; 800×).

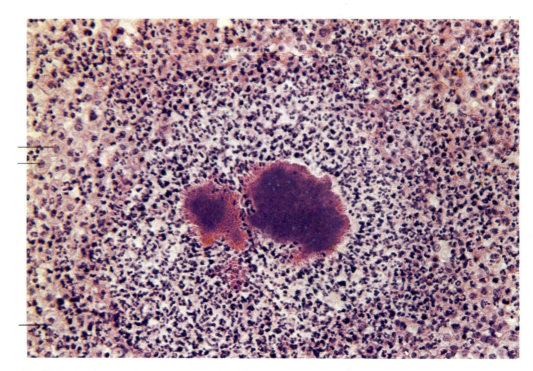

Fig 15–8.—Actinomycosis (hematoxylin-eosin; 300×).

Aspergillosis (Figs 15–6, 15–7, 15–9). Aspergillus *is a fungus of worldwide distribution. The various species produce changes in the lungs and mucous membranes. Less frequently, there is hematogenous spread to other organs. The fungus is a saprophyte, like* Candida *and the Phycomycetes. Aspergillosis occurs frequently in animals, especially birds. The infection is established mostly by inhalation of spores. The mycosis often is seen secondarily in patients whose power of resistance has become greatly reduced (malignant tumors, steroid-antibiotic-cytotoxic treatment, or x-irradiation).*

The diagnosis is based on the demonstration of septate forms (→in Fig 15–6) and dichotomous branching of hyphae (Fig 15–6), which form a network (mycelium). They can penetrate the walls of vessels and other hindrances. In addition, conidia are found (Fig 15–7). If only conidia are observed in tissues stained with Grocott stain, they can easily be confused with the yeast forms of *Candida* or *Pneumocystis*. The conidia are indented and wrinkled (→ in the illustration) similarly to *Pneumocystis carinii*. So-called fruiting bodies (Fig 15–9) occur in infections with *Aspergillus fumigatus*, particularly in areas of the body that receive oxygen (lungs, mucous membranes). The fruiting bodies develop on the end of the hyphae, bear sterigmata, and also are known as conidiophores (→ Fig 15–9). From the sterigmata, conidia (×) are formed, which then fall from them and lie free in the tissue.

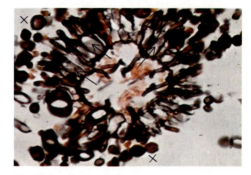

Fig 15–9.—Fruiting body of *Aspergillus fumigatus* (Grocott stain; 450×).

The tissue reaction is predominantly nonspecific but can be in the form of a granuloma showing eosinophilic leukocytes and giant cells. Not uncommonly, a tuberculous or bronchiectatic cavity becomes secondarily infected and filled with a so-called fungus ball which may resemble a tumorous mass and for this reason is called an "aspergilloma." Hematogenous spread can lead to involvement of practically all organs (brain, meninges, kidney, spleen, heart, etc.).

Actinomycosis (Actinomyces sp.) (Fig. 15–8). *In man, the disease is caused chiefly by* Actinomyces israeli, *and in cattle by* Actinomyces bovis *(anaerobic). The portal of entry is usually a break in a mucous membrane (e.g., in the oral cavity after a tooth extraction), the lungs, or the gut (appendix). Further spread results from either bloodstream invasion (e.g., liver, bone marrow) or lymphatic invasion.*

The bacteria occur in conglomerations and form so-called nodules with characteristic raylike runners to the periphery. Figure 15–8 shows bacterial masses in the center of an abscess (polymorphonuclear leukocytes and tissue destruction). Granulation tissue containing numerous foam cells (→1) with cytoplasmic fat droplets (foam cells) forms a wall around the abscess. In this way, the abscesses become confluent and form fistulous tracts (especially common, for example, in infections of the mandible). Yellow granules, which contain the nodules, may be demonstrated in the secretion of the fistulas.

Macroscopic: Hard, brawny induration of the skin with numerous fistulas. Sulfur-yellow abscess wall (granulation tissue with foam cells).

Mycetoma (Madura foot) occurs principally in the tropics and is a tumor-like, circumscribed skin lesion, usually in an extremity. It contains masses of bacteria. There are eumycetomas, caused by various sorts of fungi, and actinomycetomas, caused by actinomycetes (*Actinomyces* or *Nocardia* sp.). Eumycetomas are resistant to therapy with antibiotics; actinomycetomas are responsive. Granules composed of masses of bacteria may also occur in botryomycosis (pseudomycosis caused by pyogenic bacteria), and rarely in other true mycoses.

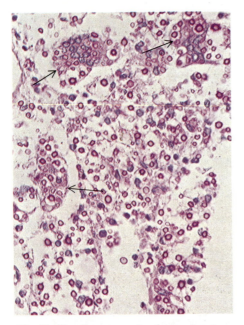

Fig 15–10.—Cryptococcosis of lung (mucicarmine; 150×).

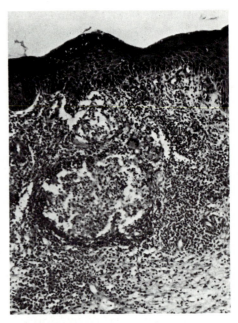

Fig 15–11.—Chromomycosis of skin (hematoxylin-eosin; 100×).

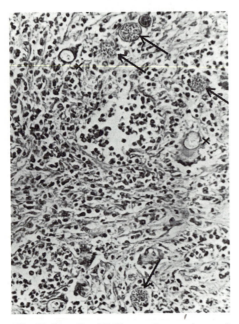

Fig 15–12.—Coccidioidomycosis granuloma of lung; sporocysts with (→) and without (×) endospores (hematoxylin-eosin; 140×).

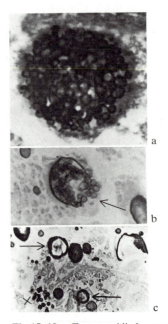

Fig 15–13.—**Top,** coccidiodes sporocyst without a membrane (hematoxylin-eosin; 130×). **Middle,** endospores released from a spherule (Grocott stain; 100×). **Bottom,** empty fungus spherule and small endospores (Grocott stain; 100×).

Cryptococcosis of the lung (*torulosis, European blastomycosis,* Fig 15–10). *Cryptococcus neoformans has a worldwide distribution. A prime source of infection is the excrement in the nesting places of pigeons. The central nervous system and, above all, the leptomeninges are favored sites for localization of the lesions, although they may occur in any organ. The portal of entry is probably the lungs, where healing results in the development of nodules.*

Figure 15–10 shows many intra- and extracellular cells. The infecting organisms appear as round bodies 4–20 μ in diameter which have a red-staining mucous capsule with mucicarmine. In massive infections, the fungi elicit only a slight histiocytic reaction. Chronic granulomatous foci contain only a few fungi. They are usually embedded in dense granulation tissue and, for this reason, often are difficult to discover and easy to confuse with foreign bodies.

Macroscopic: Gelatinous foci which look like a myxomatous tumor when many fungal cells are present in the tissues. Often the lesions resemble caseating tuberculosis macroscopically.

Chromoblastomycosis (Chromomycosis) (Figs 15–11, 15–14). *The causative fungus has an intrinsic dark brown color, hence the designation. There are five species of Phialophora and Cladosporium which may produce this mycosis. Localization occurs in the skin, particularly of the lower extremities. Seldom does lymphatic spread occur and only exceptionally hematogenous dissemination, usually to the brain and meninges. Chronic verrucous, ulcerated, and crusted lesions of the skin may result in considerable deformity of the extremities and invalidism. the mycosis is found in many tropical and subtropical countries, primary in farm workers.*

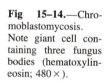

Histologically, the corium shows microabscesses composed of numerous granulocytes and marginal granulation tissue containing giant cells (Fig 15–11). Tuberculoid granuloma may also be produced. As in American blastomycosis, the overlying epidermis is hyperplastic. The brown, round fungus cells (Fig 15–14) frequently are septate, have a diameter of 5–12 μ, and often lie within giant cells.

Fig 15–14.—Chromoblastomycosis. Note giant cell containing three fungus bodies (hematoxylin-eosin; 480×).

NOTE: Many grossly similar skin lesions occur, particularly in the tropics.

Coccidioidomycosis (*San Joaquin Valley fever*) (Figs 15–12, 15–13). *The disease occurs most frequently in California and Arizona and certain parts of Central and South America, particularly where deserts exist. A large part of the population in an area may be infected. Coccidioides immitis occurs in dusty soil, attacks the lungs, and mostly produces a benign disease. Much less frequently, spread occurs to internal organs, which is often fatal.* Figure 15–12 shows a pulmonary granuloma with numerous fungus cells, some of which are phagocytosed by giant cells (×). The sporocysts contain endospores (→) or are empty. So-called coccidioidoma has been described, which shows extensive necrosis and, in contrast to histoplasmosis, only a slight tendency to calcification. Macroscopically, the lesions are similar to tuberculosis, which is true also of many other "deep" mycoses.

The fungus shows so-called dimorphism (as do *Histoplasma capsulatum, Blastomyces dermatitidis,* etc.), that is, it grows in saprophytic form both in its natural habitat and in cultures grown at room temperature (as hyphae with arthrospores), but also grows in parasitic form in animals and humans (large spherules or sporocysts with numerous endospores which are expelled from the spherule or mother cell). The sporocysts (Fig 15–13) measure 30–60 μ in size and are round. The endospores are extravasated from the fungus cells (→ in Fig 15–13, middle) and can attain the size of a white blood cell. Empty sporocysts (Fig. 15–13c →, × endospores) can be confused with *Blastomyces dermatitidis,* and endospores (Fig 15–3, middle and bottom) with *Histoplasma capsulatum* and *Cryptococcus neoformans.*

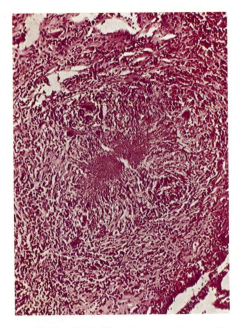

Fig 15–15.—Fresh *Histoplasma* granuloma in the lung (hematoxylin-eosin; 105×).

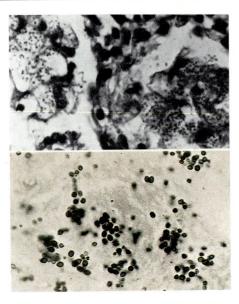

Fig 15–16.—(Top): Alveolar epithelium with *Histoplasma* (hematoxylin-eosin; 160×).
Fig 15–17.—(Bottom): Yeast form of *Histoplasma capsulatum* (Grocott stain; 320×).

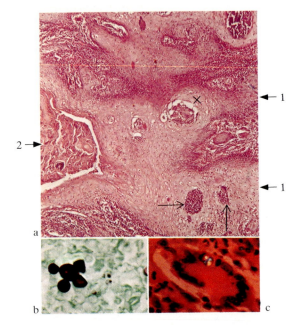

Fig 15–18.—a, paracoccidioidomycosis (South American blastomycosis) of the skin (hematoxylin-eosin; 655×). b, multiple budding of *Paracoccidioides brasiliensis* in tissue (Grocott stain; 520×). c, fungal cell *(Paracoccidioides brasiliensis)* in a giant cell under polarized light. Note the so-called Maltese cross (hematoxylin-eosin; 550×).

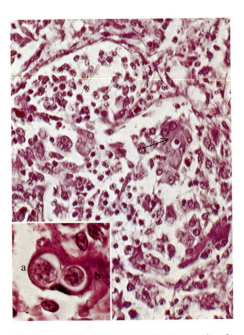

Fig 15–19.—North American blastomycosis of the lung (hematoxylin-eosin; 525×). *Inset:* Solitary bud of *Blastomyces: a,* mother cell; *b,* daughter cell (hematoxylin-eosin; 1,050×).

Histoplasmosis (Figs 15–15, 15–16, 15–17). *Histoplasmosis is one of the most widely distributed mycoses. In the United States, it is estimated that more than 30 million persons have been infected. The clinical and pathologic similarities to tuberculosis and the predominantly benign course prevented its recognition for a long time, with the result that most of the significant features of this mycosis have been recognized only in the past 30 years. Spontaneous cases are rare in Europe. The disease also occurs spontaneously in animals.*

Histoplasma capsulatum (Darling) *grows best in the soil of chicken houses, is spread apparently through the air, and causes a primary lung infection. Most cases heal with a residue of focal calcification in the lung and hilar lymph nodes, where fungi can be demonstrated for a long time. Seldom, and only under special conditions, does the disease in the lung become generalized and have a fatal outcome, particularly in children and adults over 40 years of age. In addition to the calcified residual foci in the lungs, cases are encountered with multiple scattered nodules, cavitation, or histoplasmomas. Extrapulmonary histoplasmosis may involve any organ, the adrenals being affected frequently.*

Histologically, the lungs show histiocytic granulomas with central necrosis, epithelioid cells, and giant cells (Fig 15–15). The tissue picture can be very similar to that of a tuberculous granuloma. In new infections the fungi are almost exclusively in the cytoplasm of histiocytes or alveolar epithelial cells (Fig 15–16, small black granules). With hematoxylin-eosin stains, the fungi are not often recognized, but with the Grocott stain (Fig 15–17), the organisms can be seen distinctly. There are also yeastlike forms 2–5 μ in diameter.

Paracoccidioidomycosis *(South American blastomycosis, Figs 15–18, a, b, c). As the name indicates, this disease occurs in South America. In Brazil, it is a major sanitary problem. Paracoccidioidomycosis is not encountered spontaneously in animals. In man, minor tissue changes attributed to the fungus have been seen in almost all organs. It has a chronic course, commonly occurs with tuberculosis, and is the only deep mycosis that responds well to sulfonamide. After attacking the lung (portal of entry) it spreads especially to the skin and mucous membranes of the upper respiratory passages. Predominately attacks men over 40 in rural areas—as does blastomycosis. The habitat of P. brasiliensis is still not known.*

Histologically, there is a combination of abscesses and granulation tissue. Calcification is rare. Figure 15–18 shows pseudoepitheliomatous hyperplasia of the epidermis with broad, deeply penetrating epidermal pegs (→ 1, → 2 surface of the epidermis with keratin scales). Within the epidermis, there are numerous microabscesses (→ in the picture) as well as granulomas (×). The diagnosis rests on demonstration of large yeastlike fungi showing multiple budding (Fig 15–18, b). Frequently, the granulomas contain giant cells with enclosed fungi appearing as Maltese crosses in polarized light (Fig 15–18, c). Dead fungus cells of all sorts decompose, leaving behind large dustlike masses of Grocott-positive particles, but surviving fungus cells are needed for diagnosis.

North American blastomycosis (Fig 15–19) *occurs practically only in North America, but recently has been seen in Africa. Frequently, secondary skin lesions appear first. The lungs are the portal of entry for the fungus and from there hematogenous dissemination occurs. Spontaneous animal infections occur (dogs).* The microscopic changes are similar to those seen in South American blastomycosis. Figure 15–19 shows granulocytes in a lung alveolus as well as a giant cell which has phagocytized a fungus cell (→). In tissues, the round, yeastlike fungi produce single daughter cells only (solitary budding). Figure 15–19 shows a mother cell and a daughter cell in a giant cell.

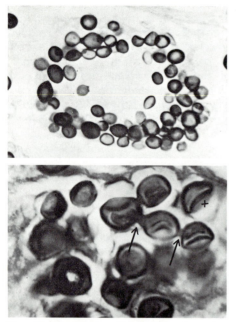

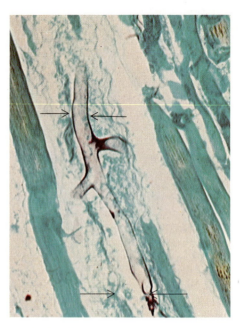

Fig 15–20.—(Top): African histoplasmosis (Grocott stain; 700×).

Fig 15–21.—(Bottom): Lobomycosis, skin (Grocott stain; 900×).

Fig 15–22.—Phycomycosis. Note broad, nonseptated hyphae in skeletal muscle (Grocott stain, 800×).

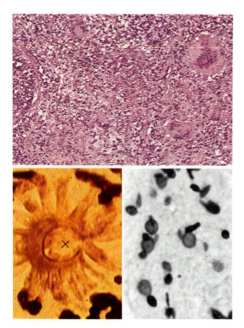

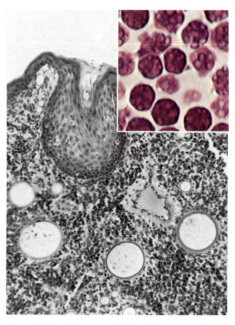

Fig 15–23.—(Top): Sporotrichosis of the skin (hematoxylin-eosin; 240×).

Fig 15–24.—(Bottom left): Asteroid bodies (hematoxylin-eosin; 950×).

Fig 15–25.—(Bottom right): Pleomorphic yeastlike form of *Sporothrix schenckii* in rat tissue (post-inoculation) (Grocott stain; 1,150×).

Fig 15–26.—Rhinosporidiosis of nasal mucosa. Note cystic fungus cells containing endospores (hematoxylin-eosin; 140×). *Inset:* Endospores in cystic fungus cells of *Rhinosporidium seeberi* (hematoxylin-eosin; 920×).

African and American Histoplasmosis (Fig 15–20). In addition to African histoplasmosis, which until now was only known to occur in man and primates in Africa, American histoplasmosis caused by *Histoplasma capsulatum* (Darling) also occurs in Europe. African histoplasmosis differs from the American variety in several essential ways. The causative agent, *Histoplasma duboisii,* is found in tissues in its typical large form—about three times larger than *H. capsulatum*—often in large giant cells (Fig 15–20). These large yeast cells must be differentiated from those of that other deep mycosis, *Blastomycosis dermatitidis,* that are similar but have only one nucleus. As a rule the nuclei of fungus cells are difficult to make out in routine sections. In addition to large yeast cells of *H. duboisii,* small forms occur in tissues (similar to *H. capsulatum*). This characteristic without a doubt makes the diagnosis of the disease more difficult. Skin and bones are chiefly attacked. The portal of entry of *H. duboisii* is *not* the lung, where the disease may be inconspicuous, (in contrast to *H. capsulatum*). The incidence of the disease at the present is not certain for so far only cases in the vicinity of academic institutions have been reported.

Lobomycosis (Fig 15–21) This is a deep mycosis limited to the skin, also called keloid blastomycosis, first described in the Amazon in 1931 by J. Lobo. It has a limited geographical distribution—from northern Brazil into Surinam, Venezuela, Colombia, and as far as Central America. It is still considered by many to belong to the paracoccidioidomycoses, although the grounds for this are not clear. The causative agent is now usually called *Loboa loboi*. In tissues the large yeast cells increase by budding, are typically arranged in chains (→) and often have depressions (×, Fig 15–21).

Phycomycosis (Fig 15–22, *mucormycosis*). Absidia, mucor, and rhizopus, as well as some other fungi grouped together under this term, cause important, deep mycoses of worldwide distribution. It was at one time called mucormycosis. The characteristic finding in tissues is the presence of broad, nonseptated fungal elements (→ in figure) or fragments of these that stain faintly with Grocott stain (Fig 15–22). In hematoxylin-eosin preparations the fungi frequently lie parallel to muscle and nerve fibers, with which they may be confused. Hyphae of *Candida* and *Aspergillus* have a different arrangement and other structural peculiarities. They penetrate the walls of blood vessels, destroy them, and cause thrombosis. It is an opportunistic infection.

Sporotrichosis (Figs 15–23, 15–24, 15–25) is a worldwide, relatively common deep mycosis of the skin. Only a few cases are known to become generalized or to have pulmonary involvement—from inhalation. *Sporothrix schenckii* causes tissue abscesses and a granulomatous reaction (Fig 15–23). The small, round or elongated yeast forms of *Sp. schencki* are only rarely met with in human tissues. In contrast, after inoculation into animal tissues they multiply well and are easily recognized (Fig 15–25). The finding of yeast cells containing asteroid bodies (×, Fig 15–24) is helpful in making a histologic diagnosis.

Rhinosporidiosis (Fig 15–26). *Rhinosporidium seeberi* is easily recognized in tissues. The fungus cells (sporangia) are large and cystic and have many small endospores (Fig 15–26). Occasionally numerous globular bodies are seen in the endospores (Fig 15–26, inset). The fungus cells resemble *C. immitis* (see Fig 15–12). A nonspecific inflammation is the usual reaction. Occasionally a foreign body reaction occurs.

The disease occurs sporadically throughout the world; it is widespread in Asia, Ceylon, and South America. Besides the nasal mucosa and mucous membranes of other facial cavities, the facial skin and particularly the conjunctiva may be affected by this disease.

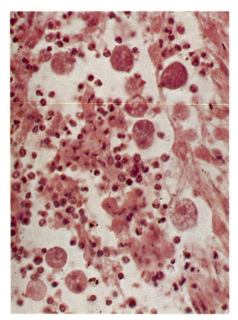

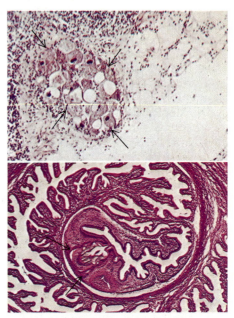

Fig 15–27.—Amebae in the submucosa of the large intestine (amebic dysentery) (PAS-hematoxylin stain; 700×).

Fig 15–28.—**(Top):** *Balantidium* dysentery (hematoxylin-eosin; 168×).

Fig 15–29.—**(Bottom):** Cysticercus (hematoxylin-eosin; 105×).

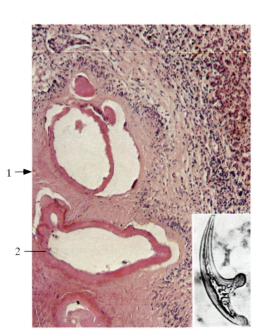

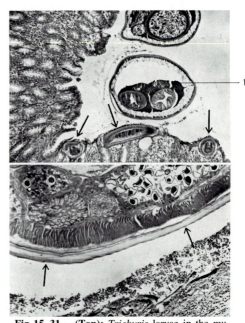

Fig 15–30.—*Echinococcus* cysts of the liver (hematoxylin-eosin; 8×).

Fig 15–31.—**(Top):** *Trichuris* larvae in the mucosa of the appendix (hematoxylin-eosin; 310×).

Fig 15–32.—**(Bottom):** Ascaris in bile duct (hematoxylin-eosin; 72×).

Amebic dysentery (Fig 15–27). *Amebic dysentery occurs chiefly in warm climates. Of the various types occurring in man, only the vegetative form of* Entamoeba histolytica *is seen in tissues. The existence of cysts and vegetative forms in the intestinal contents does not of itself signify disease.*

The intestinal lesions are usually confined to the colon. Amebae actively penetrate the intestinal wall and have both cytologic and histolytic effects. At first, there is extensive necrosis of tissue, with formation of crater-like ulcers with undermined margins. **Histologically,** the base of the ulcers shows fibrin, necrotic tissue, and many granulocytes. Careful inspection is necessary to discover the amebae in the submucosa of the large intestine. They appear as round cells with an eccentrically placed nucleus (Fig 15–27). The cytoplasm is distinctly red with PAS-stain; with hematoxylin-eosin, the protozoa can be easily overlooked or confused with reticulum cells, macrophages, or ganglion cells. Figure 15–27 shows, in addition, infiltration of tissues with round cells and granulocytes.

Peritonitis from perforation is a complication, along with dissemination of the amebae through the portal vein to the liver and other organs, where abscesses may form.

Balantidium dysentery (Fig 15–28). Balantidium coli *occurs in man and animals independently of climatic influence.* The pathologic changes in the tissues are similar to those of amebic dysentery. The living etiologic agent has no histolytic effect. Inflammation is produced primarily by the presence of a large number of dead balantidia and, as is perhaps also true in amebic dysentery, the disease is mainly the result of associated bacterial infection. Figure 15–28 shows balantidia (→) in a lymph vessel in the periphery of a lymph node in the mesocolon.

Cysticercosis (Fig 15–29). *This implies the seeding of larvae* (Cysticercus cellulosae) *of the swine tapeworm* (Taenia solium) *in the various organs of man or swine after oral ingestion of eggs. Cysticercus is found in eastern Europe, Asia, South America and Central America. The larvae are found predominantly in the central nervous system, eyes, skin, and skeletal muscles.* **Histologically,** the larvae are found enclosed in a vesicle arising from invagination. Often, the head end with hooks is visible (→). The diameter of a cysticercus seldom is larger than 1.5 cm. The shape is variable. After the worm dies, a foreign body reaction occurs. Secondary calcification (x-ray) and the development of epilepsy, if the central nervous system is involved, provide clues for clinical diagnosis.

Echinococcosis (Fig 15–30). *The larvae of* Taenia echinococcus *(dog tapeworm) pass through the portal vein into the liver, where they form cysts (hydatid cysts).* The figure shows cysts. The wall of each consists of a ring of collagenous fibrous tissue (→ I) on which rests a homogeneous, lamellar red chitinous layer (cuticle → 2). Scolices are often seen near the cuticle. The inset in the lower right in Figure 15–30 shows a single hook. The adjacent liver shows atrophy and lymphocytic infiltration.

Macroscopic Echinococcus granulosus (98% of echinococcosis in humans): Either a large unilocular cyst or several cysts filled with daughter cysts. They are especially common in the right lobe of the liver. *Echinococcus alveolaris* (2% in humans): multiple small cysts bounded by a capsule of connective tissue (60% liver, 30% lung).

Intestinal worms (Figs. 15–31, 15–32). In tropical countries, *Ascaris, Necator,* and *Trichocephalus* frequently are found in the lumen of the intestine. Their adult forms usually cause only bleeding. Hookworm *(Ancylostoma duodenale* and *Necator americanus)* causes severe anemia and wasting, which often lead to death in children. Larvae of *Trichuris trichiura* (Fig 15–31) occasionally penetrate into the mucous membrane of the intestine. In Figure 15–31, two larvae are seen covered by a layer of intestinal epithelium (→). A transversely sectioned worm in the intestinal lumen contains numerous eggs (→ 1). *Ascaris lumbricoides* (Fig 15–32) sometimes causes severe disease with eventual ileus or intestinal perforation and can also lodge in other organs. Figure 15–32 shows a longitudinally sectioned ascaris (→ cuticle) in a bile duct. The duct wall is inflamed and the worm contains ascaris eggs (→). This patient died of multiple liver abscesses.

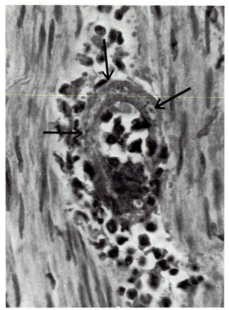

Fig 15–33.—Larva migrans and cellular reaction in the intestinal musculature (hematoxylin-eosin; 630×).

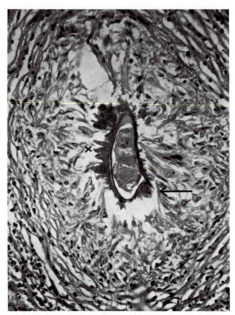

Fig 15–34.—*Schistosoma* granuloma in the liver (hematoxylin-eosin; 300×).

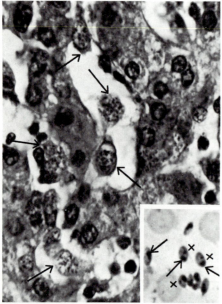

Fig 15–35.—Kala-azar in liver (hematoxylin-eosin; 450×). *Inset: L. donovani* in peritoneal exudate in hamster (Giemsa stain; 1,150×).

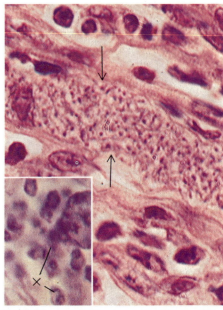

Fig 15–36.—Acute Chagas myocarditis in child (hematoxylin-eosin; 980×). *Inset: Tr. cruzi* in Chagas encephalitis (hematoxylin-eosin; 1,500×).

Larva migrans (Fig 15–33). *This includes all conditions in which larvae and microfilariae, especially of nematodes such as* **Strongyloides, Ancylostoma,** *Ascaris lumbricoides suum* as well as *Toxocara canis* and *cati* *invade the skin and internal organs. The disease occurs mostly in children and causes symptoms of a general infection with fever and, in addition, shows blood eosinophilia.* In **Toxocara** infection, man is a secondary host and the disease is known as visceral larva migrans. The larvae elicit a tissue reaction consisting of eosinophils and granulomas. The parasites are not ordinarily detected in the tissue (→). In most cases, exact classification is difficult.

The microfilariae (→), morphology of which does not easily lend itself to ordinary classification are distinguished from tissue fibers by their stippling (Fig 15–33); difficult to recognize in cross section. They elicit an eosinophilic reaction (not always) and eosinophilic granulomas, which in the tropics occur chiefly in internal organs. Microfilariae are frequently not found.

Schistosomiasis (*Bilharziasis*, Fig 15–34). *Schistosoma belong to the* **trematodes.** *Three types are found in man.* **Schistosoma haematobium** *occurs in Africa and bordering countries,* **Schistosoma mansoni** *in Africa and South America, and* **Schistosoma japonicum** *in Asia. The worm spends its youth in the outside world. Snails act as the intermediate host. Infection is the result of contact with infected water. Adult schistosomes are found in the paravesical tissues* (Schistosoma haematobium) *and mesenteric veins* (Schistosoma haematobium *and* japonicum). *The tissue changes and symptoms of the disease are caused by the eggs of the Schistosoma, which have characteristic structures that allow diagnosis of the type of parasite causing the infection. In* Schistosoma hematobium, *the eggs are found in the urinary bladder, ureter, and genital organs (occasionally rectum and lungs).* Schistosoma mansoni *and* japonicum *eggs occur particularly in the walls of the intestines and liver.*

The eggs of trematodes cause a granulocytic or eosinophilic reaction in the earliest stages. Later, a typical granuloma forms which heals with calcification and connective tissue scarring. Complications are carcinoma of the urinary bladder, hepatic cirrhosis, cor pulmonale, and, in the central nervous system, focal symptoms, depending on the site. Figure 15–34 shows a *Schistosoma* granuloma in the liver. In the center, there is a *Sch. mansoni* egg with a lateral, pointed spine (→), which has important diagnostic significance. Externally, particularly on the other long side, the egg has a layer of prickly material that stains red with hematoxylin-eosin (×). This is protein formed by the host and indicates an immune reaction (Hoeppli-Splendore phenomenon). Such a tissue reaction may also be caused by other microorganisms.

Kala-azar (visceral leishmaniasis, Fig 15–35). *The name comes from India and means "black disease." It occurs also in Asia, Africa, southern Europe, and South America. The protozoan* Leishmania donovani *produces visceral changes, as opposed to* Leishmania tropica *and* brasiliensis, *which produce only skin and mucous membrane lesions (mucocutaneous Leishmaniasis). Natural infection occurs in dogs, foxes, and jackals, and the etiologic agent is transmitted by Phlebotomus (sand fly).* Clinically, there is hepatosplenomegaly with fever, pancytopenia, and increase of plasma globulins. The cytoplasm of cells of the reticuloendothelial system contains the causative organisms, 2–5 μ in size. In Figure 15–35 numerous Leishmaniae are seen in the Kupffer cells of the liver. The typical Leishmaniae blepharoplasts are difficult to see in tissue, but are conspicuous in smears (Fig 15–35, inset: → nucleus, × blepharoplast). Diagnostically, knowledge of the organ involved is important since the organisms of Chagas disease and of mucocutaneous Leishmaniasis look alike in tissues. Histoplasmas, which resemble Leishmania in hematoxylin-eosin stains (cf. Fig 15–16), can be differentiated with Grocott stain.

Chagas disease (American trypanosomiasis, Fig 15–36). The causative agent, *Trypanosoma cruzi,* is transmitted by the barbeiro (Triatoma and related Reduvüdae) and is found only in blood. In tissue they lose their flagella and look like Leishmaniae. They occur chiefly in heart muscle fibers in the form of nonencapsulated nests (→). In routine tissue sections blepharoplasts are hard to see. In the inset of Figure 15–36 (Chagas encephalitis) they appear as rod-shaped structures within the Leishmaniae (×).

Involvement of heart muscle causes myocarditis. In acute cases the nests of parasites can be found and the diagnosis is relatively easy. In chronic myocarditis the organisms are found only rarely. If they are not found, these chronic cases present a diagnostic problem since the cardiac hypertrophy and mural thrombosis is similar to that found in Fiedler's idiopathic myocarditis or in viral myocarditis. Investigators in Brazil suggest the parasitic infection of the autonomic nervous system may lead to development of large organs.

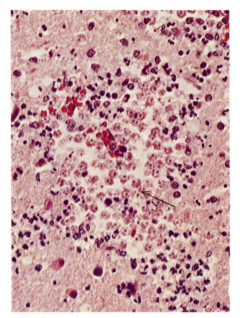

Fig 15–37.—Acanthoamebiasis. Note numerous Hartmanella amebae in brain (hematoxylin-eosin; 240×).

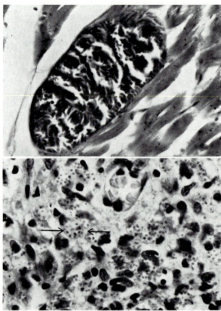

Fig 15–38.—**(Top):** Sarcosporidiosis. Note cysts in heart muscle (cattle) (hematoxylin-eosin; 320×).

Fig 15–39—**(Bottom):** Mucosal Leishmaniasis. Note numerous, predominantly intracellular *L. brasiliensis* (hematoxylin-eosin; 420×).

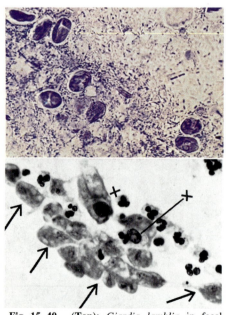

Fig 15–40.—**(Top):** *Giardia lamblia* in fecal smear from child (hematoxylin-eosin; 240×).

Fig 15–41.—**(Bottom).** *Trichomonas* in vaginal smear (Papanicolaou stain; 320×).

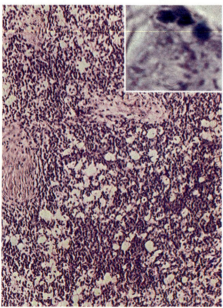

Fig 15–42.—Rhinoscleroma. Note numerous pale Mikulicz cells (hematoxylin-eosin; 130×). *Inset: Klebsiella rhinoscleromatis* in Mikulicz cells (Giemsa stain; 1,800×).

Acanthoamebiasis (Fig 15–37). In recent years infections due chiefly to acanthoameba (Hartmannella) have appeared in Europe, America, and Australia. The amebae ascend through the nasal passages, along the fibers of the olfactory nerve and cause purulent meningoencephalitis. Most patients contract the disease from swimming pools.

The amebae of this group have a different structure from that of *E. histolytica*. They are round, vesicular (→), and do not stain with PAS or Grocott stains (Fig 15–37). The pathogenesis has been established in animals. After hematogenous dissemination the organisms die in other organs without eliciting a tissue reaction.

Macroscopic: Purulent basal meningoencephalitis with abscesses.

Sarcosporidiosis (Fig 15–38). Infection with the various forms of sarcocystis is of minor significance. It is more frequent in animals than in humans *(S. lindemanni)* and affects skeletal and cardiac muscle fibers, largely without an inflammatory reaction. The parasitic cysts are easily recognized in heart muscle in hematoxylin-eosin stains. The comma-shaped trophozoites are easily differentiated from *T. gondi* and the leishmania of *Tr. cruzi.*

Cutaneous and mucocutaneous Leishmaniasis (Fig 15–39). In Asia and Africa the lesions occur only in the skin and are caused by *L. tropica* and are called oriental boil. In South America the facial mucous membranes are attacked in addition to the skin. The pathogenesis of the mucous membrane lesions is not entirely clear. Apparently they develop from a skin lesion (which may be completely healed) by secondary hematogenous spread to mucous membranes. Organism and disease are named according to the country of occurrence. Infection with *L. brasiliensis* is the most common. Figure 15–39 is not typical in that so many intracellular organisms (→) are seen only exceptionally. In most cases the diagnosis must be based on the quite characteristic tissue reaction—without evident organisms. A granulomatous reaction, often only hinted at and without a necrotic tuberculoid granuloma, points to the diagnosis. Other infections must be differentiated by the use of special stains. Skin lesions may also occur in Kala-azar.

Macroscopic: nodular thickening, frequently ulceration only.

Giardiasis (Fig 15–40). *Giardia lamblia,* a flagellate, is a very common inhabitant of the small intestine in all tropical countries, particularly in children. It causes mild intestinal disturbances. The organisms apparently occasionally penetrate the upper mucosal layers but elicit practically no tissue reaction. They are Grocott positive and scanty in routine sections, but are easily seen in smears (Fig 15–40). The paired flagella are not recognizable.

Trichomoniasis (Fig 15–41 and 16–5). Is a worldwide infection which causes vaginitis, urethritis, prostatitis, and vesiculitis. The Grocott-positive causative agents are often found in routine smears of exfoliative cytology (→in Fig 15–41). They must be differentiated from epithelial cells (×) and granulocytes. The nuclei and flagella, however, are not easily seen. Infection may cause epithelial cell atypia but has no causal relationship to cancer.

Rhinoscleroma (Fig 15–42). Because lesions not only may occur in the nose, but also in the mucous membranes of the bronchi this disease is sometimes called "scleroma." It occurs in East Europe, Africa, Asia, and South America, but nowadays chiefly only in tropical regions. The histologic diagnosis is simple: in addition to plasma cells with Russell bodies there are numerous typical pale, so-called Mikulicz cells (Fig 15–42). The fresh bacilli *(Klebsiella rhinoscleromatis)* are seen only occasionally (insert, Fig 15–42). The pale Mikulicz cells, however, must be differentiated by special stains from pale cells in other infections. Treatment is still unsatisfactory.

Macroscopic: Firm, nodular or diffuse thickening of the mucous membranes of the upper respiratory passages which may result in stenosis.

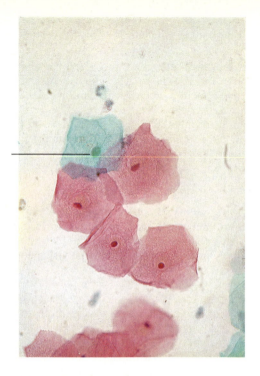

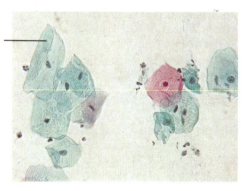

Fig 16–1.—Papanicolaou stain (vaginal smear, proliferative phase) (800×).

Fig 16–2.—May-Grünwald-Giemsa stain; normal thyroid epithelium (800×).

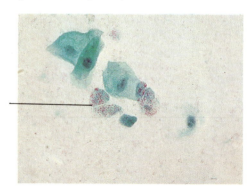

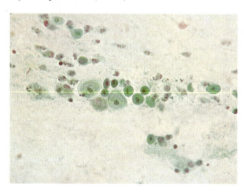

Fig 16–3.—Secretory phase, vaginal smear (Papanicolaou stain; 200×).

Fig 16–4.—Senile involution of mucosa, vaginal smear (Papanicolaou stain; 200×).

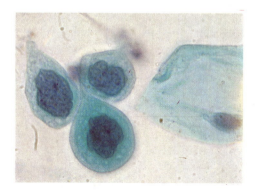

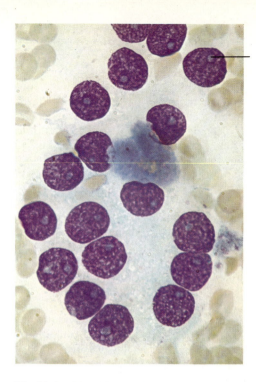

Fig 16–5.—*Trichomonas* in vaginal smear (Papanicolaou stain; 320×).

Fig 16–6.—Dyskaryosis in cervical smear (Papanicolaou stain; 800×).

16. Cytodiagnosis

Cytodiagnosis is a diagnostic method which is employed ever more commonly, particularly for the separation of tumors from inflammatory or degenerative lesions. The advantages of this method lie chiefly in the ease of obtaining material (ambulatory patients without anesthesia), the saving of time, the little technical equipment required, and the ease of execution (smear → staining → report). These advantages also permit repeated control investigations of a large patient population, e.g., in cancer detection. With suitable experience and good technique cytodiagnosis has a high degree of reliability.

Material suitable for cytodiagnosis is of two sorts: 1. **Exfoliated cells** that have detached themselves or been scraped from the surface of an organ with the help of an instrument (wooden spatula). Exfoliated cells may also be obtained from effusions (e.g., ascites) or secretions (e.g., sputum or urine). 2. **Needle biopsy,** which involves sampling a solid or cystic mass with a hollow needle. Cell fragments are loosened from the tissue being sampled and are aspirated.

Cytologic technique. Material obtained from exfoliation or by needle biopsy is smeared on a microscopic slide. Preparations for *Papanicolaou staining* are fixed with alcohol (spray). Smears from *May-Grünwald-Giemsa staining* are air fixed.

Papanicolaou stain (Pap. stain, Fig 16–1) is to be preferred when cytoplasmic structures need to be clearly shown. Figure 16–1 shows a cervical smear from a sexually mature woman **(proliferative phase of menstrual cycle)** with predominantly *superficial cells* that have acidophilic cytoplasm and pyknotic nuclei. The single *intermediate cell* from the midlayers of the mucosa has cyanophilic (greenish) cytoplasm and a vesicular nucleus (→).

May-Grünwald-Giemsa stain (MGG stain, Fig 16–2) gives good rendition of nuclear details such as chromatin structure and nucleoli. Figure 16–2 shows a group of normal thyroid epithelial cells with finely lumpy chromatin and a rather small nucleolus (→).

Cervical cytology (Figs 16–3 through 16–6) is chiefly concerned with the exfoliated squamous epithelial cells obtained from the external cervix and the cylindrical cells from the cervical canal (endocervix). It permits diagnosis of the status of the sexual hormones *(functional diagnosis: menstrual cycle and hormone activity),* of the vaginal flora *(identification of the causative organisms of inflammations),* of precursors of cancer *(dysplasia, carcinoma in situ),* and of malignant tumors *(squamous cell carcinoma).*

Fig 16–3 shows a smear from a sexually mature woman **(secretory phase).** The arrangement of superficial and intermediate cells with distinct cytoplasmic folding (→) in small groups is typical. With age **mucosal involution** occurs (Fig 16–4). There are epithelial cells from the deeper cell layers. The cells are essentially smaller (cf. Fig 16–3, taken at the same magnification).

Cytologic examination frequently reveals the causative agent of an inflammation. In this case it is *Trichomonas* (Fig 16–5), which shows the characteristic reddish granules (→). Next to the organisms there are cyanophilic intermediate cells.

Dyskaryosis (Fig 16–6). Cells with large, hyperchromatic and polymorphic nuclei and still preserved cytoplasmic structure. Their presence suggests the early stages of dysplasia, carcinoma in situ, or precancer. This finding must be confirmed by further diagnostic and therapeutic means, e.g., by cervical conization. In the field of cancer detection, preventive cytology has led to reduction in frequency of cervical carcinoma, which today is less frequent than corpus carcinoma.

On the basis of cytology the following classification of cervical lesions has been proposed by Papanicolaou: Pap. groups I and II are nonsuspicious, group III is doubtful, group IV comprises dysplasia and carcinoma in situ, and group V, invasive carcinoma.

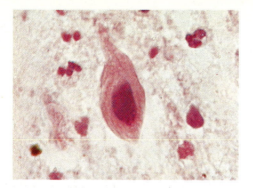

Fig 16–7.—Squamous carcinoma cell, sputum (hematoxylin-eosin; 800×).

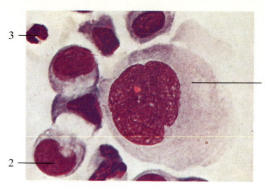

Fig 16–8.—Carcinoma cell in ascitic sediment (MCG stain; 800×).

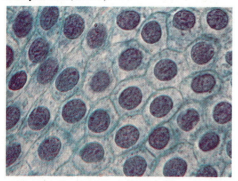

Fig 16–9.—Normal prostate (Papanicolaou stain; 800×).

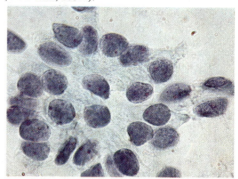

Fig 16–10.—Well-differentiated prostatic carcinoma (Papanicolaou stain; 800×).

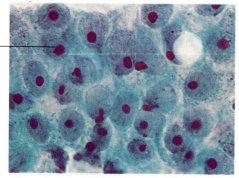

Fig 16–11.—Moderately well-differentiated prostatic carcinoma (Papanicolaou stain; 800×).

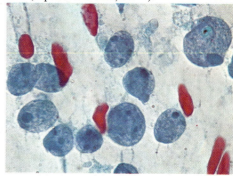

Fig 16–12.—Undifferentiated prostatic carcinoma (Papanicolaou stain; 800×).

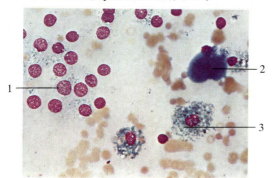

Fig 16–13.—Colloid goiter with cystic change (MGG stain; 320×).

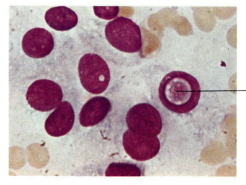

Fig 16–14.—Thyroid carcinoma, papillary type (MGG stain; 800×).

Sputum cytology (Fig 16–7). Cytologic investigation of sputum is of great value in the diagnosis of bronchogenic carcinoma. It makes possible detection of centrally placed tumors with a high degree of accuracy. Figure 16–7 shows a **tumor cell from a squamous cell carcinoma.** The nucleus is especially large and hyperchromatic. The nucleus/cytoplasm ratio is shifted in favor of the nucleus.

Exfoliative cytology of effusions (Fig 16–8). The etiology of an effusion is a common clinical question—is it or is it not from a malignant tumor? Figure 16–8 shows a **carcinoma cell** ($\rightarrow$ 1) recovered from the sediment of ascitic fluid. The size and structure of the nucleus of the carcinoma cell distinguish it from benign cells of the peritoneal lining ($\rightarrow$ 2) and from leucocytes ($\rightarrow$ 3).

Cytology of prostatic needle biopsy (Figs 16–9 through 16–12). The diagnostic value of this is well recognized today, particularly in surveys of large groups of patients (early cancer detection). Transrectal aspiration biopsy with a thin needle (obtaining a sample from multiple sites in the prostate) commonly yields a higher rate of correct diagnosis than histologic examination of a single punch biopsy specimen. Cytologic investigation of a prostatic carcinoma also allows assessment of the grade of the tumor, which is important for treatment.

Figure 16–9 shows a smear from **normal prostate.** The cells and nuclei are of uniform size and have distinct cell boundaries—signs of a benign nature (*so-called beehive structure:* occurs also in adenomyomatosis). In **well-differentiated prostatic carcinoma** there are so-called *microadenomatous structures* (Fig 16–10): a circular arrangement of cells showing essentially no nuclear changes but having faded, indistinct cell borders. In **moderately well-differentiated prostatic carcinoma** (Fig 16–11) nuclear changes are dominant. The nuclei are of different sizes, overlap one another, and have large nucleoli ($\rightarrow$). In **undifferentiated prostatic carcinoma** (Fig 16–12) the cells are isolated and *cellular dissociation and polymorphism predominate* and the nuclei show distinct variations in size.

Needle biopsy of the thyroid (Figs 16–12, 16–13, and 16–14). Cytologic study of the thyroid permits separation of a colloid goiter from inflammation or the different sorts of carcinomas. It contributes to clarification of ''cold nodules'' discovered by scintillation detectors. In Figure 16–13 **(goiter showing degenerative cystic changes)** there are typical thyroid cells ($\rightarrow$ 1, cf. also Fig 16–12), a fragment of colloid ($\rightarrow$ 2), that is uniformly dark blue with MGG stain, and macrophages ($\rightarrow$ 3). Figure 16–14 shows **tumor cells from a papillary adenocarcinoma** of the thyroid, in which can be seen the typical intranuclear cytoplasmic invagination.

Exfoliative and needle biopsy cytology are also of value in other organs, e.g. the gastrointestinal tract. By taking the sample with a brush, large areas of a suspicious organ can be examined. By combining these investigational methods with histologic gastric suction or snip biopsies it is possible to attain nearly 100% accuracy of diagnosis. Needle biopsy of the breast also is highly reliable, particularly when it is used in conjunction with mammography. It permits not only separation of benign and malignant tumors but also grading of a tumor.

Index